HOSPITAL ORGANIZATION
AND MANAGEMENT
A BOOK OF READINGS

Jonathan S. Rakich
Associate Professor
of Management

The University of Akron

THE CATHOLIC HOSPITAL ASSOCIATION
St. Louis, Missouri 63104

Copyright © 1972
by
The Catholic Hospital Association
St. Louis, Missouri 63104

Library of Congress Catalog Card No. 79-190548

ISBN 0-87125-001-2

TO MY FAMILY, PAST AND PRESENT

PREFACE

The purpose of this book is to provide students and other individuals interested in the area of hospital administration with a compilation of classic, current and controversial readings dealing with the hospital organization and its management. It is oriented toward the voluntary hospital system with particular emphasis given to the administrative subject areas of organization, management of personnel, labor relations, decision making, planning, and social responsibility. Specifically, this book treats the hospital organization from a managerial point of view.

The format used in presentation consists of the categorizing of the subject material into the following five parts: (1) THE HOSPITAL AS AN ORGANIZATION, (2) THE MANAGEMENT OF PERSONNEL IN HOSPITALS, (3) LABOR RELATIONS IN HOSPITALS, (4) QUANTITATIVE DECISION MAKING, and (5) HEALTH CARE POLICY AND TRENDS. Within each part there are multiple sections which provide for the breakdown of the subject material into logical units. Each part is prefaced with an editor's introduction and each section within each part is preceded with a brief editor's abstract of the readings included. This style was adopted for two reasons. First, the introduction to each part provides a means of interconnecting the various sections within it. Second, the abstracts provide the busy reader with sufficient information so that he can select those readings pertinent to his immediate interests.

While this work is not totally comprehensive, it does provide, in one volume, classic and current material. In addition, where the subject material permits, controversial points of view are included.

J. S. Rakich

Detroit, Michigan
March, 1972

ACKNOWLEDGEMENTS

The first acknowledgement is made to my wife who provided the moral support which made this work possible. Second, acknowledgment is made to Sam Barone of Saint Louis University and Thomas R. O'Donovan, Administrator of Detroit's Mount Carmel Mercy Hospital, for providing the assistance which lead, directly and indirectly, to the completion of this manuscript. Third, special acknowledgment is made to the HOSPITALS, HOSPITAL ADMINISTRATION, HOSPITAL PROGRESS, and MODERN HOSPITAL journals for allowing their respective articles to be reprinted along with G. P. Putnam's Sons for permission to excerpt material. In addition, appreciation is expressed to the authors represented in this volume for their cooperation. Finally, mention must be made to those who assisted in the preparation of this manuscript. Specifically, Dean R. Ito of The University of Detroit who provided support while the author was a member of the faculty and, Miss Diane Pierce who provided typing assistance, Mrs. Krieger and Mr. Pollock of the Catholic Hospital Association, and Mrs. Norlene Chadwick.

CONTENTS

PART II. THE MANGEMENT OF PERSONNEL IN HOSPITALS

Part I

THE HOSPITAL AS AN ORGANIZATION

The purpose of this part of the book is to acquaint the reader with the hospital as a functioning organization. The first section, STRUCTURE, presents the hospital as an organization, its functions, a description of its unique characteristics, and the delicate authority relationship among the institution's managing triad. The presentation of the overall organization structure provides the setting for the following three sections treating, in turn, the managing groups of the hospital. Those groups are the board of trustees, the administrator and the medical staff.

The second section, THE BOARD OF TRUSTEES, provides a description of their functions and responsibilities. The board has ultimate responsibility for the efficient and effective operation of the hospital. Consequently, its membership composition is important. In this section differing points of view are presented with respect to the issue of administrator - medical staff membership on the board.

The third section, THE HOSPITAL ADMINISTRATOR, presents his evolving professional role as it relates to the internal functioning of the hospital organization as well as his external influence on the health care system. The administrator's internal role consists of running an organization that is a major business requiring the application of modern managerial techniques. The external role focuses on the fact that the professional administrator is currently one of the central leadership figures who is instrumental in the shaping of community and national health care delivery.

The fourth section, THE MEDICAL STAFF, presents its functions and responsibilities. Due to the centralized role of today's hospital, the medical staff can no longer view the hospital as a self-service vehicle. Professional leadership is now necessary in order to cope with increased responsibilities. As the providers of health care, cognizance must be given to the issue of suboptimization which is frequently caused by ignoring the needs and requirements of the service facility within which the medical staff works. One suggestion presented is the adoption of modern management and organization techniques along with a results oriented philosophy.

The fifth section, HOSPITAL SYSTEMS, presents the hospital organization from a contemporary point of view. The hospital organization has a set of formal activities and functional areas which are interdependent with and inter-related to each other. The formal organizational system of the hospital requires the efficient functioning of all component parts. Its description provides a frame of reference whereby the impact resulting from the ineffective operation of any one component part can be perceived on all other interrelated parts. While it is not the only means to solving the hospital organization's problems, the systems concept provides the administrator with the opportunity to view the hospital as a whole rather than as disorganized parts.

Structure

The hospital is an organization that has unique characteristics which differentiate it from other institutions. This section presents the hospital as a functioning entity. In particular, its unique purpose, peculiar structure, and managing triad which consists of the board of trustees, administrator, and medical staff.

In the first reading, *THE HOSPITAL AS AN ORGANIZATION*, the community general hospital is presented as a humanitarian, quasi-bureaucratic, quasi-authoritarian organization with a mission of patient care. The organization is further described as one with extensive division of labor, specialization of work, and the requirement for adequate coordination.

The delicate balance of power, characteristic of the hospital organization, is presented in *WHO'S ON TOP? WHO KNOWS?* The scalar, functional, and informal status relationships between the board of trustees, administrator, and medical staff are described.

The awkward governance arrangement of the hospital triad is discussed in *STRICTURES AND STRUCTURES*. It is contended that the accommodation arrangement of running the hospital on compromise is in need of change due to the altered role of the hospital. A call for a governance system designed to coalesce the diverse interests, within and without the hospital, is made.

The Hospital as an Organization

BASIL S. GEORGOPOULOS, PH.D. AND FLOYD C. MANN, PH.D.

Basil S. Georgopoulos, Ph.D., is Program Director of the Survey Research Center and Professor of Psychology at the University of Michigan. Floyd C. Mann, Ph.D., is the director of the Center for Research on Utilization of Scientific Knowledge at the University of Michigan.

The community general hospital is an organization that mobilizes the skills and efforts of a number of widely divergent groups of professional, semiprofessional, and nonprofessional personnel to provide a highly personalized service to individual patients. Like other large-scale organizations, it is established and designed to pursue certain objectives through collaborative activity. The chief objective of the hospital is, of course, to provide adequate care and treatment to its patients (within the limits of present-day technical-medical knowledge, and knowledge of organizing human activity effectively, as well as within limits that may be imposed by the relative scarcity of appropriate organizational resources or by extraorganizational forces). Its principal product is medical, surgical, and nursing service to the patient, and its central concern is the life and health of the patient. A hospital may, of course, have additional objectives, including its own maintenance and survival, organizational stability and growth, financial solvency, medical and nursing education and research, and various employee-related objectives. But, all these are subsidiary to the key objective of service to the patient, which constitutes the basic organizing principle that underlies all activities in the community general hospital.

There is little ambiguity, if any, about the main organizational objective of the community general hospital. Unlike many organizations, the hospital is able to make the role it performs in the larger community psychologically meaningful to its members. And most of its members try to give unstintingly of their energies to perform the tasks assigned to them. Many doctors and nurses look upon their profession as a sacred calling. Others find working in the hospital deeply satisfying of needs that they cannot easily express in words. They see the hospital as a nonprofit institution dedicated to works of mercy, and they sense their mission in life to give of themselves in order to help others. Immediate personal comfort and satisfactions, and even material rewards, are defined by most members as less important than giving good care to the patient and meeting a higher order of obligation to mankind. Serious conflicts regarding material rewards, such as those found in organizations where profit is the chief motive, are virtually nonexistent in the hospital. For all these reasons, motivating organizational members toward the objectives of the organization is much less of a problem in the hospital by comparison to other large-scale organizations. The goals of individual members and the objectives of the organization are considerably more congruent in the case of the hospital.

EXTENSIVE DIVISION OF LABOR

To do its work, the hospital relies upon an extensive division of labor among its members, upon a complex organizational structure which encompasses many different departments, staffs, offices, and positions, and upon an elaborate system of coordination of tasks, functions, and social interaction.

Work in the hospital is greatly differentiated and specialized, and of a highly interactional character. It is carried out by a large number of cooperating people whose backgrounds, education, training, skills, and functions are as diverse and heterogeneous as can be found in any of the most complex organizations in existence. And much of the work is not only specialized but also performed by highly trained professionals—the doctors—who require the collaboration, assistance, and services of many other professional and nonprofessional personnel. In addition to the medical staff, which itself is highly specialized and departmentalized, there is the nursing staff, which includes graduate professional nurses in various supervisory and nonsupervisory positions, practical nurses, and untrained nurses' aides. In addition to the nursing staff and the medical staff, which are the two largest groups in the community general hospital, there are the hospital administrator and a number of administrative-supervisory personnel who head various departments or services (e.g., nursing, dietary, admissions, maintenance, pharmacy, medical records, housekeeping, laundry) and are in charge of the employees in these departments. There are also a number of medical technologists and technicians who work in the laboratory and X-ray departments of the hospital, as well as a number of miscellaneous clerical and secretarial personnel. And apart from all these staffs and professional-occupational groups, there is a board of trustees which has the overall formal responsibility for the organization, and which consists of a number of prominent people from the outside community. The trustees offer their services to the hospital without remuneration and are not employees of the organization. In short, professionalization and specialization are two of the hallmarks of the hospital.

HIGH INTERDEPENDENCE OF SERVICES

Because of this extensive division of labor and accompanying specialization of work, practically every person working in the hospital depends upon some other person or persons for the performance of his own organizational role. Specialists and professionals can perform their functions only when a considerable array of supportive personnel and auxiliary services is put at their disposal at all times. Doctors, nurses, and others in the hospital do not, and cannot, function separately or independently of one another, Their work is mutually supplementary, interlocking, and interdependent.

In turn, such a high interdependence requires that the various specialized functions and activities of the many departments, groups, and individual members of the organization be sufficiently coordinated, if the organization is to function effectively and attain its objectives. Consequently, the hospital has developed a rather intricate and elaborate system of internal coordination. Without coordination, concerted effort on the part of its different members and continuity in organizational operations could not be ensured.

It is also interesting and important to note here that, unlike industrial and other large-scale organizations, the hospital relies very heavily on the skills, motivations, and behaviors of its members for the attainment and maintenance of adequate coordination. The flow of work is too variable and irregular to permit coordination through mechanical standardization. And the product of the organization—patient care—is itself individualized rather than uniform or invariant. Because the work is neither mechanized nor uniform or standardized, and because it cannot be planned in advance with the automatic precision of an assembly line, the organization must depend a good deal upon its various members to make the day-to-day adjustments which the situation may demand, but which cannot possibly be completely detailed or prescribed by formal organizational rules and regulations. This is all the more essential, moreover, if one takes into account the fact that the patient, who is the center of all activity in the hospital, is a transient rather than a stable element in the system—in the short-stay hospital, he comes and goes very rapidly.

HOSPITALS: AUTHORITARIAN-DEMOCRATIC?

Fundamentally, then, the hospital is a human rather than a machine system. And even though it may possess elaborate and impressive-looking equipment, or a great variety of physical and material facilities, it has no integrated mechanical-physical systems for the handling and processing of its work. The patient is not a chunk of raw material that passively goes through an ordered progression of machines and assembly-line operators. At every stage of his short stay in the hospital, he is mainly dependent upon his interaction with the people who are entrusted with his care, and upon the skills, actions, and interactions of these different people. All of these factors necessitate heavy reliance upon the members of the organization to coordinate their activities on a voluntary, informal, and expedient basis.

Paradoxical as it may seem, however, the hospital is also a highly formal, quasi-bureaucratic organization which, like all task-oriented organizations, relies a great deal upon formal policies, formal written rules and regulations, and formal authority for controlling much of the behavior and work relationships of its members. The emphasis on formal organizational mechanisms and procedures and on directive rather than "democratic" controls, along with a number of other factors, gives the hospital its much talked about "authoritarian" character, which manifests itself in relatively sharp patterns of superordination-subordination, in expectations of strict discipline and obedience, and in distinct status differences among organizational members.

MAINTAINING AUTHORITARIANISM

The authoritarian character of the hospital is partly the result of historical forces having their origins at a time when professionalization and specialization were at a primordial stage, and when nursing, medicine, and the hospital were all closely associated with the work of religious orders and military institutions. The absence of substantial professionalization and specialization characteristic of hospital personnel at those times, along with the emphasis of religious and military institutions on social arrangements in which the occupant of every position in the organization presumably knew "his place," and kept to his place by strictly adhering to specified rights, duties, and obligations, had much to do with the hospital's adopting a strict hierarchical and authoritarian system of work arrangements. But, the advent of professionalization and specialization, the gradual independence of hospitals from religious and military institutions, and the impact of an increasingly secular culture have greatly reduced the authoritarian character of the hospital. As Lentz has noted, within the last 50 years the hospital has undergone marked changes, dropping some of its authoritarian and paternalistic characteristics and taking on those of a bureaucratic, functionally rational organization.

Today's community general hospital, however, still has some of its traditional authoritarian characteristics along with its emphasis on rational organization. Moreover, it is unlikely that it will rid itself of all authoritarianism in the near future. There are several major counterforces at work, in this connection. First, there is the fact that the hospital constantly deals with critical matters of life and death—matters which place a heavy burden of both secular and moral responsibility on the organization and its members. When human life is at stake, there is little tolerance for error or negligence. And, if error and negligence can be prevented by adherence to strict formal rules and quasi-authoritarian discipline, such rules are important to have and obedience cannot very well be questioned (although blind obedience is mitigated because the hospital increasingly relies on the expertness, judgment, and ethics of professionals who, while abhorring regimentation, are presumably capable of a good deal of self-discipline). Second, there is the great concern of the hospital for maximum efficiency and predictability of performance. In the absence of mechanically regulated workflows, this concern virtually forces the organization to use many quasi-authoritarian means of control (including rigid rules and procedures, directive supervision, rigorous discipline, etc.), in the hope of: (1) attaining some uniformity in the behavior of its members, (2) regulating their interaction and checking deviance within known limits of accountability, and (3) appraising their performance. Third, there is the temptation to adhere to traditional, familiar ways of doing things which, coupled with the lack of apparently equivalent or superior alternatives that could be employed to ensure clarity of responsibility and efficiency and predictability of performance, also serves to perpetuate organizational reliance upon customary directive means of control.[1]

HISTORY OF REGIMENTED BEHAVIOR

In brief, while historical forces might account for the origins of the authoritarian characteristics of the hospital, it is not likely that some of these characteristics would continue to persist (especially within the context of a highly secular culture) unless

[1] Incidentally, the apparent unavailability of equivalent or superior organizational alternatives is partly the result of our inadequate knowledge about how best to organize and manage human activity in a situation such as that of the community general hospital, and partly the result of the inability of hospitals to utilize the findings of modern research to best advantage.

they were more functional than not. And this clearly appears to be the case. In the first place, as in any organization designed to mobilize resources quickly in order to meet crises and emergencies successfully, a good deal of regimented behavior is required in the hospital. Lines of authority and responsibility have to be clearly drawn, basic acceptance of authority has to be assured, and discipline has to be maintained. In the second place, the hospital is expected to be able to provide adequate care to its patients at all times, with the precision of a machine system and with minimum error, even though it is a human rather than a machine system. It is expected to perform weil continuously and to produce a machinelike response toward the patient, regardless of such things as turnover, absenteeism, and feelings of friendship or hostility among its personnel, or other organizational problems that it may be experiencing. It is also expected to be responsive to the health-related needs and demands of its community, and to meet a variety of medicolegal requirements. Because of these expectations, the hospital places high premium on being able to count upon and predict the outcome of the performances of its members. And predictability of performance can be partly attained through directive, quasi-authoritarian controls which, in the absence of apparently superior alternatives, are rather tempting to the organization.

PUBLIC DEMANDS EFFICIENCY

Coupled with this great concern for predictability of performance, moreover, there is an increasing concern that the hospital operate as efficiently and economically as possible. As the hospital has become a resource for all members of the community, and not just the indigent and the impoverished, the public has come to expect of it the best medical and nursing services that can be offered. These services, however, are quite costly, as are the facilities, equipment, supplies, and medicines that are required. And while the public may be willing (though not necessarily able to afford) to pay for these essential costs of hospital care, it also expects the best care possible at reasonable cost or even at least cost. At the same time, it is neither willing to tolerate nor prepared to pay any costs that may result from inefficient operations, poor administration, duplication of services, waste, negligence, and the like. It expects its hospitals to reduce to a minimum or eliminate altogether costs of this latter type and to operate with maximum economy. The hospitals themselves are quite aware of these and other pressures for efficiency, and have come to place very high emphasis on greater efficiency. Great emphasis on economic efficiency, however, is not entirely compatible with the hospital's traditional humanitarian orientation and objective of best service to the patient; the "best" service is not always or necessarily the most economical. Furthermore, this concern for efficiency is resulting both in progressive rationalization of hospital operations and in the institution of more rigid controls within the organization. Such controls, incidentally, serve to maintain the remaining authoritarian characteristics of the community general hospital.

NEEDED: ORGANIZATIONAL COORDINATION

But, efficiency of operations and predictability of performance in the hospital could not possibly be attained only through directive and quasi-authoritarian controls. In fact, if carried to extremes, such controls would in the long run be inimical both to efficiency and to predictability. Efficiency and predictability of performance are also, and perhaps primarily, attained through a number of other factors, which are essential to effective organizational functioning. Probably the most prominent of these factors in the case of the community general hospital are organizational coordination and professionalization.

Because of the high degrees of specialization and functional interdependence found in the hospital, coordination of skills, tasks, and activities is indispensable to effective organizational performance and its predictability. The different specialized, but interacting and interdependent, parts of the organization must fit well together; they must not work at cross purposes or in their own separate directions. If the organization is to attain its objectives, its different parts and members must function according to each other's needs and expectations of the total organization. In short, they must be well coordinated. But, as we have already pointed out, the hospital is dependent very greatly upon the motivations and voluntary, informal adjustments of its members for the attainment and maintenance of good coordination. Formal organizational plans, rules, regulations, and controls may ensure some minimum coordination, but of themselves are incapable of producing adequate coordination, for only a fraction of all the coordinative activities required in this organization can be programed in advance.

THE SUBJECT OF PROFESSIONALIZATION

The other relevant factor that we wish to consider here, in addition to coordination, is that of professionalization—professionalization being one of the major distinctive features of the community general hospital. The majority of those who hold the principal therapeutic and nontherapeutic positions in the hospital are trained as professionals. The doctors, through their training, have been schooled in certain professional obligations, ethics, and standards of appropriate behavior, and have acquired a number of common attitudes, shared values, and mutual understandings about their work and work relations with others. The same is true about the registered nurses. Other groups in the organization are also on the road to professionalization: the administrators, the medical librarians, the medical technologists, the dietitians, and others in paramedical positions.

COMPLEMENTARY EXPECTATIONS

This high degree of professionalization among those entrusted with the care of the patient has developed along lines of rational, functional specialization, and has had the effect of inculcating many complementary expectations and common norms and values in the members of the principal groups of the hospital—values, expectations, and norms that are essential to the integration of the organization. These include the norms of giving good care, devotion to duty, loyalty, selflessness and altruism, discipline, and hard work. This normative structure underpins the formal rational structure of the organization, and enables the hospital to attain a level of coordination and integration that could never be accomplished through administrative edict, through hierarchical directives, or through explicitly formulated and carefully specified organizational plans and impersonal rules, regulations, and procedures. However, increased professionalization and specialization have also had the effect of sharpening some of the status differences among the people working in the hospital—and sharp status distinctions bespeak of some authoritarianism.

Among other things, increased professionalization in the hospital has helped guarantee that certain minimum levels of competence and skill would exist in the organization, thus having a direct impact upon performance and organizational effectiveness. Similarly, professionalization and specialization have contributed to greater public confidence in the hospital, and to a wider acceptance of the hospital as a resource for the health needs of all people, for high professionalization and specialization imply expertness and knowledge. Increased professionalization has undoubtedly resulted in improved patient care and, in so doing, it has also raised the expectations of the public for both high-quality care and high efficiency in hospital operations. More and more of us go to the hospital for our various health needs nowadays but, because of improved service, we stay there for a shorter and shorter period of time. In the last 30 years, the average length of stay for adult patients in general hospitals has decreased by about a third, from 12.6 to 8.6 days—making it increasingly appropriate to refer to the community general hospital as the short-stay hospital.

NO SINGLE LINE OF AUTHORITY

Another of the distinctive characteristics of the community general hospital, closely related to professionalization and specialization, is the absence of a single line of authority in the organization. This feature has already been the subject of considerable discussion by Smith and others, but is important enough to warrant some brief observations here. Essentially, authority in the hospital is shared (not equally) by the board of trustees, the doctors, and the administrator—the three centers of power in the organization—and, to some extent, also by the director of nursing. In the hospital, authority does not emanate from a single source and does not flow along a single line of command as it does in most formal organizations.

A formal organizational chart of the hospital shows the board of trustees as having ultimate authority and overall responsibility for the institution. The board delegates the day-to-day management of the organization to the hospital administrator. In turn, the administrator delegates authority to the heads of the various nonmedical departments (including the director of nursing, who also wields a different kind of authority that originates in her professional expertness). The heads of these departments, in turn, have varying degrees of authority over the affairs of their respective departments and personnel. In the formal organizational chart, the medical staff, its officers, and its members are not shown as having any direct-line responsibility; they are outside of the lay-administrative line of authority. Yet, as is well known both within and outside the hospital, the doctors exercise substantial influence throughout the hospital structure at nearly all organizational levels, enjoy very high autonomy in their work, and have a good deal of professional authority over others in the organization. Over the nursing staff and over the patients, their professional authority is dominant. And although the board of trustees is in theory shown as the ultimate source of authority, the board actually has very limited *de facto* authority over the medical staff. Partly because the doctors are not employees of the hospital (they are "guests" who are granted practice privileges), partly because they enjoy high status and great prestige, partly because they have almost supreme authority in professional-medical matters, and partly for other reasons, they are subject to very little lay-organizational authority.

THE DIFFICULTIES THAT ARISE

Professionals in staff capacities in business corporations—lawyers, doctors, accountants, and others—have little or no authority to be involved in the activities of the line; they mainly serve as consultants and advisors. But this is not so in the case of the hospital. The absence of a single line of authority in the hospital, of course, creates various administrative and operational problems, as well as psychological problems having to do with the relative power and influence on organizational functioning on the part of doctors, trustees, administrators, and others. For one thing, it makes formal organizational coordination rather difficult. For another thing, it allows for instances in which it is not clear where authority, responsibility, and accountability reside. Similarly, it allows for a situation wherein a large number of organizational members, particularly members of the nursing staff, must be responsible to and take orders not only from their supervisors but also from the doctors. The lay authority and the professional authority to which nurses are subject, of course, are not always consistent. The absence of a single line of authority also makes for difficulties in communication, difficulties in the area of discipline, and difficulties in resolving problems that must be resolved through cooperative efforts on the part of both the lay-administrative and medical-professional sides. Frequently, the administrator, feeling that the responsibility for the overall management of the organization is his, and feeling that doctors through their power and pressures interfere in the discharge of his responsibilities, is motivated or actively attempts to circumvent the medical staff on various matters, and this, too, is apt to lead to problems. (The doctors, in turn, are likely to try to circumvent the administrator.) For the same reasons, the administrator is likely to be prone toward more and more bureaucratization in the hospital. And increased bureaucratization of organizational operations is likely to be fought and resented by the doctors, for it eventually means a reduction in their influence.

DELICATE BALANCE OF POWER

In general, multiple lines of authority require the maintenance of a very delicate balance of power in the organization—a balance of power that is rather precarious. On the positive side, multiple lines of authority may serve as a system of "checks and balances," which may prevent other kinds of possible problems, such as organizational inflexibility and authoritarianism, or may serve to lighten the burden of responsibility in situations where responsibility may be too great for any single group or individual to shoulder. Regardless of the advantages and disadvantages of a system of multiple lines of authority, such a system is an integral part of the community general hospital. Not only is it an integral part, moreover, but also a part that is virtually inevitable for an organization such as this. This is because much of the work in the hospital is performed by influential professionals and not by low-status workers, and because of the high degrees of both professionalization and specialization characteristic of the organization. As Parsons has aptly observed, "The multiplication of technical fields, and their differentiation from each other . . . leads to an essential element of decentralization in the organizations which must employ them." For this reason, he goes on to explain that, unlike business and military organizations, "A university can not be organized mainly on a 'line' principle. . . ." In this respect, the community general hospital is very similar to a university. (Hospitals and universities have a number of other interesting characteristics in common, but here we are interested only in hospitals.)

In summary, the community general hospital is an extremely complex social organization that differs from business and other large-scale organizations on a number of important characteristics. Among its main distinguishing characteristics, the following are worth reemphasizing:

MAIN DISTINGUISHING CHARACTERISTICS

1. The main objective of the organization is to render personalized service—care and treatment—to individual patients, rather than the manufacture of some uniform material object. And the economic value of the organization's products and objectives is secondary to their social and humanitarian value.

2. By comparison to industrial organizations, the hospital is much more directly dependent upon, and responsive to, its surrounding community, and its work is much more closely integrated with the needs and demands of its consumers and potential customers. To the hospital and its members, the patients' needs are always of supreme and paramount importance. Moreover, there is high agreement about the principal objective of the hospital among the members of the organization, and the personal needs and goals of the different members conflict little with the objectives of the organization.

3. The demands of much of the work at the hospital are of an emergency nature and nondeferrable. They place a heavy burden of both secular-functional and moral responsibility upon the organization and its members. Correspondingly, the organization shows great concern for clarity of responsibility and accountability among its different members, and very little tolerance for either ambiguity or error.

4. The nature and volume of work are variable and diverse, and subject to relatively little standardization. The hospital cannot lend itself to mass production techniques, to assembly-line operations, or to automated functioning. It is a human rather than a machine system, with all the attributes this entails. Both the raw materials and end products of the organization are human. And, being human, they participate actively in the production process, thus having a good deal of control over it.

5. The principal workers in the hospital—doctors and nurses—are professionals, and this entails various administrative and operational problems for the organization.

6. By comparison to industrial organizations, the hospital has relatively little control over its workload and over many of its key members. In particular, it has little direct control over the doctors and over the patients—two of its most essential components. In the short-stay hospital, the patients are not only a very heterogeneous

and very transient group, but are also, mainly and ultimately, in the hands of their doctors, who are not employees of the organization.

7. The administrator has much less authority, power, and discretion than his managerial counterparts in industry because the hospital is not and cannot very well be organized on the basis of a single line of authority. The simultaneous presence of lay, professional, and mixed lay-professional lines of authority in the hospital creates a number of administrative and other problems, which business organizations are largely spared.

8. The hospital is a formal, quasi-bureaucratic, and quasi-authoritarian organization which, like most organizations of this kind, relies greatly on conventional hierarchical work arrangements and on rather rigid impersonal rules, regulations, and procedures. But, more importantly, it is a highly departmentalized, highly professionalized, and highly specialized organization that could not possibly function effectively without relying heavily for its internal coordination on the motivations, actions, self-discipline, and voluntary, informal adjustments of its many members. Coordination of efforts and activities in the hospital is indispensable to organizational functioning, because the work is of a highly interactional character—the activities of organizational members are highly interlocking and interdependent, and the various members can perform their role only by working in close association with each other.

9. The hospital shows a very great concern for efficiency and predictability of performance among its members and for overall organizational effectiveness.

10. Finally, the community general hospital is an organization which is important to us all, and which is becoming increasingly important. Several basic social trends tend to ensure this: the accelerating accumulation of new medical knowledge, new medical, surgical, and nursing procedures, and new drugs and medicines; rising levels of family income in the nation; increased use of the general hospital for numerous different diseases and health needs; and a growing demand by the general public for the best possible quality of medical-surgical and nursing care.

It has been the purpose of this section to introduce the reader to some of the key characteristics and organizational problems of the community general hospital. (Many of these will be examined in detail in subsequent chapters.) The characteristics and problems discussed above, along with many others to be dealt with throughout the book, show how complicated an organization the hospital is, and lead one to suspect that increased understanding of such problems and characteristics might help ease some of the management difficulties and perhaps also improve the organizational effectiveness of our hospitals.

Who's on Top?
Who Knows?

RICHARD T. VIGUERS

When we try to draw a chart to illustrate the organization of a hospital, we come out with either a neat, clear chart which bears no relationship to the actual organization, or else we produce a complex pattern of squares, lines and boxes that no one can understand. Every author produces a different type of chart, and each graphically illustrates one aspect of the hospital organization, but none of them shows the varied and complex and different relationships of the hospital organization. Perhaps the reason for this is that any one chart, or at least any two dimensional chart, cannot show the different organizational relationships that exist in the hospital. If we are to deal more effectively with the relationships of the various people in the hospital working together to serve the patient, we need a better understanding of the organizational relationships or status systems of the hospital. There is not just one organizational structure, but several distinct status systems which are the basis of the way in which the hospital really operates.

Chester A. Barnard, in 1946, wrote a thoughtful article which he called "a report of a preliminary inquiry into the nature and functions of systems of status in formal organizations." Mr. Barnard points out two kinds of status systems, one which he designates as *scalar* and another as *functional.* These are relatively similar in business corporations, which Mr. Barnard considers, but they are quite different in hospitals.

The scalar status is the one with which we are all familiar and is what is shown on the usual hospital organization chart. It shows the chain of command in the formal organization of the hospital. This scalar chart of hospitals was borrowed from the business or industrial corporation.

There are at least as many different scalar charts of hospital organization as there are hospitals, but a general pattern is illustrated in Chart 1, which shows a line and a staff organization. Here we have the usual pattern of authority emanating from a board of trustees to the administrator and from the administrator to the department heads: nursing, dietary, medical records, accounting, maintenance, housekeeping and so on. In a unique position is the medical staff of the hospital—responsible to the administrator in certain matters and also reaching the trustees through the joint liaison or similar commitee, consisting of representatives of the staff, several trustees and the administrator.

CHART 1–HOSPITAL SCALAR STATUS

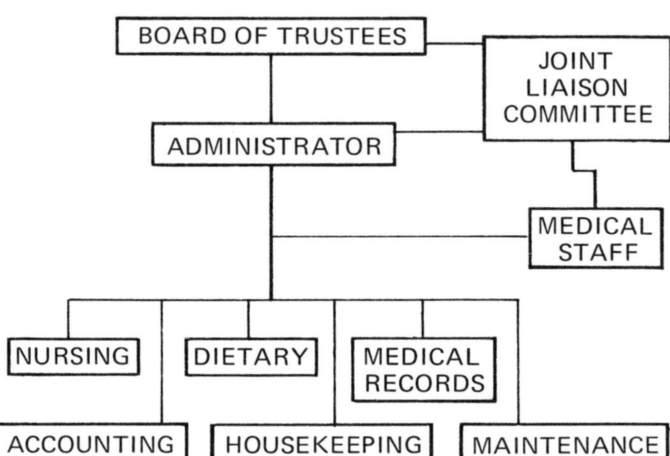

This scalar pattern deals with matters of general policy, financial aspects of the hospital operation, and employes, and is charged with carrying out the rules and regulations of the hospital.

The second kind of organization in the hospital is the functional. It is in this functional organization that the doctor assumes the top position of command and authority. He does this not because of the scalar organization but because in the care of patients the doctor, by his education, training, skill and responsibility, must assume this top position in the functional organization of the hospital.

This functional status system does not depend on authority and jurisdiction as in the scalar organization. Leadership in this functional organization depends upon the skills, the training, and the ability to carry out the specific objective.

Harvey L. Smith, a sociologist at the University of North Carolina, discussed this functional organization in his article, "Two Lines of Authority Are One Too Many," in **THE MODERN HOSPITAL** for March 1955. Thirty years ago, that remarkable student of administration, Mary Parker Follet, discussed it. What has been here called "scalar status" she called "position authority," that is, authority stemming from the position in the hierarchy, and pointed out the growing importance in industry of "functional authority." (See also "The Give and Take in Hospitals" by Burling, Lentz and Wilson. G. P. Putnam's Sons, New York, 1956.)

To illustrate this functional organization we can look at the army, which is the supreme example of the scalar organization, but still you can find special situations illustrating the functional organization. I remember a language class consisting of officers, ranking from captains to brigadier generals, which was taught by a corporal. The corporal stood at the top of this functional organization because he was a specialist in linguistics and had the special knowledge and skill necessary to teach the langauge. The fact that he was only a corporal was irrelevant. He taught the class, directed, corrected, and guided the officers. The corporal teaching this language class is an example of functional organization or functional status.

In the army the functional organization is unusual and unimportant, but in the hospital it assumes a position of primary importance. The physician in carrying out the direct care of the patient assumes the position of leadership in this functional situation because of his professional knowledge, skill and training.

In Chart 2 is shown the functional organization or status of the hospital. Here the doctor steps into the primary role of direction and leadership. It is the doctor who decides whether the patient should have aspirin or cortisone. In this position the doctor tells the nurse, the dietitian, the housekeeper, and the administrator what to do. The doctor occupies the top position in these matters dealing with the direct care of the patient, and the paramedical personnel and other hospital employes follow his directions.

CHART 2—HOSPITAL FUNCTIONAL STATUS

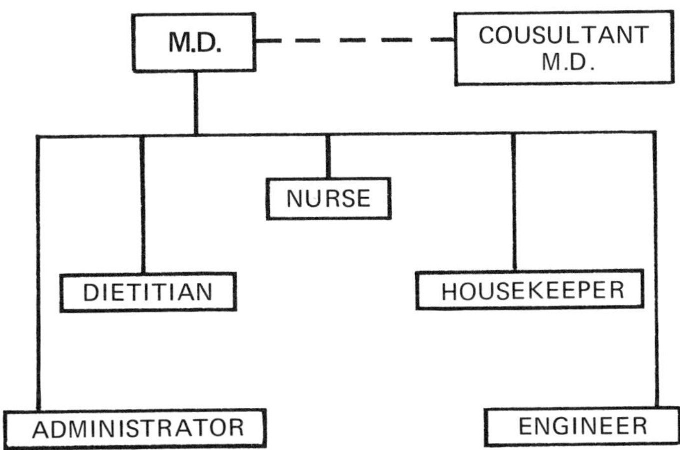

WHO'S BOSS HERE?

Consider several situations which illustrate the two separate and distinct organizations—scalar and functional. Suppose the hospital has a rule that no elective surgery can be begun after 3 p.m. Surgeon "A" has a case which he says is not an emergency, but he wishes to do the case today and will start the case at 3:30 p.m. This situation falls under the scalar organization, and the operating room supervisor, the director of nursing, or the administrator has the authority and the responsibility of telling Surgeon "A" that he cannot do the case.

Now suppose that at 4 p.m. Surgeon "B" says that he has a patient requiring immediate surgery. This now shifts the situation to the functional status. Surgeon "B" now assumes the top position, and he directs the nurses, the technicians, the administrator, and other hospital employes in what they must do to assist in providing optimal care for the patient. As long as Surgeon "B" is dealing with the care of this patient and as long as he operates within the scope of his appointment by the trustees and within the general rules and regulations of the hospital, all the persons involved follow the directions of Surgeon "B." This includes not only the nursing care, medication and treatment, but the type of food, necessary equipment and supplies, and even administrative regulations such as visiting and the like.

If Doctor "C" calls the administrator and says, "I have a polio patient who is 6 feet 9 inches tall and I need an eight-foot bed and a special long respirator," the administrator, purchasing agent, or responsible administrative officer immediately tries to get the necessary equipment. This is part of the functional organization, and the doctor directs the activity. Of course, if the policy of the hospital is not to accept polio patients, then there is a shift back to the scalar organization, and the responsibility of the administrator is to enforce the policy of the hospital and direct the admission of the polio patient elsewhere.

The operation of the hospital breaks down when those who work in the hospital fail to work within the proper structure. When the administrator (M.D. or not) tells Doctor "A" that his patient should have aspirin and not cortisone, disaster is likely to result. Or if Doctor "A" reminds the administrator that he knows where smoking is dangerous and that he will decide when and where to smoke, or if Doctor "A" states that he will decide whether or not a medical record is necessary for his patient, only chaos can result.

Those who say that the doctor must always be boss and those who say that the doctor is never the boss are both ignoring the realities of hospital organization. In the scalar organization the doctor is not the boss, and in the functional organization the doctor must be the boss.

The nurse is put in a particularly difficult position as she works sometimes in a functional status and sometimes in a scalar status. Working with the same people and in the same situation, the nurse frequently has to change positions. For example, consider the scrub nurse working with Surgeon "B." As the operation proceeds the nurse follows the directions of the surgeon. But suppose the surgeon says: "It is not necessary to send this tissue to Pathology. Put it in the incinerator." Since the rule of the hospital is that all tissue removed in surgery must be sent to Pathology, the nurse must now change her role, assume authority under the scalar organization, and not only refuse to carry out the order to destroy the tissue but must give a contrary order that the tissue be sent to the pathology laboratory. It is this sort of a situation which can lead to such explosive results and which is so difficult for all the personnel involved.

PERSONALITY PLAYS A PART

Having discussed the scalar and functional status systems in the hospital, now let us look at a third status system—the *informal status* in a hospital. This status system depends upon personal relationships. This organization emerges because in every situation there are individuals who, because of their personality or activities, assume a position of leadership or influence. This has nothing to do with the person who is appointed as a department head or supervisor; rather it is the person who naturally emerges and is accepted by others as a leader with special contacts and influence with other personnel. We administrators are often unaware that an informal organization exists in our hospital, but every time a study is made, we always find that one does exist, and hospital employes who do not have top positions in the scalar organization are usually well aware of the informal status pattern in the hospital and know how it operates.

CHART 3—HOSPITAL INFORMAL STATUS

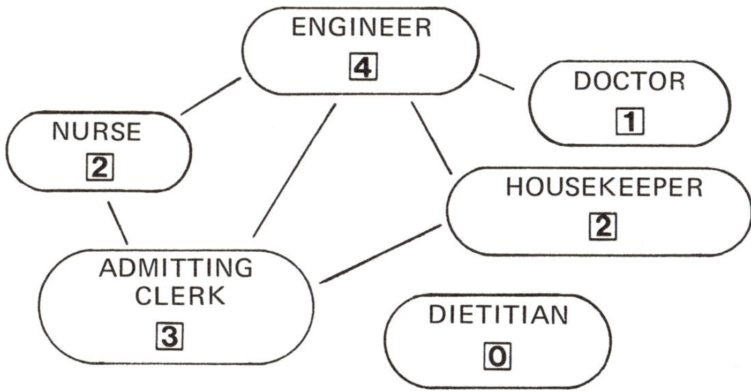

Chart 3 gives an example of an informal status pattern. In this hospital, the engineer is an efficient, valued employe who has been on the job for many years and is a friendly, helpful person, liked by everyone. This engineer knows the nurse very well since they have worked together for many years. He is likewise on close, friendly terms with the admitting clerk and housekeeper, and has been for some years friendly with the doctor who has taken care of the engineer's family without charging a fee. The nurse, in turn, knows the admitting clerk, who is an older nurse, and they often eat lunch together. The admitting clerk is a close friend of the housekeeper, and the dietitian is not particularly friendly in this social group. On the chart the arrow-heads by each individual show these relationships, and the engineer is designated as a *(4)*, the nurse as a *(2)*, the admitting clerk as *(3)*, the dietitian as *(0)*, the housekeeper as *(2)*, and the doctor as *(1)*.

This is only one informal grouping within the hospital and there are likely to be others in which these individuals bear different relationships. For example, the dietitian might be a *(5)* in another informal status pattern, and the engineer might be a *(2)*.

MRS. JONES GETS A BED

As an illustration of how this might work, suppose the doctor comes into the hospital in the morning and meets the engineer. As he stops to talk in the basement corridor the engineer thanks the doctor for having taken care of his little girl and asks the doctor how things are going. The doctor comments, "Very well, except that old battle-ax admitting clerk will not get a free bed for my patient, Mrs. Jones." The engineer says he will see what he can do about it and takes off for the admitting office. The engineer then says to the admitting clerk: "Where's that radio you want fixed? I think I can fix it up for you and it won't cost you anything." As the admitting clerk is thanking the engineer for this favor, the engineer mentions poor old Mrs. Jones, whom he says is a friend of his and he certainly thinks the hospital should admit her to a free bed. The clerk says, "Well, since you put it that way, I'll make the arrangements to admit Mrs. Jones." The engineer then arranges to catch the doctor before he has left the hospital and tell him that he has arranged it, and that they are going to be able to find a bed for Mrs. Jones.

Later in the day the engineer, having fixed the radio for the admitting clerk by getting a new tube from the hardware store which will be billed to the hospital as "miscellaneous screws and bolts," takes the radio back to the admitting clerk and completes this cycle.

However, at this time the admitting clerk starts chattering about the hospital and comments that the food is "terrible." Well, the engineer is duly concerned about this, so as he passes the nurse he mentions the fact that he has heard the food is terrible, and the nurse says, yes, she guesses it is. The engineer also makes it a point to tell the doctor that the patients all think the food is terrible and that something should be done about it. In the next day or so, word also goes to the housekeeper over the lunch table that the food is terrible. Not so long afterward, the administrator all of a sudden gets complaints from the doctor, the nurse, and the housekeeper that the food is terrible and that something should be done about it. In most cases the administrator will assume that he is doing a good job in coordinating the reports which come to him, and so he proceeds to tell the dietitian that the food is terrible and something must be done about it, etc., etc., etc..

This informal organization is an important part of the hospital status structure. It is a part of the way a hospital operates and, depending upon the department head's or administrator's relationships with the key individuals in the informal structure of the hospital, the policies of the administrator or department head can be assisted or, to a large extent, they can be blocked. We are not concerned here with what an administrator should do about this informal organization, but are merely pointing out that it exists and that the informal organization has as important effect upon the hospital's operation.

SOCIAL STRATA EXIST

We have discussed the scalar, functional and informal statuses in the hospital, but there are other status systems which have an important, although less obvious, bearing on the hospital operation. In Chart 4 we see the sociological status of the hospital.

This status system is based on the social traditions and mores of the community. It is a rigid pattern and new groups in the hospital organization find that they do not easily fit into the pattern.

<h2 style="text-align:center">CHART 4—HOSPITAL SOCIOLOGICAL STATUS</h2>

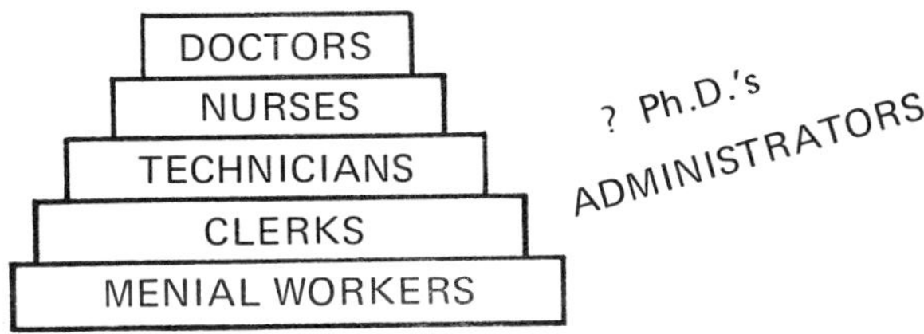

At the top of the sociological organization are the doctors. Under the doctors, and going down the ladder, are the nurses, then the technicians who are followed by the clerical personnel and, finally at the bottom, are the menial workers.

A new group coming into the hospital finds it difficult to establish its status in the sociological pattern. For example, the Ph.D.'s, the biophysicists, biochemists, statisticians and sociologists, who are playing increasingly active roles in hospitals, have no clear social status. They do not feel that they should be classed with the technicians and they are not accepted, as yet, into the medical staff category.

The administrator as a representative of a distinct professional group is a " johny-come-lately" and has no clear-cut niche in the sociological structure. If the administrator has a background as a doctor, a nurse, a technician, or an accountant, he tends to remain with this group sociologically. But if the administrator has no such background or if he has not served in such a capacity in that hospital, then he does not fit comfortably into any of the social strata.

The position of the individual in the community outside the hospital has an important influence on his social standing in the hospital structure. An administrator who has a high econimic, social or political position in the community tends to move up to the top of the social ladder in the hospital, and conversely, a low economic, social or political position in the community moves the administrator down the social ladder in the hospital. A technician or a bookkeeper who is the wife of a doctor on the hospital staff tends to move up the ladder as does the menial worker who is related to a doctor or a nurse.

The sociological structure of a hospital is a fascinating area but it cannot be developed here. It has been discussed only to bring out the fact that a sociological structure exists in the hospital; it is an important status structure, and, as every administrator knows, it often causes complex and difficult administrative problems.

We have looked at four status systems within the hospital—scalar, functional, informal, and sociological. Now let us look at a fifth status system—the psychological — which operates quietly but sometimes with devastating results.

FATHER-CHILD RELATIONSHIPS

When a trustee or an administrator becomes a patient of one of the doctors on the staff (and sooner or later everyone becomes a patient), if there is a serious illness or if emotional elements are an important aspect of the illness, a relationship often results which can be described as a child-father relationship. This child-father relationship between the patient and the doctor does not imply anything derogatory to the patient or the doctor; it is merely a psychological fact. If a trustee, administrator, nurse or any other employe is carried through a serious illness, especially one with strong emotional aspects, there tends to develop a child-father relationship between the patient and the doctor. This same relationship can also develop indirectly; for example, between a father and the doctor when the doctor is caring for the child.

CHART 5—HOSPITAL PSYCHOLOGICAL STATUS

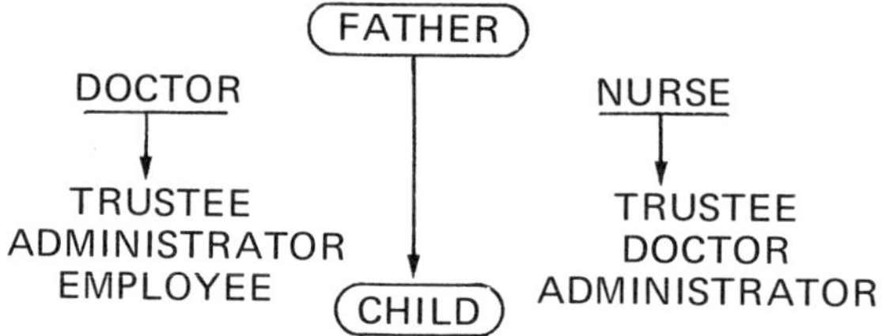

This child-father relationship can be, and sometimes is, exploited by the physician for personal advantage or for ends which the physician believes are in the best interests of the hospital. But even if this relationship is not exploited, there is an emotional bias which tends to distort decisions being made by a trustee, an administrator, a nurse, or any other hospital employe.

Independent and separate psychological relationships may be developed in any formal organization, but they are developed to a unique and significant degree in hospitals. It is true that the trustee, administrator or other hospital employe may develop a situation where he becomes the father and the doctor the child in the relationship. This will create special problems, but it is not the typical situation.

In the hospital psychological status the typical pattern is to find some trustee, the administrator, or some key employe in the relationship of child to father with some member of the medical staff. This situation almost always causes difficulties and sometimes has disastrous results. The trustee, administrator or other employe in this child-father relationship is emotionally motivated in his decisions and actions to the detriment of other physicians, the hospital, and the patients.

This discussion of status systems in the hospital does not pretend to give any specific answers as to how to administer a hospital. It is hoped that it will give a basis for the understanding of some of the complex relationships in the hospital organization, for understanding is the basis of cooperation, and we must all work together—the medical profession, allied groups, and the public—if we are to advance in the area of medical care.

Strictures and Structures

RAY E. BROWN

Ray E. Brown is Executive Vice President of the McGraw Medical Center of Northwestern University.

The governance of the American hospital has always been elusive, amorphous, and confusing. Bewildered students of management have been able to find no theories to fit the apparently headless enterprise and have dismissed the situation as an enigma in much the same manner as aerodynamics engineers have treated the notion of the bumblebee flying. Hospitals had to coordinate too many diverse parts and divergent interests to remain organizationally inexplicable, however, and so they invented their own explanation. Because hospitals weren't anxious to admit to the organizational anomaly of a headless enterprise—and even less anxious to face up to the confrontation of the interests at contest by establishing a clear-cut hierarchical structure—they retreated to the other end of the anatomical scale and created the concept of the multilegged organization. Thus was born the presently existing organizational model with no avowed head but three proclaimed legs—trustees, administrator, and medical staff. This organizational arrangement has served the same purpose as the Soviet troika by ensuring an uneasy standoff between the three principal contenders for organizational authority. But it provided capabilities more for legwork than headwork. It also was magnificently designed to ensure that the hospital could move in three different ways without going in any direction.

The awkward and fragmented governance arrangement of the hospital is an inheritance from its past. The hospital was originally conceived as an agency dedicated to doing good rather than well. It was little more than a home away from home for the sick poor. The physicians didn't need the hospital in the beginning and the hospital didn't need management. Money was almost the sole problem of the early hospital and it was not a serious one. The persons who put up the needed sums of money thereby solved the major problem. These persons were the trustees, and they sat alone in the governance saddle because they were responsible for the saddlebags. That arrangement was natural and appropriate and it still persists in many welfare agencies whose purpose is assistance rather than operations. Sitting on top was neither too difficult nor too threatening to others as long as hospital trustees were sitting largely on their own funds.

SOME CHANGES MADE

Scientific medicine changed the seat on which hospital trustees were sitting, however. Scientific medicine changed the nature and the traditions of hospitals and brought both the doctor and his private patients into the hospital. The hospital became the depository of the community's medical resources and, with that change, the hospital trustee began sitting on the doctor's professional and economic prerequisites. At the same time, the hospital trustee started sitting on the hospital patients' funds rather than his own. He also began sitting on top of a complex, expensive, and multipurpose operating enterprise. All this produced a need for management in large doses. It also spelled dependency for a very independent medical profession and it necessitated operational disengagement by deeply engaged hospital trustees.

The present model of fragmented, divergent, and indecisive governance of the hospital represents a stalemate between the aspirations, the fears, and the needs of the three principal participants in that governance. It is more a result of compromise than of organizational logic. In a real way it can be described as a product of organizational treaty rather than organizational treatise.

NOT TOO DAMAGING

The accommodation arrangement under which hospitals have been governed for the past half century was not too damaging to hospital effectiveness. In some ways it was highly effective. If one discounts the frustration experienced by the participants, and the occasional abortive upheaval that has occurred in a few hospitals, the individual hospital has fared well. Reviewing this apparent paradox, one sees several reasons for it. Foremost is the rapid growth in utilization and support that hospitals have experienced. It is hard to go wrong when everything is going right. Also, the momentum of growth helps an enterprise run away from its deficiencies and run over its problems. In another vein, the very rapidity of change along all environmental fronts has served to both lay the dust over hospital miscues and lay the path for them to follow. Perhaps most importantly, the expertness in brinkmanship developed by all three components of the hospital governance triad enabled the hospital to hold together and to maintain a course. Perceptivity regarding how far one can go in bucking the crew or the tide preserves sufficient order to keep things moving. In the case of the hospital, this has meant a large unity of effort, instead of large dissension, despite the diffusion of authority.

CHANGING CIRCUMSTANCES

The governance by sufferance that has characterized the hospital to date is not being challenged by changing circumstances and by other claimants to a piece of the governance. Running hospitals to suit the compromised notions of trustees, administrators, and doctors is being attacked on both organizational grounds and on public policy grounds. There is mounting concern and criticism from various groups and organizations that hospitals are not running well nor running in the right direction.

The concerns and criticisms reflect in part the changing circumstances in which hospitals find themselves. Inflation, medical advances, and increasing utilization have caused hospital costs to rise precipitously and have raised questions regarding the operating efficiency and quality of hospital management. Third-party payers are now picking up most of the tab for the hospital, meaning that hospital costs and hospital programs are concerns of the paying public—whether through private sector or governmental third parties. Social policy, now committed to adequate medical and hospital care for all members of the population, denotes governmental responsibility to redeem this commitment. At the same time, those to whom the commitment was made are asserting a right to help determine how the commitment will be met. So, the long-standing obscurity in the governance of the hospital is further clouded by the strong claims of third parties, government, and organized community groups to have an input in that governance.

It is not simply a question of adding the new claimants as legs to a three-legged entity. The present three legs have themselves become restive because of the criticism and the threats of the new claimants. Each entity is asking for a clearer definition of its role and a better structured mode of role expression. A multitude of court decisions and a host of private and governmental approval and regulatory agencies are making similar demands.

As hospitals become more expensive, involved, and committed, the need for restructuring of their governance becomes imperative. The demand for this will grow increasingly loud and incessant by all parties at interest. The organizational model that is developed must provide strength in both program determination and in operations. It also must afford a proper amount and mode of input into the governance process from each of the interest groups. Most of all, the governance must be designed to coalesce rather than to checkmate the diverse interests represented. The present governance arrangement provides an easy means for everyone to say "no" and very little means for the hospital to say "yes." The central position hospitals now have in the total medical care program of the community requires positive leadership on the part of the hospital. This does not mean that it is supposed to be easy prey for all claims made on its program or resources. It does mean that if it is to program effectively, and operate efficiently, it must have an effective governance arrangement for making up its mind and carrying out its decisions.

The Board of Trustees

This section is devoted to the board of trustees. As the major policy making body in the organization, the board members are responsible for the total well being of the hospital. Changing patterns of medical care, demand for services, and technologies have thrust greater responsibilities on this governing body. As a result, the functioning of the board is taking on increased importance.

Membership composition of the board and its responsibilities are discussed in *BOARD OF TRUSTEES.* In addition, the board's operational relationship to the other two groups within the triad, the administrator and medical staff, is presented. As the public guardians of the hospital organization, the board serves an increasingly important function.

The issue of "Inside" board membership is raised in *SHOULD ADMINISTRATORS SERVE ON HOSPITAL BOARDS?* The analogy of corporate officers serving on their organization's board is made along with the identification of the advantages and disadvantages of having the administrator serve on the hospital's board of trustees.

The question of having physicians serve on the board of trustees is raised in *SHOULD DOCTORS BE ON YOUR BOARD?* It is contended that organization effectiveness is dependent upon more physician involvement in policy making.

A different point of view and convincing argument is made for not having the physician serve on the board in *THE DOCTOR AS A TRUSTEE.* Since the doctor's function is to devote his time to healing, maximization of human resource effectiveness is achieved when the management of the hospital is left to the administrative experts.

The Board of Trustees

TEMPLE BURLING, M.D., EDITH M. LENTZ, PH.D. AND ROBERT N. WILSON

The responsibility of the hospital trustee for the general policy of the institution cannot be understood without some conception of the voluntary nature of the role. The spirit of voluntarism in America has traditionally supported the idea that men can willingly band together for a common purpose without governmental controls. Thus outstanding citizens freely devote time and energy to a nonprofit enterprise from which they can derive no personal gain except community prestige and inner satisfaction. Trustees serve, for the most part, because they are genuinely interested in the quality of hospital care and feel some obligation, as favored members of the society, to give their voluntary service. When a loose association of men governs a complex organization, innumerable problems of authority, specialization, and definition are created. The advantage of such control is that it is responsive to local community interests and preserves the flexibility essential to meet a swiftly changing situation.

WHO ARE THE TRUSTEES?

Trustees are usually chosen from among the more prominent members of the community, and in the hospitals we observed they tended to have attained high status in business or the professions. Representatives of old families with inherited wealth are often found on hospital boards. More recently, however, trustees seem to be chosen more for community influence or unique ability than for social position alone. A businessman who can lend his prestige to fund appeals or policy decisions is valuable. So is an advertising executive who can contribute expert talents in the field of public relations. The strategic position of a prospective board member in the community at large is generally given first consideration. Does he hold a place from which power can be wielded in the hospital's favor? Is he likely to be able to influence the press, the city government, or the private donors to hospital funds? In one hospital the local newspaper editor and the president of the women's auxiliary of the hospital were elected to the board although neither was wealthy nor conspicuously successful. The editor was chosen because he could arrange favorable treatment to news stories and provide much free publicity through editorials. The president of the auxiliary was chosen because the board thought that her presence would insure liaison between the trustees and the volunteer hospital workers, and add a feminine voice to an otherwise male board.

The vice president of a board in a small hospital explained the membership composition of the board in this way:

> I feel the board should include representatives from the top business and professional people and those that can really do something for the hospital. Some people think we should get some boys from the other side of the tracks, but if we did, they would just talk and not *do* anything, because they haven't any influence.

Another board president, after describing his work in fund raising for the hospital and explaining how important a personal chat could be in obtaining a large gift, said:

> Our auxiliary does well too. Their main trouble is that they don't ask for *enough* money when they try to raise funds.

Although certain board members recognize the need for bringing the young community leaders in, it is probable that boards tend to be heavily weighted with older citizens because of the qualifications demanded for membership. It takes time to develop into a successful, prominent community leader and in a man's early career he is perhaps too busy getting ahead to occupy himself with public service. Since age and high income tend to be associated with conservatism, it is to be expected that a board of trustees is usually conservative. Many harassed administrators and eager research-minded medical men would agree that one of the functions of the board seems to be to "drag its feet," especially when finances are an issue.

It is not always easy to get good members for the board. The hospital in a small town, especially, may be handicapped by scarcity of citizens qualified for and interested in board service. Many otherwise outstanding people do not have the largeness of view, particularly in fiscal matters, which a board needs if it is to set far-reaching policy.

The composition of a hospital board almost inevitably reflects the characteristics of the surrounding community, since the members are leading products of that setting. A board can be a mirror of community social relationships. It cannot assume a character or set goals which are radically different from those of the city in which it is enmeshed. This is not to say that trustees cannot exercise creative leadership, but the hospital is closely bound up with other institutions and with prevailing patterns of behavior.

RESPONSIBILITIES

The board holds the hospital in trust. A private voluntary hospital is a gift of private donors to serve a community need. It is the responsibility of the board to provide and maintain an institution which will serve these needs according to the wishes of the donors. It has a responsibility both to the terms of the trust and to the community which the hospital serves. In order that it may fulfill this trust, it must be the ultimate source of authority. Individual trustees differ widely in the amount of responsibility that they exercise. Some attend the board meetings once a year merely to confirm policies which have been determined by others, while some take an active, detailed interest in hospital problems. Boards as a whole also differ from one hospital to another in the degree to which they participate in the formation, as compared to the ratification, of policy.

We pointed out in the introduction to this section that much of the initiative for major policy comes from outside the board itself, because so many choices are grounded on specialized knowledge which the trustees do not have. This seems to be an increasing trend. But because they are in a sense outsiders to the hospital system, they are able and are often called upon to mediate between the goals of competing groups within it. The board's relation to hospital policy can be of three sorts:

> (a) initiation of policy
> (b) transmission of policy
> (c) mediation of policy

(a) There are times when the board must *decide* upon some important change and work to carry it through. Excellent examples occur in the reorganization of smaller hospitals which have fallen on grim days. The major difficulty may be financial, but just as frequently it is an internal disorganization of one sort or another, especially the sort found when the administrator and medical staff are at loggerheads. At one such institution the president described his first steps after being chosen to head the board:

> First I fired the superintendent and brought in somebody I thought could do a good job. This place was saddled with debts. There were many months of bills outstanding and some creditors were getting worried about the hospital's ability to pay. The first thing I did was to go down to the bank and borrow $25,000 to pay off the worst debts. The doctors had been fighting among themselves. There were two factions on the medical staff, and their battles had split the whole town. Our hospital had a bad reputation and the public was beginning to lose confidence so I called the leaders of the factions together—they're both younger than I am—and told them that they would have to get together and end this open warfare. Then I started a fund raising campaign and forced the doctors to contribute first. I told them they were benefiting from the hospital as much as anyone else.

(b) The board may be called upon to transmit policy when an outside agency puts pressure on the hospital to improve its standards or run the risk of losing accreditation.[1] The various accrediting agencies do not actually determine policy but the penalties for losing their stamp of approval are serious for the hospital. The trust imposed upon the board members cannot be fully met if minimum standards are not maintained. The trustees pay attention to these agencies and will fight hard for suggested changes that did not originate with the board.

(c) When a suggested policy change is developed from within the hospital, as it often is, the trustees must monitor the proposal and attempt to resolve divergent aims. One interesting type of conflict involves the relative emphasis to be placed on research on the one hand and regular medical care on the other. Here, although the root of the difference is probably a philosophic disagreement as to the hospital's proper function, it may be brought to the trustees as a technical argument; e.g., whether a particular type of research investigation is feasible. The board must then attempt to choose on information supplied by others. A group of generally informed laymen is thus called upon to decide between technically informed experts.

---

[1] Accrediting agencies are voluntary in character. Member hospitals submit to regular inspection as a means of self discipline. In this way, adequate standards are maintained and regular improvements are encouraged.

RELATIONS WITH THE ADMINISTRATOR

In a large industry, the board of directors exerts its authority mainly through a hired president or executive. The situation of the hospital administrator differs from that of the company president in two ways. First, hospital administrators are usually given much less discretionary power than a corporation president. They have been on the whole much more closely tied to the board and its wishes, and consult with it more frequently in decision-making. In the second place, the board of directors of a factory is in a position to delegate to the president authority over all workers, but, as we have pointed out in Chapter IV, the hospital board is not able to delegate effective authority over the doctors.

The board itself occupies a unique position in hospital affairs which sharply distinguishes it from the business situation. While it lacks the proprietary interest of directors who have a financial stake in an organization, there is often a feeling of responsibility exceeding anything found in other enterprises. A hospital board has a keen sense of pressure stemming from responsibility for human life. This makes for difficulty in the delegation of authority, as trustees responsive to patient needs strive eagerly to be certain those needs are met. Reluctant to assign authority in matters which may touch life-or-death, they sometimes become directly involved in hospital operations.

The amount of discretionary power which the board does delegate to the superintendent varies widely. Many administrators feel strongly that the board should limit its activities to the formulation of general policy, but should stop short of detailed supervision in the day-to-day life of the hospital. Yet they express a desire that the board be interested and involved. Perhaps one cannot have deep presistent commitment without inviting occasional "meddling."

The board president whose sympathetic understanding of the difficult position of his hospital superintendent was noted earlier,[2] when he remarked on how hard it is for a full-time executive to be supervised by part-time trustees, nevertheless said at a later time:

> Did you notice the color Jenkins [the administrator] put on the front hall? He went right ahead without asking anybody. I should have kicked his pants for it, but I didn't because it's unimportant.

One administrator writes as follows about the general problems:

> On the negative side there is something more to expect. I want my trustees to know what not to do. Many of my colleagues dread the interference of trustees in the routine administration of the hospital. This interference is generally conceded to be the greatest single threat to the authority of the administrator.[3]

A very important feature of the obligation of the board both to the donors and to the public is to insure the permanence of the hospital and its services. This imposes on the board a very clear responsibility for financial management and most people probably think of this first, as the trustees' job. A prominent feature of nearly every report from the hospital administrator or his staff to the board is a balance sheet showing what part each specific department or activity plays in the hospital's economic structure.

[2] Introduction to Part Two, p. 36.

[3] E. M. Bluestone, M.D., "What I Expect of My Board," *Hospital and Modern Society,* Bachmeyer and Hartman, eds. Cambridge: Harvard University Press.

The board considers the effect of every proposed policy decision on the financial stability of the institution. If it failed to do so, it would be unfaithful to its trust. This is obvious, but the necessary concern of the board with means is one of the commonest sources of misunderstanding between it and those who are primarily concerned with ends. It should also be pointed out that attention to financial problems of the hospital has its constructive side. Very often it induces the administrator or the medical staff to re-examine certain of their goals and to clarify their own thinking. The board is the great asker of questions in the hospital. Why build a new wing? Why purchase new equipment? Why raise the salary of maids? The close questioning often irritates enthusiastic proponents of an idea, but it can be a safeguard against hasty or ill-examined actions. Furthermore, close attention to the budget is more than a banker's concern for neatly balanced ledgers. The board may use financial management as a means of directing the hospital to certain goals, rather than make it simply an end in itself. Money problems often symbolize underlying cross-purposes in conflicts which seem at first to have little relation to dollars and cents.

Though all boards in discharging their responsibility must concern themselves actively with financial matters, they differ widely in their attitudes toward hospital finances, as the following quotations indicate:

> We have developed a research philosophy in this hospital. Our trustees once were very anxious about the balance sheets but they have educated themselves to accept the deficit as the price for intensive research work. They recently expressed remarkable attitude and insight for a group of businessmen. We were considering a candidate for the administrator's position, since I will soon retire. This young fellow came up here and brought with him the books from his current hospital. He was very efficient and very proud of his balanced books. Our board rejected him as a candidate because he showed *too much black ink* in his books. They felt that he couldn't be recording these beautiful surpluses if his hospital were doing all that it *ought* to in the way of medical care and research.

—An administrator

> All that board cares about is how much will it cost. They pondered and pondered over the problem of buying a new deep therapy machine. I explained to them that if they bought the equipment and didn't like it they could turn around and sell it at a profit the next day. . . .Finally they put up the funds. They just can't look ahead of the immediate costs and what a hole it makes in their books. They don't see the long-range value of spending money in certain ways.

—A staff surgeon

Human relations inside the hospital are influenced by the attitude of the top policy-makers toward monetary decisions. In a hospital where the board allowed the administrator fairly wide discretion in the purchase of equipment, nurses spoke in warm terms about how promptly their most urgent needs were met. Little doubt seemed to exist that money policies were well tailored to medical requirements.

RELATIONS WITH DOCTORS

The board and the organized medical staff seldom deal with each other directly as formally constituted groups, although liaison committees may be created to act in an advisory capacity, and as we pointed out, informal relations between individual doctors and individual board members often have far-reaching effects on the hospital.

Although it was once common for one or two older physicians to be appointed to the board, both trustees and doctors have come to feel that this practice is generally undesirable. It is held that such an arrangement fosters a possible conflict of interests, since the doctor is himself subject to the judgment of the board, and his membership on it might give him an undue economic or policy-making advantage. As a noted surgeon put it:

> We doctors have no part in management, and I am sure that that is only right. We do plenty of griping about management but it is better that we should not have responsibility in management.

Since the board has little direct authority over the doctors except its power to appoint or refuse to appoint them to the staff and since even this authority is limited in practice, it must to a considerable extent depend on the self regulation of the medical group. However, when this fails the trustees often try to push the doctors toward accepting a new code of standards and practices. Sometimes they try to do so through the administrator, instituting regulations which he is expected to enforce. At times they persuade the medical staff to tighten its own self regulation. Dealings between the trustees and the doctors were greatly facilitated in the hospitals we studied if the medical staff itself was well organized. A board has no effective, established way of exerting pressure unless it can do so through a chief of staff who has definite authority. A board president took note of this in the following comments:

> Discussion of cases with our liaison committee usually ends up in a pleasant evening's conversation. The doctors say, "Oh, we'll take care of that," but that's as far as it goes. There is no clear line of responsibility shown. I was asking the staff about a new anesthetic that had been used on a patient who had died on the table. They couldn't give me a good explanation. I feel that if there were a head of surgery appointed by the board of managers, we could go to him and say, "Look, you're responsible for this case, we want to know what happened."

Just as in its relations with the administrator, the line between guidance and meddling by trustees in medical problems cannot be clearly drawn. No one can say just how deeply the trustees should penetrate into medical affairs. The medical staff can often use its special competence as a lever to extend its influence into nonscientific areas and to block trustee investigation. A board president recounted that in discussions with the doctors about economic practices, as in the case of salaried medical specialists, a certain physician always lectured the trustees about interfering with "the sacred doctor-patient relationship."

Yet medical topics are legitimately reserved for those qualified to discuss them. The dividing line cannot be drawn in advance but must be worked out in give and take between the two groups and this calls for mutual understanding of the other's point of view. But that this understanding is not always complete is shown by the following quotations:

> I don't like the way the board always goes so slow. We should have a full-time pathologist, but you have to get them used to the idea gradually. It's the same with equipment. How do you get them to see the medical necessity?

> —A doctor

> The board must watch expenses. Doctors will buy anything, all sorts of new gadgets, and never care how much it costs. Once they were all excited about those glass boots for stimulating circulation. We bought them, and I'll bet you can still find a few around the hospital, but they were never once used to my knowledge.

> —A board president

Many trustees believe they must take a broader view of hospital affairs than doctors can be expected to. These board members tend to see the medical staff as a group of experts whose interests are largely confined to medical matters. The comments of two different board presidents are illustrative:

> Doctors you might say are technicians. What we need are not technicians but coordinators. People who bring all the different techniques together. As I see it, that's what the board of managers is supposed to do at the hospital. The first duty of the trustee is to help preserve the patient's identity. Doctors get case-hardened, can't see the patient as an individual.

> Our publicity committee has to censor the things doctors say for publication. Doctors will do foolish things in public if you don't watch them.

RELATIONSHIPS WITHIN THE BOARD

Trustees vary greatly among themselves. Any single board, despite the common characteristics described earlier, will have members who differ in the interest and the amount of time they devote to the hospital. An "active board" is not necessarily one in which every member digs eagerly into hospital affairs. One board president stressed that certain trustees who don't participate fully should nevertheless be retained:

> Some members who don't appear at meetings can still be very important. I know their telephone numbers. I called on a business executive the other day and before we were through he had given me $10,000 for the hospital out of a clear sky.

A major problem is age and retirement. Unless individuals are elected for a specific tenure, the board may become weighted with inactive members.

> Some of them don't do anything. I'm sure some haven't been inside the hospital for over a year. We have one old lady who has been an invalid for five years, but still hangs on. They stay until they die. I am trying to get some of the dead wood off of the board. We have a committee set up now to ask one member per year to retire.

> —A board president

Factionalism may of course interfere with the board's effectiveness. The members, perhaps because of their success in the outside world, tend to be individualists and to hold their opinions with some firmness. The stress which they place on values may diverge at many points. The familiar conflict between financial means and humanitarian objectives which is a source of stress among other hospital people sometimes divides board members as well.

Since trustees have the major task of threshing out a working philosophy for the institution, it is not rare for them to disagree, particularly on the policies to be adopted toward the other two powers, the administrator and medical staff. One board president described his effort to induce the other board members to have chiefs appointed to the medical departments. His board refused to back him in this proposal, arguing that, "We cannot do medicine. You can't get away with that." Similarly we have known boards which debated long and hard the problem of replacing an authoritarian director of nurses with a more democratic one.

RELATIONS WITH THE PUBLIC

Trustees are an important link, perhaps the most important, between the hospital and the community. They are normally active in the community and can exercise much influence by explaining the hospital's position on controversial issues such as costs. They (and the patients) *are* the public within the hospital.

While the trustees represent the public interest, they serve without compensation. This adds weight to their impartial position. However, their very eminence as community leaders, which makes them alert to certain key values and attitudes, may separate them from the average citizen. The board is in some sense insulated from the currents of mass opinion, and may have to make special attempts to discern that opinion.

Trustees recognize that part of what the board holds in trust is the hospital's reputation and they are usually zealous to preserve its good name. They work toward this end in two ways. First, there is a formal explicit effort to hold public favor. There is often a publicity committee of the board which concentrates on this problem. One such committee was set up under the leadership of an advertising executive and charged with the supervision and censorship of all news releases. It is interesting that in this case the committee began to act only after a premature release of research findings had brought censure to the hospital.

Perhaps more vital than planned effort to promote understanding is the informal influence of the board. Through their day-to-day activities in the community, trustees can learn what the public opinion is and do much to sway influential persons. A casual word dropped by a powerful trustee can often accomplish much more than months of routine work.

The hospital's position and policy have become the object of so much public attention in recent years, and its problems are so enormous, that some board members have nearly a full-time job smoothing public relations. Constant interpretation of the hospital's situation to the surrounding community is essential for both financial support and intelligent public use of hospital resources. Then, too, the growing public awareness of medical standards has made the board more sharply aware of responsibility for explaining those standards, and defending hospital practices in the forum of community opinion. In particular, complaints about the high costs of medical care and anxieties about its quality as compared to the ideal or to standards in other cities have forced trustees to become self-conscious about the relation of hospital to community. Finally, the board has come to protect the hospital against unwarranted pressures of outside groups eager for a policy-making voice.

The success of the board in its public relations has a direct bearing on human relations within the hospital. The employees soon learn the local reputation of the hospital. Their pride and spirit are strongly influenced by what others think of their job. These in turn have a significant effect on their attitudes and relationships to one another.

SUMMARY

The board of trustees is the bridge between the hospital and the local community. Its members are the responsible public guardians of the hospital organization. Beyond their corporate trust in the financial realm, the board members act as general policy-makers. Their degree of supervision over the administration varies, but it is generally agreed that they should not concern themselves with the details of routine management. The division of the responsibility between the two varies widely from one hospital to another. The board deals chiefly with the administrator and the medical staff. In both cases, the relationship poses the fundamental problem of lay versus expert authority. The board members' prestige and formal power in the community are usually at least as great as that of the physician and therefore they are better able than anyone else to maintain a balance between technical scientific claims and other interests. Relations between board, medical staff, and administrator are complex and rest finally on mutual understanding and accommodation rather than formal lines of organization. This triad of human relations affects more than the three top agents. It profoundly influences the internal relations of the hospital as a whole, as well as its ties with the outside world.

Should Administrators Serve on Hospital Boards?

J. A. ROSENKRANTZ, M.D.

J. A. Rosenkrantz, M.D., was formerly Executive Director of Beth Israel Hospital in Newark, N.J. He is now with the United States Government.

Traditionally, hospital operation has been based upon close cooperation among the board of trustees, the administrator, and the medical staff. This triad has been the backbone of administration and still is an effective organization, providing there is close communication and harmony among the component parts. Unfortunately, in some hospitals this triad is not as well integrated as it should be and becomes more like the "eternal triangle."

Changes are occurring in the field of medicine, in social welfare, in administration, and in the utilization of hospitals. What was good for hospitals 30 years ago may not be good today. It is time to pause and take inventory of organizational procedures that may have become archaic. An audit of current operations and functions may or may not indicate a need for alterations. However, where conditions indicate that changes will improve the efficiency of operation, outdated techniques must be eliminated.

BIG BUSINESS

Those who make their careers in the broad areas of administering health services proudly and rightly proclaim that hospitals are big business—they constitute the fourth largest industry in the country. To support this position, statistics show that in 1965 there were about 29 million patients admitted to 7123 hospitals at a cost of about $13 billion.[1]

Hospitals no longer function with funds derived substantially from voluntary contributions. Modern business methods are being applied, and an effort is being made to relate charges to costs. Many patients rely on third parties to help pay their bills, necessitating communication with health insurance agencies. Government is providing more funds for the aged and the indigent; for research; and for the construction of hospitals, medical schools, and nursing schools. Government also makes available long-term loans at low interest rates for building dormitories to house student nurses, interns and residents. Endowments and grants from industry and private foundations aid in the operation, modernization, and expansion of hospitals. Labor unions have moved into the hospital field and tend to involve administration in labor-management relations. If hospitals are big business, why don't they act the part?

Consider the common practices in the industrial world. The chief executive is named the manager—or more commonly in larger industries, the president of the board—with full management authority. The titular head of the governing board is the chairman, who is responsible for policy that subsequently is carried out by the president and other officers of the board. Although the chief executive is salaried, this does not impede his effectiveness. He is a member and integral part of the board and as an internal director, he helps provide good management.

One authority points out that inside directors of industry have a good technical background; demonstrate leadership ability through long service with a specific organization; are available immediately for both routine and emergency sessions; are completely dedicated to the organization; and have a keen comprehension of the wants and attitudes of the company's rank-and-file, the stockholders, and the customers.[2]

Other authorities reinforce these opinions[3]—they hold that the inside board member usually is intensely loyal to his organization; the firm is his chief interest and main source of employment and income; and he usually can expect better support and cooperation from fellow executives. Furthermore, they contend that inside directors understand the internal human relations of the firm better than outside directors, and they can deal with exceptional organizational problems better than outside directors can. How accurately these conclusions concerning the inside director fit the position of the hospital administrator!

How far have hospitals come in electing the administrator as a member or officer of the board? What are the advantages and disadvantages of having the administrator serve in the capacity of an internal director?

TABLE 1.—NUMBER AND PERCENTAGE OF ADMINISTRATORS SERVING AS MEMBERS OR OFFICERS OF BOARDS OF TRUSTEES OF HOSPITALS IN NEW JERSEY, NEW YORK, AND PENNSYLVANIA.

Number of beds	*New Jersey*					*New York*				
	Total	*Yes*	*Per Cent*	*No*	*Per Cent*	*Total*	*Yes*	*Per Cent*	*No*	*Per Cent*
Under 100	6	1	16.7	5	83.3	52	4	7.7	48	92.3
Under 200	22	6	27.3	16	72.7	42	4	9.5	38	90.5
Under 300	9	2	22.2	7	77.8	39	6	15.4	33	84.6
Total	37	9	24.3	28	75.7	133	14	10.5	119	89.5
Under 400	12	9	75.0	3	25.0	14	3	21.4	11	78.6
Under 500	3	0	0.0	3	100.0	8	2	25.0	6	75.0
Over 500	7	3	42.9	4	57.1	14	6	42.9	8	57.1
Total	22	12	54.5	10	45.5	36	11	30.6	25	69.4
Grand total	59	21	35.6	38	64.4	169	25	14.8	144	85.2

Number of beds	Pennsylvania					Composite Totals				
	Total	*Yes*	*Per Cent*	*No*	*Per Cent*	*Total*	*Yes*	*Per Cent*	*No*	*Per Cent*
Under 100	33	4	12.1	29	87.9	91	9	9.9	82	90.1
Under 200	34	7	20.5	27	79.5	98	17	17.3	81	82.7
Under 300	25	4	16.0	21	84.0	73	12	16.4	61	83.6
Total	92	15	16.3	77	83.7	262	38	14.5	224	85.5
Under 400	11	5	45.5	6	54.5	37	17	45.9	20	54.1
Under 500	8	2	25.0	6	75.0	19	4	21.1	15	78.8
Over 500	17	10	58.8	7	41.2	38	19	50.0	19	50.0
Total	36	17	47.2	19	52.8	94	40	42.6	54	57.4
Grand total	128	32	25.0	96	75.0	356	78	21.9	278	78.1

HOSPITAL SURVEY

In an attempt to answer these questions, the author conducted a survey of hospitals in the states of New Jersey, New York, and Pennsylvania. Questionnaires were sent to administrators of all hospitals in these states, but were not sent to nursing homes, rehabilitation centers, and other specialized facilities. An analysis of the 356 hospitals that responded is shown in Table 1. Following is a summary of the findings:

1. Of the total number of hospitals responding to the questionnaires, 22 per cent of the administrators are members or officers of the board of trustees.

2. In analyzing the responses by hospital size, the number of administrators who serve on the board increases markedly as the hospital size increases; this is consistent with the trend in industry. About 42 per cent of the hospitals with over 300 beds have administrators who are on the board, as compared with 14.5 per cent of administrators in hospitals with fewer than 300 beds.

3. In New Jersey, where 59 hospitals responded, about 35 per cent of the administrators are either members or officers of the board. In hospitals with over 300 beds, about 54 per cent of the administrators serve on the board as compared with about 24 per cent in smaller hospitals.

4. In New York, where 169 hospitals responded, about 15 per cent of the administrators are either members or officers of the board. In hospitals with over 300 beds, more than 30 per cent of the administrators serve on the board as compared with about 10 per cent in smaller hospitals.

5. In Pennsylvania, where 128 hospitals responded, 25 per cent of the administrators are either members or officers of the board. In hospitals with over 300 beds, about 47 per cent of the administrators serve on the board, compared with about 16 per cent in smaller hospitals.

PATTERNS OF HOSPITAL ADMINISTRATIVE ORGANIZATION

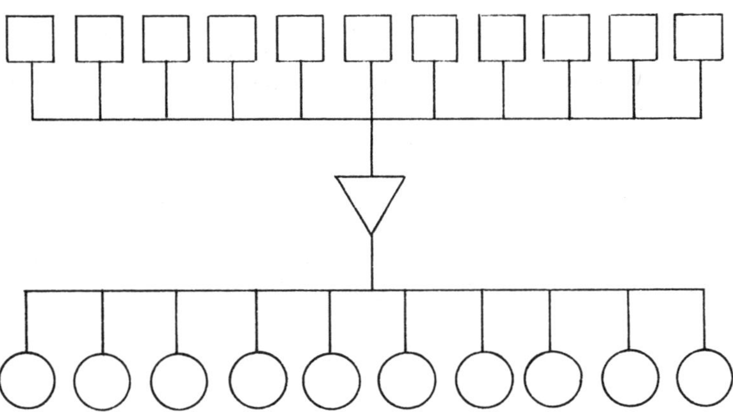

PATTERN A—This pattern prevails in the majority of hospitals. The administrator, as the operational head, is interposed between the board of trustees and the department heads.

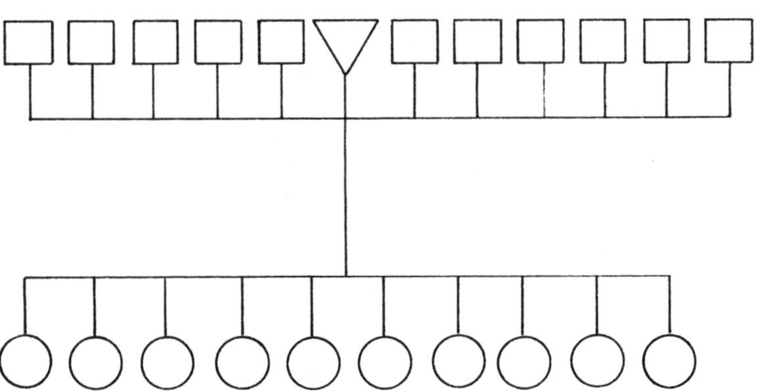

PATTERN B—In a growing number of hospitals, the administrator has become a member of the board, but retains direct operational control of the hospital.

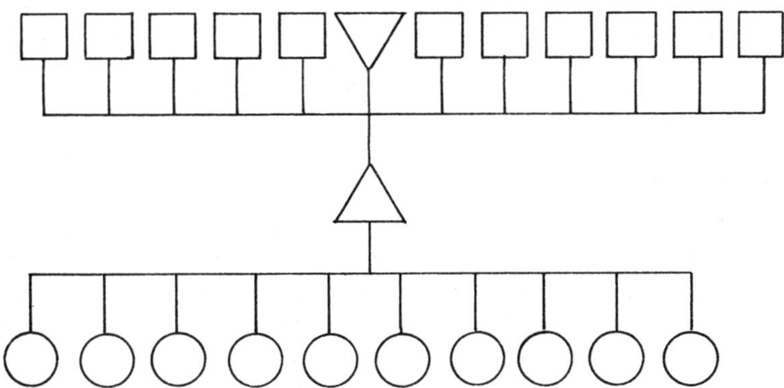

PATTERN C—In some hospitals, the responsibilities of the administrator who is a board member have been broadened, with a new title reflecting this broadening, and an operational administrator has been added to the administrative roster.

6. The most common office to which the hospital administrator is elected is that of secretary or assistant secretary of the board. A lesser number serve as executive vice president; however, seven administrators hold the office of president of the board of trustees.

Only a few of the respondents indicated that there were any disadvantages in having the hospital administrator serve as an internal director, and these adverse factors could be eliminated easily by reeducation, adequate communication, and revision of the bylaws. Peculiarly, many administrators who are not members or officers of the board indicated that there were many advantages to serving on the board and hoped to influence their boards to change their policy in this regard.

ADVANTAGES

The administrators surveyed noted the following advantages in serving as an internal director of the hospital:

1. Having the administrator on the board is the most direct method of ensuring implementation of policy decisions. It gives the administrator the privilege of proposing policy, and because he is professionally trained and has extensive experience he can be of great benefit to the board.

2. Having the administrator serve as an internal director minimizes any division between board and management, promoting greater harmony and unified planning. Some administrators experience some difficulty in getting boards to accept their plans. As a nonmember of the board, an administrator, being an outsider, cannot press his point beyond certain limits and then must yield to the board. As a member or officer of the board, an administrator can be more insistent; he can act on an equal level with board members, and as part of the board, he can plan with them.

3. Making the administrator an officer of the board is legally efficient in that the administrator can affix the corporate seal, sign documents and checks, correct minutes, and expedite record keeping on behalf of the board. Frequently, official forms require the signature of an officer of the board. These often are routine matters in connection with grants, licensing agencies, or reporting bodies. If the administrator serves as an officer of the board, time is saved and inconvenience is avoided in getting the forms signed.

4. Being part of the board gives the administrator a greater leadership role and increases his prestige in the eyes of the medical staff and the community.

5. Hospitals are big business and as such, they must project an image of sound corporate organization and management. In business and industry, if the executive of the corporation is to speak responsibly for the organization and represent it with authority before the public, he generally is an officer of that corporation. The same policy should apply to hospitals.

6. The medical staff point of view is ensured a place in board discussions and decisions. Where boards do not have a representative of the medical staff at the meetings, and where a member of the medical staff most commonly is not and should not be a member of the board, the administrator must represent the interests of the medical staff. Accordingly, if an administrator has been involved in planning with the medical staff and supports an idea that should be presented to and passed by the

board, the administrator as a member of the board has greater strength in his discussions and will ensure that the medical staff's point of view will be well represented.

7. Members of the board generally are able to communicate to each other their reasons for wanting to adopt certain policies. The administrator then is in the best position to implement policy, to see that it not only is carried out as intended, but that the execution of the policy is followed to the letter.

8. Serving on the board provides an added protection for the administrator in the event that a legal suit is brought against the hospital and members of the staff. Often a legal suit against the hospital includes a separate suit against the administrator. If a state still has total exemption or limited exemption, up to $10,000, for example, the administrator still is sued as an individual for an amount over and above the exemption. If the administrator is a part of the board, it is possible, although not absolutely certain, that he will have added protection against such a situation.

9. For business-oriented trustees who know and understand management corporate structure, the administrator is placed in proper perspective. Administratively, hospitals in many ways function similarly to colleges and industrial organizations, which are headed by presidents acting as the executive.

10. The increasing complexities of hospital organization demand clear-cut patterns of organization. As an officer of the board, the administrator can prevent outside forces from breaking down lines of authority, causing confusion and lowering morale. In some hospitals, individuals often circumvent the administrator and deal with individual members of the board. As an officer of the board, however, the administrator can prevent such incidents.

11. Being an officer of the board may be helpful to the administrator in fund raising and public relations because he would be more closely identified with the board.

The advantages listed above are those reported by the respondents. Some persons might question whether or not the administrator can effectively represent the medical staff in board meetings, as stated above. They might argue that the interests of the medical staff might be served best by having physicians on the board. However, unless the physician selected for board membership has unusual qualities, his decisions might be biased. On certain decisions, such as appointments and promotions, he might show favoritism.

Although the subject of having members of the medical staff serve on the board is somewhat removed from the present discussion, a few comments seem to be appropriate. Elsewhere it has been suggested that boards would do well to put medical staff members on their committees.[4] In brief, the board cannot be informed on all matters pertaining to advances in medicine, research, education, the application of social sciences, and accreditation problems. Physicians may offer constructive advice and establish a closer liaison. Furthermore, the president and past president of the medical staff might be invited to sit in on all board meetings. They would be readily available for a first-hand interchange of information. Certainly by being present at all board deliberations, the physicians would develop a deep respect for the responsibilities of the board—consideration of the safety of patients, the quality of medical care, the financial solvency of the hospital, and other matters.

Thus, if the medical staff is represented on board committees and on board meetings, it would have a voice. This does not necessitate appointing physicians as full voting members. In hospitals where such a procedure cannot be implemented and where the administrator has a good working relationship with the medical staff, the administrator can adequately represent the physicians.

DISADVANTAGES

The following disadvantages to being members of the board were recorded by some administrators:

1. If the administrator develops a close association with the board, he might take advantage of this relationship.
2. There may be a tendency for other officers of the board to expect the administrator to perform duties for which trustees usually are responsible.
3. The administrator's dual responsibilities may create an incompatible situation.
4. The hospital might lose its tax-free status.
5. The medical staff may think that they are being excluded because the administrator and board are one and the same.
6. The propriety of an administrator voting on his own recommendations might be questioned.
7. A loss of checks and balances might destroy the relationship that normally exists between administration and board. It eliminates the triad of board, administrator and medical staff.

CONCLUSIONS

It is apparent from this survey that the election of hospital administrators as officers of the board has been increasing in New Jersey, New York, and Pennsylvania. This reinforces the opinion that hospital boards should continue to employ practices used by industry. Comments by administrators clearly express sentiment in favor of the advantages of being an officer of the board. Certainly the disadvantages reported can readily be overcome.

Because the governing body determines policy, the administrator as an officer is in an excellent position to act as an advisor. His training and experience qualify him for that position. Although the administrator is part of the board, the governing body still can require him to carry out policies, keep the board informed of all activities, and be responsible for the management of the hospital.

The author concurs in the conclusions of those who contend that whatever title is given the head of the board, the title doesn't raise or lower the degree of accountability.[5] The escalation in titles has become prevalent since World War II, with the addition of vice presidents, senior vice presidents, and executive vice presidents. In some large organizations, the chairman is responsible for corporate service functions and the president is responsible for operations.

During the same time period, hospital organizations have undergone parallel changes. Administrative residents and assistant and associate administrators have been added, and more recently, administrators have been elected to office on the board. The addition of the administrator to the top board level provides a two-man combine. In industry, a two-man combine makes it possible to segregate more neatly the chairman's reserved responsibilities and give them greater emphasis and attention.

REFERENCES

1. The nation's hospitals: a statistical profile. *Hospitals, J.A.H.A. Guide Issue* 40:427 Aug. 1, 1966, Part 2.
2. Vance, S. Do boards of trustees need surgery? *Mod. Hosp.* 104:105 June 1965.
3. Kennedy, R. E. and West, R. H. Board of directors: its composition and significance. *Advanced Manage.* 24:8 Nov. 1959.
4. Rosenkrantz, J. A. and Lucchesi, P. F. Albert Einstein Medical Center puts medical staff members on governing board committees. *Hosp. Manage.* 87:45 May 1959.
5. Stieglitz, H. and Janger, A. When the chairman is chief-executive. *Bus. Manage. Rec.* 25:7 Aug. 1963.

Should Doctors be on Your Board?

C. JEROME JORGENSEN

C. Jerome Jorgensen is Executive Director of Stormont - Vail Hospital in Topeka, Kansas.

Recommendations for involving physicians more directly in hospital management are being heard with increasing frequency and greater force from national and state medical societies and hospital associations, from the Joint Commission on Accreditation, from such authoritative groups as the Barr Committee which reported its findings on hospital effectiveness directly to the President.

Some agencies suggest involvement of doctors in the highest decision level—the hospital governing board. Others merely say, "We encourage more meaningful involvement of doctors in policy-making councils of the hospital." But the reasons for the recommendations seem more important than the suggestions themselves, for they reflect changing attitudes and the use of new concepts of management.

The clamor for more physician involvement has not necessarily arisen because the physician is *not* "involved" in most hospitals but because there are contemporary demands for rethinking this concept. It appears that there is a need for *renewal* of present relationships and the role that physicians must play within the hospital setting and in revising the form of delivery of health care services.

REASONS FOR PARTICIPATION

Let's explore some of the reasons given for greater doctor participation and what objectives may be achieved. Presumably, doctors should become more involved in the *hope* of helping to improve the health-care system and because without them some problems cannot be solved.

One primary problem is spiraling hospital costs. Because quality and cost of care decisions are inseparable, governing boards and management will find it difficult to bring about fundamental changes or effective controls without including the patient's purchasing agent—the doctor—someplace in the deliberations. More frequently, hospitals and physicians on many issues are not judged separately but as a single entity.

Reprinted by permission from *Hospital Administration: Quarterly Journal of the American College of Hospital Administrators,* Chicago, Vol. 15 (Fall, 1970), 6-13. Copyright 1970 by the American College of Hospital Administrators. All rights reserved.

The increased cost problem cannot be taken lightly. It threatens to profoundly change the entire voluntary health-care system which hospital leaders want to see continue. This dual system of responsibility for patient care can no longer be continued. We must all get on the same team. As a further aggravation, technological improvements in medical care usually do not reduce costs—they increase them. This is contrary to the technological change in most industries. Numerous examples can be cited of expensive duplications of highly complicated and expensive equipment and personnel. There also are duplications in unsophisticated services. Cooperation, not competition, must be emphasized in planning and physicians will be needed to bring about sound decisions.

THE CHARLESTON CASE

The second reason for greater physician participation in hospital management is the legal principle established in the Charleston Case—that the hospital board is responsible for the quality of professional care provided by the institution. The hospital is now seen as *one* organization designed to deliver the highest quality of care which clearly points out that the division of medical staff and administration objectives has been conceptually and legally eliminated.

The development of professional care standards is a shared responsibility. Hospitals and boards of trustees are legally required to maintain the medical staff structure for advising and recommending professional standards of care and to insure that these standards are enforced. This does not dilute control for medicine because this is a shared responsibility between administration and medical staff. To insure that the institution effectively controls care, it will be necessary to integrate the physician even more completely within the authority and responsibility structure of the hospital.

The third major reason is that federal and third-party interest in health care is creating greater public scrutiny. Medicare, comprehensive areawide planning, Regional Medical Programs, and various commissions and committees established to evaluate the delivery of care can be cited as compelling areas of activity requiring greater doctor involvement.

The fourth reason is the need for fundamental changes in the delivery of health care, such as progressive patient care, neighborhood health centers, areawide planning councils, and expanded preventive health programs. If these fundamental changes are to be made in the near future, participation by all providers is essential. Physicians should be included to help shape the process.

A fifth point is the medical centering of the hospital. It has been said that the hospital will no longer be merely a facility but will become a facilitating agency providing the leadership and direction for the development of comprehensive and continuous services. Most likely it will play a central role in the organization of health services, not necessarily providing them, but providing centrality to a nebulous system of health care delivery. It must provide functional and organizational relationships to the farious facets currently providing health care.

INCREASED USE OF EMERGENCY ROOMS

One example of the centrality of this role is increased utilization of hospital emergency rooms all across the United States. The solution to this problem is complex and will require all of the skills and thinking of the entire health care establishment to provide proper solutions. The physician must lead the way in assisting with solutions.

Another factor is most basic to all—the patient-physician relationship. After all, the relationship between the patient and the physician will remain regardless of the organization of health service. It is only natural that those serving the patient most directly should be involved in structuring the setting for delivery.

The complexity of hospital operations is another factor. Hospitals can no longer afford monolithic decision processes. The successful hospital will use participative management and integrative organization theory to administer the health care program. Elimination of separatism, establishing mutual trust, and developing a clear understanding and appreciation of the role of all individuals within the hospital operation must be a common goal.

These reasons are all substantial. There may be more. There are also reasons cited why physicians shouldn't be involved. Fear of diminishing the role of the hospital administrator, having one more group or person to counsel, lack of trust, alleged lack of improvement in the decision-making process are a few that might be cited. I would suggest renewed thinking about present and more effective participation by physicians be considered before judgments are made regarding its success.

ACHIEVING MEANINGFUL INVOLVEMENT

How can this be done? How can more meaningful involvement be achieved? In many hospitals good physician representation within the organizational structure already exists. The question is, "Is this meaningful participation?" Increased involvement is a two-way street. There must be an interest in having physicians participate and physicians must be interested in participating in a positive fashion. I would suggest that there are three steps to achieve meaningful involvement of physicians within hospitals: (1) education and information, (2) present performance, and (3) future participation.

Let's examine each step.

EDUCATION AND INFORMATION

First, education and information. In order for anyone to become effective in his performance or participation, he must be educated regarding the nature of the problem and what can be done to help. I suggest there is not enough education of medical staff or of individuals within the staff toward the problems faced by the hospital. How many administrators have conducted cost seminars? How many have really tried to explain why hospital costs are what they are, and found some way to justify their increased spiraling? What innovative and creative ways have been tried to bring this message across? Physicians must be brought into the picture to the extent that they become aware of their influence on unit cost and total patient cost. The physician must be equipped with proper information, not only to assist in making judgments but to assist in interpreting hospital and medical problems to his patients and to the community. I was recently informed that one hospital adminstrator sends copies of the patient's bill to his attending physician upon dismissal. The effects were astounding. Immediately, staff physicians became acquainted with the costs of the services they were ordering and became concerned about the high prices the hospital had to charge. I am not suggesting this be done to open the door to criticism but it is a technique that can develop enough interest to open ears so the message regarding costs will be heard.

Education about the management function is also important. Costs cannot be viewed separately and apart from planning, management, and financing of hospital care. Informal day-to-day communication by the administrator with individual doctors and in-depth discussions with staff leaders also can be extremely helpful in bringing to bear the opinions and judgments of physicians on any single problem. There must be a formal education program aimed at board and staff—seminars, medical staff meetings, reading material, retreats, and national conferences for physicians and trustees.

PRESENT PERFORMANCE

The second step I labeled "present performance." Currently there exist within the hospital framework many legitimate areas for effective and meaningful physician involvement. It seems to me that performance of these activities ought to be improved before we begin talking about new patterns or new relationships to be superimposed upon an already complex situation. The management structure for physicians is the medical staff organization. It is not separate from the hospital organization. You say you have that? But, is it effective? Does it function using good principles of organization and management? It is, after all, the agency of the *board* for managing medical practice.

Professional practice within the hospital in the future will need to hold up under public scrutiny. Frequently there are weaknesses of hospital staff organization, bylaws, meetings, discipline, patterns of practice, etc.

Within the medical staff organization several committees are concerned with hospital costs and can provide the physician with an opportunity to become involved in the management process.

Utilization review is an excellent area for committee function evaluating and controlling the quality and use of hospital services. Under the purview of this committee any department of the hospital or any patient activity can be scrutinized on some regular basis. Many tools are available to permit this committee to function effectively and it can become a real strength for management if used properly—tools such as HAS, PAS, and MAP. Blue Cross-Blue Shield and state hospital associations can also provide useful hospital data.

The Nursing Liaison Committee is another example of where new services can be evaluated, with reference to both improved patient care and costs. The Adjunctive or Professional Services Committee involving physician evaluation and direction to pharmacy, physical therapy, inhalation therapy, and other paraprofessional departments is an excellent opportunity for physicians to assist in the process of drug inventory and control, understanding the problems of quantity purchasing, and becoming involved in cost and quality-related decisions in patient care departments.

And not to be forgotten is the Joint Conference Committee which in many hospitals is made up of either the officers of the staff or other selected physicians to meet on a regular basis with members of the board of trustees. If these committees are viewed properly and the functions defined, all of them can be reoriented and *renewed* with broadened objectives and new emphasis and functions to provide for a more direct relationship between physician-patient decisions and effective management decisions based upon cost information.

FUTURE PARTICIPATION

The third area I labeled "future participation." Numerous references indicate it is no longer enough to merely have physicians sitting in various meetings of the hospital. They argue that in order to be truly effective in decision- and policy-making there must be a full and complete involvement which would include voting privileges.

What about having physicians on the board? At our hospital we have had a physician on the board for many years. Personally speaking, it is very helpful and in the future will be even more essential. He is selected just as any other member of the board. In addition, the president of the medical staff attends all meetings of the board and reports on activities of the staff. When considering the various ways in which physicians can become involved directly in policy- and decision-making, this is the most direct and least difficult since the board of trustees is a legally constituted body which is formed for policy- and decision-making. Decisions made by other groups within the hospital can cause problems.

It is suggested in the Barr Report that physicians be *involved in the development* of the budget and operating plan and in the achievement of financial and service objectives as budgeted and planned. Presumably, at some point, the recommendations of the Barr Committee may become the law of the land. Also, already within the State of Kansas the Department of Health, in its new regulations soon to be published, has specified that "the governing authority shall demonstrate evidence of liaison and close working relationship with the medical staff."

Another area of physician participation can be the long-range planning committee of the board. This group can be constituted with members of the medical staff or physician members of the board or both. Certainly the Joint Conference Committee is an effective mechanism in existence in most hospitals to achieve close liaison with the medical staff.

NOT THE WHOLE ANSWER

Greater physician involvement is not the whole answer to improving the hospital cost picture, but it's a beginning. The case for involvement will not necessarily result in improved effectiveness. The dichotomy of the present approach must be diminished and physicians must have more responsibility.

Education and information are the forerunners to more effective physician involvement and this should lead the way to improved staff performance in the present organizational patterns. Meaningful involvement cannot be achieved without an understanding of the complexity of hospital management and a delineation of the role the medical staff as well as individual physicians must play. Once this is achieved, the way is paved for involvement in other levels of hospital policy-making situations. With this approach and informed perspective, the physician can make his greatest contribution to the balance of quality care and costs. Physicians' involvement is a change in attitude and process rather than a change in pattern or structure.

THIS IS THE BOX SCORE FOR KANSAS

A 1968 survey by the Kansas Hospital Association, based on replies from 122 of 154 hospitals in the state, reveals the extent of physician involvement in Kansas hospitals:

	Yes	No	No Answer or Answer Unclear
1. Do you have one or more physicians on your Hospital Board?	16	106	0
(The 16 indicating "Yes" reported a total of 23 doctors as Board Members.)			
2. Do you have one or more physicians on your Hospital Advisory Board?	26	88	8
3. Do you have a Joint Conference Committee?	69	48	. . .
4. Do physicians who are not Board Members attend your Board Meetings?	52	63	. . .
5. Does your hospital have the medical staff or a physician group review any of the following:			
a. The Budget?	16	100	6
b. Cost and/or Financial Statement?	27	87	8
c. Staffing Needs?	63	51	8
d. Need for New Services?	100	21	1

REFERENCES

1. Crosby, Edwin L., M.D. "The Physician's Place in Health Care Administration," *Hospitals, J.A.H.A.,* Vol. 42, Part I (August 1, 1968), pp. 47-49, 121.
2. Eisele, C. Wesley, M.D. "How Changing Times are Changing Staffs," *The Modern Hospital,* Vol. 108, No. 5 (May, 1967), pp. 127-128.
3. Kansas State Board of Health, Hospital Facilities Division. *Hospital Regulations,* 4th ed., 1958.
4. U.S. Department of Health, Education, and Welfare. *Report of the Secretary's Advisory Committee on Hospital Effectiveness* (Washington, D.C., U.S. Government Printing Office, 1968).

FURTHER READING SUGGESTED BY THE AUTHOR

"The Physician's Place in Health Care Administration," Edwin L. Crosby, M.D. (*Hospitals, J.A.H.A.,* Vol. 42, Part 1, August 1, 1968, pp. 47-49, 121).

"How Changing Times are Changing Staffs," C. Wesley Eisele, M.D. (*Modern Hospital,* Vol. 108, No. 5, May, 1967, pp. 127-128).

Report of the Secretary's Advisory Committee or Hospital Effectiveness. (U.S. Department of Health, Education, and Welfare, Washington, D.C., U.S. Government Printing Office, 1968).

"The Practicing Physician's Role in Hospital Management—a consultant's view," Albert W. Snoke, M.D. (*Hospital Progress,* Vol. 50, No. 11, November, 1969, pp. 57-59, 84).

The Doctor as Trustee

E. M. BLUESTONE, M.D.

E. M. Bluestone, M.D., is a practicing physician in Tucson, Arizona.

With very few exceptions, doctors do not qualify for trusteeship in hospitals. One of the reasons you do not see them oftener on hospital boards is that they are naturally preoccupied with their professional work and willing to let others build and maintain their workshops for them. It certainly is more profitable to them that way; they wisely prefer not to look a gift horse in the mouth in the knowledge that architects, builders, engineers, merchants and businessmen generally are more likely to be generous and do a better job with the hospital than are doctors, who are notoriously unworldly in almost all but their immediate tasks of healing the sick. By unwritten law, policy making in a hospital is a joint undertaking, with enough credit for both—the philanthropist and the doctor.

SHOULD NOT BE HAMPERED

Members of the medical staff of a hospital do better by limiting their activities to professional matters of scientific interest only. They should not be hampered, or have their precious time consumed, by practical business matters of hospital administration. They are there to serve the patient and they must, in turn, be served by governing board and hospital executive alike. They are the middlemen through whom philanthropy distributes its bounty to the sick in hospitals.

The presence of a doctor on a governing board places him on two levels of authority and often displeases more people than it can possibly please. It gives him a preferred position, hampers the lay group in its decisions and is therefore distasteful to his medical colleagues who are on the outside as well as to his lay colleagues who are on the inside. In problems of medical discipline he exercises a privileged vote and this often protects a colleague who may be under fire. The governing authorities cannot expect from a doctor a recommendation that may injure the standing of another doctor.

IT'S INVITING TROUBLE

You cannot burden a medical man with administrative responsibilities without inviting trouble and the exceptions prove the rule. In the administration of a hospital medical men must be given an opportunity to express themselves, but this means medical men as a group and not one or two favored medical members, or a small group of them which enjoys special governing privileges.

The practice of medicine is an arduous profession. There is little time left to the medical scientist to deal with extra-clinical problems. He is, indeed, impatient with them as a rule and is willing to put up with them to protect himself or his colleagues from a possible lack of sympathy or friendship on the part of a governing group that might be lacking in understanding. As a result, physicians seldom have the time, nor do the best of them have the requisite ability, to serve in the field of hospital administration. A distinguished surgeon recently complained that the time was when his activities were confined to the preoperative, the operative and the postoperative care of the patient; he was now burdened with a fourth responsibility—committees!

A group of sympathetic and understanding lay trustees is more likely to be impartial in appointing men to the visiting staff, or retaining them, than physician-trustees themselves would be likely to be. In any case, the lay trustee is not as easily influenced by personal or professional relationships with applicants for appointment and is, therefore, in a better position to canvass the field thoroughly and to obtain the best available men. He has no other debt to discharge to the candidate than his obligation to the patient himself.

MUST TAKE COUNSEL

In such technical matters the lay trustee should, of course, be advised by medical experts and it is for this reason that a medical board has been established in hospitals. In well organized hospitals, where a high grade of friendly teamwork prevails, and where each side takes counsel with the other whenever necessary, such a medical board can become, for all practical purposes, a legislative body. The board of trustees must be free, however, to take counsel elsewhere if this should become necessary to meet the requirements of impartiality. Hospitals must take counsel wherever they can in their search for the best.

Nonpartisan trusteeship should be sought as a conscious goal in every hospital and the staff doctor is wise who leaves management to those who are expert at it. We all know medical men who are first rate executives, but most of them are to be found in hospital administration, not in the wards.

The Administrator

This section is devoted to the role of the hospital administrator. As the chief executive officer, his duties and functions can vary depending upon the size of the institution he represents. Being the central figure in the organization triad, his de facto authority is also greatly influenced by the other two groups.

A description of the administrator's changing role within the hospital is offered in *THE HOSPITAL ADMINISTRATOR - HIS EMERGING ROLE.* The fact that today's hospital has been forced to adopt an administrative structure commensurate with its importance as a major business and social institution is presented. Furthermore, the necessity of applying lessons from organization theorists and management science techniques is emphasized. The administrator must expand his role toward minimizing costs, furthering research, as well as promoting effective interaction with physicians and the board of trustees.

The external professional leadership required by the hospital administrator is presented in *A NEW ADMINISTRATIVE MODEL FOR HOSPITALS.* The administrator is emerging as the central figure in the determination of the hospital's role in the community. It is stipulated that the professional administrator should function as a policy maker, innovator, and initiator of medical care programs to meet community and society health care needs. He is the logical health professional to assume this leadership role.

The Hospital Administrator
His Emerging role

BRIGHT M. DORNBLASER

Bright M. Dornblaser, is Director of the Graduate Program in Hospital Administration at the University of Minnesota.

To participate in the preservation of health is a valued opportunity for those of us in the health administration field. "The hospital is one of the pillars on which all of society and Western civilization rest. It is taking its place with the courts, the schools, and the churches as an essential institution of a good society."[1]

Our concomitant responsibility is to do our job so as to meet Alfred North Whitehead's standard of "the habitual vision of greatness." The quality of our efforts unquestionably has an essential impact upon the quality of the health services, which are and will be provided.

It is therefore appropriate that we consider the hospital administrator's emerging role. It is also timely to do so. The role is in transition, because the institutions and society we serve are in transition.

THE "GOOD" ADMINISTRATOR

As might be expected, we see in transition a variety of roles. Probably no one role by itself is a panacea for the future. A variety of ingredients is still needed to answer the smorgasbord of new and changing situations with which the administrator will be confronted. In each case, the results must meet the nutritional needs and demands of those we serve. These needs are expanding with the multifaceted growth of our society.

A model can be useful to examine our emerging role. Let us consider the case of a hospital administrator whose objective of the administrative process is the improvement of patient care and support of the hospital's school of nursing and the medical residency programs. He has established objectives for each department of the hospital in the better care of general acute inpatients and private outpatients, and some clinic outpatients. He delegates authority as well as responsibility and controls by reviewing

[1] Inaugural Address, Philip D. Bonnet, M.D., president, American Hospital Association, September 1, 1965, San Francisco.

---

the results. As an agent of the board of trustees, he stresses cooperation and communication with the autonomous medical staff. He is liked by most of the medical staff. He has a Master's degree in hospital administration, and usually attends one institute and/or a national hospital meeting annually. He is considered a likable person and an able administrator, both inside and outside the hospital. He serves on civic and state hospital association committees. He readily exchanges information with colleagues about hospital operation in local hospital council meetings. The hospital annually funds building depreciation, and is planning a building program to expand inpatient beds, and diagnostic and emergency department space.

Many additional similar attributes could be ascribed, but with these already listed there might well be agreement that the role of a "good" administrator has been described. We can readily recognize that his role is different from those played by administrators in the past. Is this a model of the hospital administrator's "emerging role"? It is not. It is perhaps a model of a role that has emerged, but it falls short as a model of the emerging role demanded by the challenges of today and tomorrow.

Without attempting to analyze all facets of the model, we can examine it from the perspective of several challenges of today and tomorrow.

PROGRAM DEVELOPMENT

Awareness of the increased, and rapidly increasing, complexity of hospital programs is inescapable. The explosion of knowledge of medical and basic sciences is increasing at what appears to be a geometric rate. Ninety per cent of all the scientists who ever lived are reportedly alive today. The trend appears to be sharply upward, rather than leveling. The hospital has been the health institution asked by society to translate medical science into programs of practical reality.

A more sophisticated and educated citizenry is expressing an increasing demand for this service to be comprehensive and coordinated, of broader scope and depth. The days are past when a hospital can provide programs limited to those of our earlier example.

The hospital's responsibility for preventive care has been given lip service, but little substance. The community hospital's role in the future may well lie primarily in this area.

Rehabilitation, in concept and concrete program reality, must pervade the hospital inpatient, outpatient, and home care services now, not in the future.

SOME PERTINENT QUESTIONS

General acute inpatient programs need continued examination as to content and organization. Long-term care programs demand at least equal weighing of time and attention. Medicare legislation may well place many community hospitals into the extended care institution business. The need to integrate mental health programs with other general acute and long-term care programs is clear.

Outpatient care has been given much attention in the literature, which has noted the increased demand for such services, and the need to coordinate them with related services inside and outside the hospital. Medicare legislation is only a recent and certainly not the last stimulus to the development and coordination of a broad, comprehensive program of coordinated ambulatory services.

Out-of-hospital services, e.g., home care, has been described as a need far more acute than action has been demonstrated. Financial support is now available, in part, to a portion of our population for such services. Despite shortages of key professional personnel, the pressure is now on hospitals to grab hold of and run with the opportunity to provide these services for which many are in need.

Hospitals very likely will not be by themselves all things to all people, from a health viewpoint. But if hospitals and all those associated with them as providers of care cannot provide a pluralistic, effective answer to society's demand for coordinated, comprehensive health care, what social institution will? Should hospitals abdicate responsibility for this role to other voluntary institutions of society with less resources for a continuing, effective concern for the quality of care of services provided? Do hospitals have a contribution to make in a continuing dialogue with government with which they are in partnership? Should hospitals and other providers of care assume a leadership role in the provision of coordinated, comprehensive care, or should the vacuum be filled by the third party payers for care?

If we conceive that the hospital as a social institution has a central role to play in the development of a broad spectrum of coordinated, comprehensive health services, if we perceive that time is rapidly running out on the hospital's opportunity to live up to these responsibilities, and if we conclude that the hospital administrator has a leadership role to play in the formation of the hospital role—then we begin to understand the expanding role of the hospital administrator.

ORGANIZATIONAL COMPLEXITY

Within the above context, and as a result, the size of the hospital organization has increased and its composition has become more complex. The hospital "has been forced to adopt an administrative structure more commensurate with its importance as a business and social enterprise."[2] This means an emerging role for the hospital administrator. This trend is apt to continue.

Georgopoulos has charged hospital administrators today with being "guilty of failure to recognize the significance of social-psychological factors for hospital functioning."[3] He goes on to note that, ". . . the fact of *inter*dependence, and the realization that hospital organization must be viewed and understood as a whole, are of fundamental importance. . . . Viewed this way, the (expanding) role of the administrator will be mainly, distinctively, and above all, a coordinative and integrative role, and not a resident director role, or a business manager role, or a universal expert role. The administrator will be *less* concerned with technical matters, bookkeeping operations, and specific work problems that can be better handled at the point of their origins. . . . The articulation of the organizational system, as such, will constitute an even more important aspect of his role."[4]

[2] George Bugbee and Andrew Pattullo, "A Foundation Views Hospital Problems," *Hospitals,* 32 (April 1, 1958), 39-43.

[3] Basil S. Georgopoulos, Ph.D., "Hospital Organization and Administration: Prospects and Perspectives," *Hospital Administration,* 9, No. 3 (Summer, 1964), 23.

[4] *Ibid.*

TECHNOLOGICAL CHALLENGES

Better understanding of organizational theory, if he has it, will be vital also to the hospital administrator endeavoring to adapt his organization effectively to technological impacts, such as that of the computer. Also vital will be the administrator's ability to apply management science with its mathematical and statistical techniques. The hospital administrator must appreciate that an important effect of new technology "is to make a man-machine system out of what was formerly an all human system—the managerial group. . . . For the first time—in industrial history at least—those who will be most affected by the change are also those who are responsible for initiating and planning the change. . . ."[5]

The expanding role, then, requires continued mastery of an expanding technological and scientific armamentarium. Other examples may be readily found in the literature.

Post-graduate education is a fundamental requirement if we are to cope with our expanding role, if we are to fulfill our expanding role. Without it, we most certainly will become professional anachronisms during our careers. With it we may be able to contribute to translating management from an art into a science.

Margaret Mead has declared that the most vivid truth of the age is that no one will live all of his life in the world in which he was born. Thus, adaptability to change is a great challenge for the hospital administrator today. He must be prepared to understand—and apply in the future—things, concepts and ideas which are non-existent—which, in fact, have never even been thought of today.

RISING HOSPITAL COSTS

Rising hospital costs have in large measure influenced the present role of the hospital administrator. This phenomenon has been well discussed and documented. Further increases in hospital costs will similarly affect his future role. How he reacts will have an important effect upon whether his role will expand or contract. For example, support of and participation in areawide planning and utilization controls will provide an opportunity for expanding leadership on the part of the hospital administrator (and also the board of trustees and the medical staff). Opposition, or nonparticipation, will create a vacuum which society will otherwise fill.

The many forces stimulating area-wide planning[6] will undoubtedly cause it to become much more widespread. The future could well find the hospital industry franchised and regulated as a public utility. The hospital administrator's (and board of trustees', and medical staff's) influence upon decisions which will be made in this changing setting may be rejected, unless we abandon the all too prevalent "corner grocery store" philosophy in our chain store age. There is evidence that participation by hospital administrator statesmen in planning board decisions is needed. Areawide planning agencies are not a panacea if uninformed or unknowledgeable decisions are made, however well intentioned. However, such involvement by hospital

---

[5] Thomas L. Whisler, Ph.D., "Executives and Their Jobs: The Changing Organizational Structure," *Hospital Administration,* Vol. 8, No. 3 (Summer, 1964).

[6] Ray E. Brown, "The Vital Framework of Areawide Planning," *Hospitals,* 37, No. 5 (March 1, 1963), 48-49.

administrators must be earned by demonstrations of attitude and capability to perform this expanded role.

"One can safely predict that the question of hospital utilization will not be finally answered by the enforcement of precise medical criteria by hospitals and prepayment, but rather by the usual interplay of social forces that determine the end of all social questions."[7] Will the hospital administrator, board of trustees and medical staff have an expanded role to play as one of the social forces? Only if earned, only if there is a willingness to abandon tenacious adherence to the status quo of the corner grocery store philosophy, only if there is a willingness to participate in the decision-making process—which will occur with or without us—and only if there is the ability to participate effectively.

Our partnership with other organizations provides only one, albeit important, example of the shift in the loci of decisions concerning the hospital to points external of the hospital. Decisions made here in many cases will be more significant for patient care than decisions made within the hospital organizations. This phenomenon greatly extends what Cordes calls the

radius of administrative responsibility . . . and requires new skills on the part of the administrator. He must be adept at winning consent from those over whom he has only persuasive influence.

To accomplish this extension of his administrative influence, the hospital administrator of today must know and understand his community, its people, their historical traditions, the value structure that is at work, the resources available, and the weaknesses to be reckoned with in any course of action. Armed with this knowledge and understanding, he must educate the community to his enterprise, its goals, its problems, its needs, and its opportunities for contribution to the community . . . .[8]

Responsibility for the expanding role which we have been discussing must be shared by the administrator in the smaller hospital,[9] as well as the larger hospital.

EDUCATION

The hospital administrator's expanding role with respect to education can be viewed in a similar fashion to his expanding role just discussed. Outside forces will be increasingly dominant whether they are represented by a professional organization with an accrediting program or an educational institution using the hospital as a clinical resource. The hospital administrator's role must expand accordingly. It should be a positive role, recognizing that high standards of care and education should and can be mutually supporting, each vital to the other. The hospital administrator should work to make this so.

RESEARCH

The hospital administrator's expanding role with respect to research also requires positive leadership. Competent administrative as well as medical research is needed.

---

[7] Ray E. Brown, "The Public's Attitude toward Hospital Use," *Hospitals,* 37, No. 17 (September 1, 1963), 35.

[8] Donald W. Cordes, "Radius of Administrative Responsibility," *Hospitals,* 38, No. 12 (June 16, 1964), 44.

[9] Elmina L. Snow, "For the Administrator, Swiftly Expanding Responsibilities," *Hospitals,* 38, No. 11 (June 1, 1964), 32.

Promulgation of research mindedness in the organization, and in some cases the actual conduct of research, is a requirement of the hospital administrator of the present and future. This is a requirement in the smaller as well as the larger hospital.

RELATIONSHIPS WITH PHYSICIANS

The administrator's role in relation to the physician also is emerging. As hospitals become large scale organizations, the physician will need to accommodate increasingly to institutional teamwork.[10]

". . . The individual physician remains the decision-maker in the care of the individual patient; but the implementation of his decisions is in large part an organizational affair, requiring the participation of many different skills and the use of a complex variety of specialized facilities."[11]

Physicians will become increasingly subject to the scrutiny of others, including the hospital administrator. This will be the result of the outside forces affecting all of us in the health field. As a result, physicians will take more interest in, and will be active in, all aspects of the hospital operation. This can be a creative and constructive force. It is the hospital administrator's responsibility and his emerging role to actively help make it so.

THE BOARD OF TRUSTEES

Some hospital administrators may say: "This is all very well, but if I attempt to assume these responsibilities, my board is going to tell me that I'm getting into their business, where I don't belong. I have enough to do taking care of the jobs I already have, and we can't afford the additional help to give me time to take on these new responsibilities."

The answer in brief is "yes," the hospital administrator's expanding role does include responsibilities that are and will continue to be those of a board of trustees. Yes, the hospital administrator has been busy enough minding the store, the corner grocery store. But we must also say that the hospital cannot afford not to provide the administrator with time to develop essential foundations for the hospital's future.

It is a key point that the public has placed hospitals and medical staffs in a partnership with third party payers. If the providers of care do not hold up their end of the partnership the public will dissolve it, by eliminating them as decision makers from it. Subsequent decisions concerning patient care might not fully weigh the patients' needs as known only to the providers of care "on the firing line."

AN INFORMED BOARD OF TRUSTEES

If we have any belief in a pluralistic society and a conviction that the hospital industry has a unique and valuable contribution to make in a dialogue on the who,

---

[10]George Rosen, M.D., "The Impact of the Hospital on the Physician, the Patient, and the Community," *Hospital Administration,* 9, No. 4 (Fall, 1964), 31.

[11]Ray E. Brown, "The General Hospital Has a General Responsibility," *Hospitals,* 39, No. 12 (June 16, 1965), 47.

what, when, where and how's of patient care—we need to show that we are responsible, effective partners.

This is not a part-time job. Our partners have many able, effective people working full time at the partnership. It is not reasonable to ask hospital boards of trustees to work full time. They are already the unsung volunteer heroes, providing judgment of inestimable value. It is reasonable to ask one person in the hospital organization to work full time, or more nearly full time than heretofore, at the level of trustee responsibility. This is not a preemptive role. It is a role essential to the board of trustees if it is to deal effectively with the really critical business of our partnership—program development; quality control; coordination of community resources for a comprehensive program; translation of the findings of medical science, social science and technology into practical reality; participation in vital decisions such as in areawide planning and utilization, which will more greatly affect hospital operation of the future than those we have been used to considering—business requiring an extended radius of decisions and skills in guiding their outcome.

Health security as an expression of social need will be a dominant issue in the political arena during the coming ten years. The opportunity before us is to join forces to help shape those patterns in the form that we believe will best meet the needs of the patient. We, the persons and groups most closely associated with patient needs, should guide decisions concerning the best means of meeting these needs. There is little time left for family quarrels. We must recognize that we are inseparably linked and that we are in an era of profound change. We must strive together to guide these changes into the course best suited not to our convenience but to the public's interest.[12]

Part of the hospital administrator's expanding role, therefore, is the responsibility of presenting to his board of trustees information about the issues and needs of our times. With this information, in most cases, we can have confidence that boards of trustees will recognize that the changing role of the administrator is necessary to meet effectively the challenges which confront us.

STATESMANSHIP IN ADMINISTRATION

In effect, what we've been saying is that there must be an element of statesmanship added to our expanding role.

By statesmanship in administration, we mean the concept pointed out by educator J. Martin Klotsche, in his address to the Sixth ACHA Congress on Administration.

If the hospital administrator does not understand his primary function to be one of creating objectives, he has no business being an administrator. His concern should, therefore, not be primarily to see how he can conduct additional tasks more efficiently, or how to implement the dubious theory that there is virtue in bigness, or how to run an enterprise that strives to be popular rather than respected. . . . The real issue in administration is how to create a climate under which constructive change and progress may be facilitated and how the creative and imaginative forces of an institution can be unleashed.

This can only occur if the administrator is a man of broad knowledge capable of original thought. Unfortunately, we have fostered the belief that the efficient administrator is one who makes fast decisions, who can accomplish changes with great dispatch, who can speed things up—in short, a man of action. Quite the contrary is the case. A good administrator is one who takes time

---

[12]T. Stewart Hamilton, M.D., "Changing Patterns in Medical and Hospital Administration," *Hospitals,* 37, No. 11 (June 1, 1963), 31.

to think, to reflect, to consult, to talk, and who keeps abreast of the best thinking of the day, not only in his own field but in broader areas as well. . . . This may appear to be a big order but statesmanship in administration requires it![13]

THE CONCEPT OF EXCELLENCE

Implicit in all our comments on the expanding role of the hospital administrator has been the concept of excellence. ". . . the wealth of a nation," according to psychologist William James, "consists of, more than anything else, the number of superior men that it harbors." We must foster our concept that dedication and high morale in our field must be continually promulgated if its growth and creativity is to answer the needs of a great society. "We must and can," as former Harvard University President James B. Conant said, "generate the qualities of mind or spirit which allow us to conceive excellence as a goal, to achieve it in some cases, but to strive to achieve it in all."

This is the expanding role of the hospital administrator.

[13] J. Martin Klotsche, Ph.D., "Statesmanship in Administration," *Hospital Administration 8*, No. 3 (Summer, 1963), 6.

A New Administrative Model for Hospitals

DOUGLAS R. BROWN, D.P.A.

Douglas R. Brown, D.P.A., is an Associate Professor of Hospital and Medical Care Administration at Cornell University.

In a society with ever increasing expectations concerning health, the hospital must continually search for new organization forms in order to meet broader demands. To this end, the author of a recent journal article provocatively questions the need for a chief executive in the hospital and goes on to suggest that consideration should be given to a dual reporting system more clearly separating the administrative and medical delegations of authority made by the hospital's governing board.[1] It is the hope of the author to bring organizational structure into harmony with actual functioning and thereby to increase the hospital's effectiveness.

Although a system of multiple authority and reporting has been formalized in Great Britain and other European countries, it seems unlikely that a similar pattern will be adopted in the typical American hospital. In fact, the trend in this country seems to be in the opposite direction. We are, in practice, placing greater responsibility for administrative and medical care services in the same hospital office. As a consequence, it would appear that the American hospital administrator is being held accountable for more and more matters, both administrative and medical. Increasingly, it is him to whom the governing board is turning for crucial advice relative to *all* hospital programs. And for the reasons discussed here, this practice seems irreversible in our environment.[2]

[1] Richard L. Johnson, "Do Hospitals Need a Chief Executive?" *The Modern Hospital,* September, 1964.

[2] Hospitals, of course, are only one of the many types of organizations attempting to deal with the problem of executive leadership and the board-administrative division of authority. For example, see Fred M. Hechinger, "Education: Who Should Run the Schools?" *The New York Times,* October 31, 1965.

Titles of executive vice president and president, relatively new to the hospital field for *operating* administrators, undoubtedly reflect the development of broader positions of responsibility. The experience of the last 25 years shows rather dramatically the changing role of the hospital administrator, in many institutions from a comparatively low-level actor in policy and decision-making to a central figure in determining the hospital's role in its community. With greater responsibilities, the hospital administrator's new role tends to emulate the position of leadership normally assumed by the university and corporation executive. Both of them have been granted a considerable amount of authority in American society.

Another writer observing the industrial and hospital administration scene would go even further and place the administrator and several other key people in the hospital on the board of trustees in a kind of "mixed directorship."[3] In general, this type of authority pattern would seem to be unwarranted and in several states the hospital's charitable status would be in jeopardy if voting members of the governing board were to receive compensation in the form of salaries.[4] However, this is not the main point of this discussion. Greater authority for the administrator does not depend on board appointment. Indeed, it is possible that appointment to the board might hamper rather than aid the development of professional hospital administration. An administrator motivated by professional concepts and values might well be recognized by the board as a source of "independent" expertise in decisions crucial to the organization. Voting membership on the board could impair such "independence."

MULTIPLE AUTHORITY

This examination is not meant to ignore in any way the multiple authority problem in hospitals—as a matter of fact, this is an attempt to alleviate the dilemma at the upper decision-making level. The two types of authority, one administrative and the other professional (the latter emanating from within the medical staff), may generate confusion and strain in the organization, in addition to causing problems in the policy area.[5] The conflict is felt most keenly at the ward level, where administrative directives can be, and often are, countermanded by those claiming medical necessity.[6] While it creates tension in the organization, this perplexing feature of the hospital may well be a source of its vitality and may contribute to its ability to change.

CHANGING POSTURES

It is interesting to note that, while hospitals are viewed as becoming more bureaucratic in our society,[7] business corporations seem to be taking on some of the

[3] Stanley Vance, "Do Boards of Trustees Need Surgery?" *The Modern Hospital,* June, 1965.

[4] See the Health Law Center, University of Pittsburgh, *Hospital Law Manual, Administrator's Volume,* Sections 2–3, 3–5, 5–10.

[5] Systematic attention is given this in Paul J. Gorden, "The Top Management Triangle in the Hospital," *Hospital Administration,* Spring, 1964, and Amitai Etzioni, *Modern Organizations* (Englewood Cliffs, N.J.: Prentice-Hall, 1964), ch. 8.

[6] Harvey L. Smith, "Two Lines of Authority Are One Too Many," *The Modern Hospital,* March, 1955.

[7] Robert N. Wilson, "The Social Structure of the General Hospital," *The Annals of the American Academy of Political and Social Science,* March, 1963.

characteristics of hospitals and other professional organizations (e.g., universities and research institutes). In the case of corporations, this professional posture is largely the result of increasing occupational specialization which has stimulated a search for new organization systems to integrate highly-trained personnel more successfully.[8] As hospitals have so readily illustrated, professionals do not take well to a hierarchical structure with its command authority. Recognition of the need for suitable alternatives to the highly structured, monistic organization is necessary if many of today's business organizations are to carry out their stated objectives and compete in the marketplace. These industrial organizations may in time rather closely imitate the professional organization despite the dysfunctions possible at the "production level" with multiple sources of authority.

Thompson and several other current analysts suggest that organizations might develop internal systems which are more task-oriented, built around the nature of the work itself. Presumably, this would result in the organization being made up of more or less autonomous clusters of diversified experts chosen for their appropriateness to the problem to be solved. In such an arrangement, the needs of the job to be done rather than any preconceived notions of status and hierarchy would determine relationships among the specialists involved. This exchange relationship of technical competence hopefully would stimulate a recognized interdependence among the group members at the same time that it promoted a kind of benevolent intellectual competition.[9]

DISTINGUISHABLE EXPERTISE

Hospitals, which are becoming increasingly bureaucratic in the sense that more professionals (particularly physicians) are becoming full-time salaried members of the organization, are also showing signs of the cluster phenomenon to a greater degree than has been true heretofore. Examples in the hospital setting, in addition to the established departments such as X-ray and laboratory, would be the open-heart surgery team and the patient research unit—wherein highly skilled physicians, nurses, technicians, etc., carry out their specific project with appreciable recognition by each member of the essential inputs made by the others. Such recognition, one may suggest, is not always found in the hospital unit. At the moment, status differences between physicians and nurses pretty much preclude an awareness of such interdependence. Probably more important, evolvement of a recognized professional interchange requires a high level of distinguishable expertise on the part of each team member contributing to the task. Unfortunately, nursing and many of the emerging medical technologies have yet to make explicit their specialized contributions on medical care teams.

Thus, according to recent literature, structural looseness, technical interdependence and group problem-solving, along with a great deal more experimentation, appear to be indicated within the *operational areas* of modern organizations (including hospitals) if they are to remain viable and innovative. At the *upper decision level,* however, it would seem that hospitals in particular would benefit from more unified, professional

---

[8] See Victor A. Thompson, *Modern Organization* (New York: Alfred A. Knopf, 1963).

[9] For an interesting discussion of conflict and creativity in organizations, see Victor A. Thompson, "Bureaucracy and Innovation," *Administrative Science Quarterly,* June, 1965.

administrative leadership than is presently the case. Internal tension and conflict properly harnessed can enhance organization effectiveness, but hospitals have amply demonstrated that divided authority at the policy level can stifle imagination and innovation. An organization that depends as much on compromise as does the hospital is at the mercy of all the sources of power at all times because of the veto power each has over new courses of action.

CHANGING MEDICAL PRACTICE

Freedom to practice unfettered by organizational restraints in order to preserve professional judgment and the fundamental doctor-patient relationship is uppermost in the minds of most physicians. There is, of course, justification for this view, for, if advancing medical technology is to be received by individual patients expeditiously and with dignity, physicians will have to apply their skills as their professional wisdom dictates. On the other hand, the practice of medicine is becoming more and more dependent on organizations.

Developments in the medical sciences, the arts of medicine, and the financing of health services have precipitated an evolutionary course which is placing limitations on the traditional solo practice of medicine.[10] There is increasing reliance on the coordinated team of skilled specialists for the provision of comprehensive medical services, and organized group practice and hospitals are evolving as the organizational frameworks for quality care. With the hospital in transition from doctor's workshop to community medical center, the need for linkage with the comprehensive group-practice team is growing more apparent.

As George Rosen has put it, "To use an analogy, one may say that the medical practitioner is being brought into the 'factory' (the hospital and the whole bureaucratic complexity of the provision of medical care) where he is being subjected to the necessary 'labor disciplines.' "[11] The numerical growth of salaried physicians in hospitals is a pointed reflection of fundamental changes affecting medical practice.[12] This organizational phenomenon has continued to place more and more authority, once held by voluntary medical staffs, in the hands of hospitals and their full-time physicians. For many reasons, some physicians view this trend with apprehension. The extent to which physicians can be drawn into organizational life—in essence the bureaucratization of medicine—without endangering the quality of medical care is a moot question which may never be answered fully.

GROWING CONSUMER INTEREST

Emerging public expectations regarding medical care and concern over rising costs are bringing about a shift in the relationship between the providers and the consumers of medical services. More and more people, and particularly the informed spokesmen

[10]See I. S. Falk, "Group Practice Is Pattern of the Future," *The Modern Hospital,* September, 1963.

[11]George Rosen, "Notes on Some Aspects of the Sociology of Medicine with Particular Reference to Prepaid Group Practice," (unpublished manuscript) cited in Robert N. Wilson, *op. cit.*

[12]Milton I. Roemer, "Growth of Salaried Physicians," *Hospital Progress,* September, 1964.

for organized consumer groups, are asking questions about the efficient integration of health services. It is evident that they want to have a voice in decisions affecting their own medical care—decisions which have been left mainly to the suppliers in the past. These forces, added to the growing conviction in our society that medical care is a matter of human right, based not on ability to pay but on health need alone, undoubtedly will enlarge the consumer's influence in the nation's health programs, at least in the short run. Intensified public interest, in turn, will probably reinforce the trend interlocking physicians and hospitals in group-practice arrangements.

PROFESSIONAL DIRECTION OF HOSPITALS

The move toward full-time medical practice in hospitals would appear to be a force shaping the professional direction of hospitals. The task of integrating a greater number of institutional physicians itself seems to point to the need for a professional type of leadership. Similarly, the emergence of other "professional" groups in hospitals would suggest a broader base of authority at the top—an authority aware of the sentiments of the specialists and respected by them.[13] Is there any doubt that practically every occupational group in the hospital will be intensifying its struggle for professional recognition in the years ahead?

While it could be inferred that only persons with a knowledge of medicine could provide the unified professional direction of hospitals, it must be pointed out that medical education alone does not prepare one for work in administration. There are problems of finance and personnel to which medical education normally does not address itself. Indeed, the intensively specialized nature of medical education may actually inhibit comprehensive administration on the physician's part by unduly circumscribing his perspective on overall medical care demands and the need for integrated planning.[14] Additionally, with the increase of new professions in the hospital, as pointed out, there is a need for a more "unencumbered" or "neutral" administration, not identified with any particular interest group.

In any case, physicians with administrative training or individuals specially trained for administrative work in medical care organizations would seem likely to be the most functional in hospital organizations. But since it is improbable that larger numbers of physicians will become interested in administrative employment—in fact, a recent study shows a declining number[15]—the burden of providing the necessary manpower would appear to fall to the programs in hospital and medical care administration. Because of the complex character of a medical care organization, it is difficult to believe that the untrained or those trained in other fields could provide, in sufficient numbers, the kind of leadership required.

[13]Specialists such as social workers, occupational and physical therapists, X-ray and laboratory technicians, inhalation therapists, etc.

[14]For the limitations of specialty training, see the discussion of "trained incapacity" in Robert Dubin, *Human Relations in Administration,* 2nd ed. (Englewood Cliffs, N.J.: Prentice-Hall, 1961), pp. 150, 193.

[15]J. A. Katzive, "The Vanishing Medical Hospital Administrator," *Hospital Topics,* February, 1965.

A PROFESSIONAL HOSPITAL ADMINISTRATION MODEL

If a broadened role for the hospital administrator continues to develop, as predicted here, the professional model for this role takes on ever increasing significance.[16] One need only contemplate the possible damage to the organization with a misguided chief executive. Moreover, if we assume that the community health center approach, with all of its ramifications, will be the hospital pattern of the future, an administrative orientation consistent with this concept would seem to be an essential ingredient. Consequently, given a larger role for the hospital, the administrative role also becomes more complex. The prototype of the administrator as custodian of the plant is a thing of the past in many hospitals. The "means-oriented" chief executive who is responsible only for financial and internal operations may become just as outdated in a relatively few years.

BROADER FIELD OF OPERATIONS

Without doubt, a number of hospital administrators in the United States are now operating in a noticeably broader context. These administrators, with or without the title of vice president or president, are often referred to as "outside men," and their major responsibilities commonly lie in the areas of policy-making, long-range planning, and representation of the hospital in the community. Hospital administrators are playing an increasing role in shaping medical care policy at state and national levels. One assumes this whole movement to be a response to the growing complexity and involvement of hospitals in our society and to the need for more knowledgeable leadership in medical care affairs at every level.

In capsule form, the administrative model proposed here views the professional hospital administrator largely as a policy-maker, an innovator, and an initiator of medical care programs to meet health needs. He is a program-planner and program-developer with a broad social role in the total community.

Such a professional orientation stresses hospital objectives related, in most instances, to the solution of overall community health problems.[17] Further, it means that the professional hospital administrator must have convictions of his own concerning the distribution and organization of medical care services in the society. No occupational group can hope for professional status if it merely executes the ideas of others—it must have values which are shared by its members and are at the same time socially useful. More specifically, it is likely that the professional hospital administrator's conceptualization will encompass social as well as medical care needs, preventive as well as rehabilitative care, long-term and psychiatric as well as short-term acute services, and so on. In short, his concern is for comprehensive, high-quality care for all people in the community.

---

[16]The whole question of professionalism with special application to hospital administration is treated most interestingly in Harold L. Wilensky, "The Dynamics of Professionalism: The Case of Hospital Administration," *Hospital Administration,* Spring, 1962, and "The Professionalization of Everyone?" *The American Journal of Sociology,* September, 1964.

[17]Specialty hospitals, of course, would define their mission in narrower terms.

GENERALIST AND SPECIALIST

Thus, according to the suggested paradigm, if one had to single out the hospital administrator's chief professional area of competence, his most exclusive expertise, it would be his ability to innovate programs and shape organizations designed to deliver medical care services more adequately to the population. His *raison d' etre* would be invention and program effectiveness rather than organizational efficiency alone, and his professional judgment in these matters would be recognized by those around him and by society in general. Successful adoption of this model perforce makes the hospital administrator a generalist concerned with formulating medical care goals and values, as well as a specialist responsible for implementing goals.

Relatively few hospitals and other local medical care administrators are operating at this level in their own communities, and fewer yet are making an impact on the formulation of state and federal health policy. While it is true that some will see this role as completely inappropriate for the hospital administrator, few will deny the need for such expertise in most sectors of the health field. Furthermore, with the hospital taking a central role in our medical care system, the hospital administrator would seem to be the logical health professional to assume leadership.

Such a professional orientation may develop as administrators begin to concern themselves more with meeting community health needs and less with adjusting to boards of trustees who sometimes view the hospital's purposes narrowly and evaluate the hospital and its administrator only in terms of the profit-and-loss statement.[18] In the long run, the hospital administrator's professional allegiance must be tied to the broader community and not merely to the board that hires him or the medical staff that provides the institution's patients. If the hospital administrator places the interests of the board or the medical staff above the interests of the community dependent on his organization for their medical care, there is little justification for his professional claim. The pursuit of community needs might result in shorter job tenure for some administrators. More frequent turnover could be dysfunctional, however, and it is interesting to note that hospital administrators are reported to have longer job tenure than business and federal executives.[19]

Some hospital boards are awakening to the realities of twentieth-century medical care and are providing leadership and support for institutional innovation. Nonetheless, the future role of hospital boards of trustees in this regard is open to question, for reasons dealt with in later paragraphs.

As the professional hospital administrator broadens his activities to include the larger community, the need for effective, internally oriented administration will in no way diminish. Unquestionably, skills of a higher level will be sought here as well if the organization is successfully to relate changing technology to patient welfare and to maintain relative internal harmony.

[18]For a perhaps rather dismal picture of board functioning, see Frederic C. LeRocker and S. Kenneth Howard, "What Decisions Do Trustees Actually Make?" *The Modern Hospital,* April, 1960, and Harleigh B. Trecker, "Who Are Board Members?" *Trustee,* April, 1960. There has been so little systematic research done on board decision-making that one may conclude that these findings probably reflect accurately the current scene.

[19]Miriam T. Dolson, "Today's Administrator: Educated, Mobile Executive," *The Modern Hospital,* June, 1964.

UNIFIED PROFESSIONAL LEADERSHIP

It is possible that some will interpret the case for an overriding administrative authority in the hospital as an attempt to undermine medical practice. Such reasoning would imply that administrative and medical goals are separate and conflicting. To the contrary, the gap between these perspectives is not as wide as often assumed. The varying viewpoints of administrators and physicians are not the result of any fundamental disparity in professional orientations; presumably both are working toward the same end—high-quality medical care for the community.

Differences that do arise largely concern the *means* for achieving this quality care. Often the differences will involve the needs of single patients versus the needs of the many. The physician's primary responsibility is to his individual patients. The administrator is concerned with the medical needs of patients in the aggregate. As the physician has a client relationship with his particular patient, the professional hospital administrator, in a sense, has clients too: all the patients and potential patients served by the organization. Consequently, when conflict does occur in the hospital, the administrator would seem well advised to draw upon persuasive skills based on the concepts of his profession relating to the rational or optimal organization of comprehensive medical care services.

MEDICAL CARE ASSESSMENT METHODS

In a similar vein, it can be asserted that the professionally oriented administrator can be responsible for the quality of care rendered in the institution, much as he is held accountable for its financial affairs. While he is unable or, in fact, unqualified to attend personally to the many specialized activities of the organization, with adequate measuring tools and reporting systems, the administrator can see that all programs receive the attention they deserve from the appropriate medical and non-medical specialists associated with the organization. The day is not far off when practical methods for the assessment of medical care will be available and utilized. In addition to placing a valuable tool for appraisal and education at the disposal of hospitals and other medical care organizations, these techniques could make possible more informed decisions for consumers seeking medical care.

In summary, the suggested professional administrative model would be all-encompassing, concerned with the total quantitative and qualitative aspects of community medical care. The physician's role in the system would be essential, of course, but within the context of comprehensive health care objectives. If medicine is thought to be subordinated in this scheme, then it is subordinate only to expanding rationality of medical care services as our society strives to meet its health needs.

Whether one is considering economic, social, and political forces impinging on health in our nation, or developments in the practice of medicine itself, all signs point to the increasing involvement of organizations in the provision of medical care services. Medical specialization, advances in technology, medical care costs, and public attitudes foreshadow no other alternative. As a result, greater authority is flowing to those equipped to mold and control organizations which meet emerging health care demands. The administrator of the central institution, the hospital, would appear to be at the threshold of broader opportunities. Whether he grasps these opportunities and contributes to society in a meaningful way will depend in large part on his professional orientation.

Should fate project the ill-equipped hospital administrator into a position of wide influence, he will likely impede rather than expedite the provision of health services. Hence, one must necessarily stress the importance of formal education, properly supervised training, and continuing self-development for the administrator. An understanding of the major social, economic, and political forces in our society and an ability to foresee and shape organizations to meet medical care needs loom as critical components of the hospital administrator's armamentarium.[20]

THE FUTURE OF BOARDS OF TRUSTEES

Earlier it was stated that the role of hospital boards of trustees will likely change. This prognostication is based on the general notion that, increasingly, important decisions in the hospital field will not be made by the same people who made them in the past. The quest for rationality in a progressively complex medical care system suggests greater reliance on emerging, highly skilled specialists in medical care organization. While boards may in fact become more representative and remain large in size, important decision-making will not reside, for all practical purposes, with such groups.[21] Decisions will gravitate to the professional hospital administrators and, as suggested in later sections of this paper, to other specialists beyond the individual hospital. The decisions being considered today are just too complicated for "part-time" people to cope with. Additionally, legislation and specific regulations of government agencies will further circumscribe the hospital board's area of responsibility. It is highly unlikely that future boards of separate hospitals will need to be concerned with matters relating to expansion of beds and services, setting charges and reimbursement formulas, and evaluating the quality of care. These decisions will be considered too important to be left to the hospital alone.

Perhaps a few board members at the local hospital or regional planning level will devote the necessary time to qualify as experts themselves. It is difficult to see how these expert board members will be able to belong to several hospital or other agency boards as is the current practice. Most board members, however, will not have the interest or will not take the time to become adequately informed; and, even though they may go through the motions of discussion, decisions of the experts will almost always prevail. With the complexities of new programs and regulations precluding the "occasional" trustee from a complete understanding, the hospital administrator, if he avails himself of the opportunity, becomes the main source of information—and the chance of the board overruling his informed judgments becomes more remote with time. What is suggested here is simply that hospital decision-making, both local and regional, is fast becoming an "expertise" function, with the hospital board of trustees being sharply curtailed in its discretionary power.

---

[20]For a discussion of the dynamics of administration with particular reference to hospitals, see Rodney F. White, "Current Trends in Administration," in J. K. Owen (ed.), *Modern Concepts of Hospital Administration* (Philadelphia: W. B. Saunders Co., 1962).

[21]The term "representative," which has recently evoked considerable interest in the health field, is perhaps a useful generalized objective or theme, but it virtually defies precise definition in the real world.

SPECIALIZATION AND CENTRALIZATION

What is becoming true for hospital services would seem to be already true for many sectors of our society. In the incredibly complex, modern industrial state, widespread participation by an informed citizenry in the many specialized fields is difficult indeed. It is just impossible for the average person to remain knowledgeable in more than a few of these areas at a time. In some instances, information is not available, and participation is not possible, even if the individual should seek it. Ours is an era of specialization, in which large-scale bureaucratic organizations, with their oligarchic power, predominate.[22] As C. P. Snow has characterized it, "One of the most bizarre features of any advanced industrial society in our time is that the cardinal choices have to be made by a handful of men: in secret:. . . ."[23]

This development, of course, presents a threat to popular control, a threat which must be reckoned with in a democratic society. Uncritical acceptance of decisions made by the few, whether they are experts or not, is a potential danger only too clear. Nevertheless, it remains to be seen whether specialization in itself is antagonistic to egalitarian values.

GOVERNMENT "SPECIALISTS"

Very recently there has been a marked growth in major medical care programs emanating from federal, and to a lesser extent, state, and local governments. President Johnson's health proposals may be considered nothing less than revolutionary and it would appear that he has the support of the American people in this regard. Federal leadership in health care has been considerably dependent on the active support and advice of specialist "types," such as elected representatives (especially legislators serving on health and welfare committees), appointed health officials, and the medical care organization experts in and out of government. There is every indication that these specialists will play an even larger role in the nation's medical care system as the many programs proposed are implemented.

With more government programs, accompanied by regulations and standards, there is less room at the local hospital level for alternative courses of action. It is apparent that crucial decisions are shifting from the individual hospital, traditionally epitomized by its board of trustees and its voluntary medical staff, to state and federal governmental agencies and quasi-public planning organizations at the regional level. While the present hospital system is characterized by independent and separate hospitals, the tendency toward centralized regionalization, with its concomitant dependence on specialists in medical care organization, is giving birth to an integrated system of medical facilities.

The centralization of hospital services is occurring at a time when there is grave concern about an enlarging government and the loss of local initiative. Some would argue that many of the European nations, even with their national health schemes, depend considerably on local participation—probably to a greater extent than we do at the moment. One could hypothesize that in the United States more centralization of

---

[22]Robert Presthus, *The Organizational Society* (New York: Alfred A. Knopf, 1962). Also, for a provocative discussion of power-holders in our society, see C. Wright Mills, *The Power Elite* (New York: Oxford University Press, 1956).

[23]C. P. Snow, *Science and Government* (Cambridge: Harvard University Press, 1960), p. 1.

hospital activities may be necessary before broad participation in hospital affairs can occur at the local level. Moreover, the emergence of specialists in medical care organization is not entirely incompatible with expanded citizen involvement. In the final analysis, however, the basic question will remain: what kind of hospital system is more responsive to the needs of a changing society? And the answer to this will depend on many diverse considerations.

While sustained popular participation in health and other matters is possible in American society, it is not likely. Even though we may go through a transitional period in realizing the "welfare state" (the "Great Society" in current terminology), which appears to emphasize direct citizen participation in community programs, the future prospect is a continuing centralization and a more complete take-over by salaried professionals. As the major problems in our society are met one by one, the ordinary citizen will become increasingly satisfied to let the different hierarchies (government, labor unions, political parties, large organizations, etc.) manage the society.[24] With this general tendency, there is no reason to believe that health services will be the exception. Therefore, in the long run, the governing of the American hospital will pass to the full-time specialists employed in the institution itself and in area-wide networks. Briefly stated, the thesis of this section is that intensified public concern is bringing about the centralization of medical care planning and is placing more authority in the hands of specialists. Eventually, a contented population will allow its concern to wane and, within rather broad guidelines, will leave most of the decisions affecting the organization of medical care to the specialists.

In time, there will be those who will look back with effusive nostalgia to bygone days when hospitals were in the "hands of the people." They will have long forgotten that these institutions in the earlier period were seldom subject to popular control, having been closely guided more often by self-perpetuating boards of trustees and self-interested medical staffs. For the immediate future, the rising interest in medical care may at least serve to clarify problems and lead to a broad definition of the limits to which we are willing to go to solve these problems.

TRIAL-AND-ERROR APPROACH

Whatever occurs on the American scene over the remainder of the century, it seems probable that the development of our hospital pattern will be, in some ways, unlike that experienced elsewhere in the world. Our penchant, and perhaps strength, is our pragmatic, trial-and-error approach to problems. Similarly, while public medical care is the form found throughout the world, "volunteerism" may remain a strong force in our society, and it hasn't often sought a governmental partnership. Consequently, about all one can conclude for certain is that the emerging system will be characteristically American—that is, peculiar to our own needs and aspirations. Perhaps we should recognize that it will be a "mixed" form and let it go at that rather than rigidly defend the voluntary or public way. Efforts would be better spent making sure that hospitals are adapting to modern times.

---

[24] A provocative discussion of citizen participation in a welfare state may be found in Gunnar Myrdal, "The Swedish Way to Happiness," *The New York Times Magazine,* January 30, 1966.

Insofar as the hospital administrator is concerned with such a plan, the contribution he makes will depend on the spirit in which he views his role.[25] If he remains technique-oriented, his impact will be limited to within the institution's walls; but, should he become goal-oriented to community medical care, his contirbution could be far-reaching. Filling the broader role will necessitate a generalist outlook to complement the hospital administrator's specialized abilities. Admittedly, such comprehensive wisdom and technical competence are difficult for any one person to achieve.

In all, it seems reasonable to assert that, from an ideal standpoint in our democratic society, the medical care system should be directed by men possessing a broad perspective as well as professional competence, men who are acutely sensitive to the health needs of the population.

CIRCUMVENTION OF THE HEALTH ADMINISTRATOR?

Of the forces examined, there is one in particular which could alter the emergence of the hospital administrator as one of the chief organizational experts in our medical care system. As regional planning spreads in the nation, its specialized agencies could evolve as the preponderant centers for hospital decision-making and its personnel as the chief organizational experts. A number of regions currently have planning agencies in operation, and several states have passed or are considering legislation which mandates and closely regulates this activity. The likelihood of further standards affecting hospital operations and the quality of care is obvious. Recently, the New York State Legislature delegated considerable authority to its State Health Department and seven regional hospital planning councils. It is difficult to see *any* aspect of hospital activity that is left untouched by this legislation.

Conceivably, the forces projecting the hospital administrator into broader authority could bypass him for the most part and concentrate at the regional and other levels. The hospital administrator's role then would become more routine and programmed, and the contention of much of this paper would have to be modified. Consequently, rather than a working partnership among the specialists at the hospital and regional levels, the regional representatives would clearly dominate. Experience with the regionalization of health services in Great Britain indicates that, while the position of the hospital secretary (the administrator) has been strengthened overall, he, along with other decision-makers in the individual hospital, has been removed to some extent from the locus of top authority.[26] Since key decisions once made by hospitals are now being made by hospital management committees (which are responsible ordinarily for several hospitals), regional boards, and the Ministry of Health, individual hospitals have noticeably surrendered their independence. In the interest of regional objectives,

---

[26]Cyril Sofer, "Reactions to Administrative Change" in Dorrian Apple (ed.), *Sociological Studies of Health & Sickness* (New York: McGraw-Hill, 1960). It is likely that, since the hospital secretary's position was comparatively low-level prior to 1948, the National Health Service, of necessity, recognized the need for an upgraded administration in the hospital despite the centralization of many functions.

[25]For a scholarly treatment of potential roles of the public executive in American society, see Alan Altschuler, "Rationality and Influence in Public Service," *Public Administration Review,* September, 1965.

rapid decision-making and freedom of independent action at the local level evidently must be sacrificed in the British experience. Inasmuch as voluntary hospitals have operated with considerable freedom in American society, outside controls will not be accepted easily.

If *systematic and controlled* regional planning becomes the rule in the United States, hospital decision-makers who are distressed by this development should ask themselves a candid question. Would decision-making at another level be necessary if coordination of health services at the community level had come a little sooner to meet obvious health problems? Perhaps, despite the virtues of the voluntary system eulogized over the years, the local approach alone was never destined to meet the broader demands for medical care in a nation growing in population, complexity, and public-private interdependence.

CONCLUSION

This paper has attempted to formulate a model for the emerging professional hospital administrator—a model which is appropriate to the changing role of the hospital in our society. It has been argued that this increasingly complex organization, serving an expanding demand for medical care, would likely benefit from unified professional direction. Additionally, it has been asserted that greater "professionalization" of the administrator, with concurrent recognition of his expertise by society, may well depend on his ability to innovate and shape medical care programs to meet health needs in the community.

If this model falls short in some respects, it may stimulate further thought and discussion of appropriate roles and values as the hospital administrator continues to seek his place in the nation's medical care system.

The Medical Staff

This section presents the role of the medical staff and its directors within the hospital setting. As the third of the hospital's major managing groups, the medical staff is responsible for overseeing the offering of medical care. By necessity its authority in the area of patient care is paramount. However, the medical staff is housed within an organization which must concern itself with financial, material, and facility resources in order to function. The administrator's responsibility of efficiently running a major organization, with all its material and human resources and the medical staff's demands on those resources, often gives rise to conflict.

Leadership, in *MEDICAL STAFF FUNCTIONS AND LEADERSHIP,* is considered to be a prerequsite of an effective medical staff. It is contended that the chief of staff, as a leader, should have a peer (authority) level equal to the administrator and the board. It is stipulated that cooperation between the medical staff and the administrator is vital in order to avoid fragmentation. It is also advocated that the medical staff and the governing board be integrated. That is, at least one physician should sit on the board of trustees. Further discussion is directed toward the functions and responsibilities of the medical staff and the necessity for effective leadership.

Changes in the delivery of medical care have resulted in the centralization of activities within the hospital organization in contrast to the historical decentralized delivery within the physician's office. In *HOW CHANGING TIMES ARE CHANGING STAFFS,* it is avered that physicians can no longer hold the obsolete notion that the hospital is merely a vehicle to be used by them in the treatment of their patients. The hospital today is a single organization where the physician's responsibility extends beyond self utilization. A call is made for the utilization of professional medical staff leaders with administrative training in order to provide effective interaction with the administrator and the board of trustees.

External and internal factors have caused the hospital to change. In *THE HOSPITAL MEDICAL DIRECTOR: AN ADMINISTRATOR'S VIEW,* it is contended that modern management techniques and organizational trends have not been developed as rapidly within the medical staff as they have within the administrative staff. Hospital medical staffs are not organized to cope with the responsibilities that have been thrust upon them. Various areas of accountability are presented along with suggestions for modernizing the management techniques of the medical staff.

Medical Staff Functions and Leadership

WILLIAM W. JACK, M.D.

William W. Jack, M.D., is a practicing physician in Grand Rapids, Michigan.

In the functioning of the medical staff of the modern hospital, leadership is the single most important factor. The leadership and administration of the medical staff are provided by the executive committee. This committee is normally composed of the officers of the medical staff and the various department chairmen, although the actual composition of the committee may vary from hospital to hospital.

The chief of staff (or the highest elected officer of the committee) and the members of the executive committee must possess essential leadership requirements if the purposes of the medical staff are to be realized. The chief of staff must be the peer of both the hospital administrator and the president of the hospital's governing board. He must be thoroughly familiar with the internal operation of the hospital, as well as with all local, regional, or national influences that affect the hospital and/or the medical profession.

In order to effectively fulfill his duties, the chief of staff needs a strong executive committee whose members are as dedicated to good staff government as he is. The physicians who make up the executive committee are department heads, and it is their responsibility to make their leadership felt at the department level. Good patient care, good continuing education programs, and good administrative practices are all essential functions of their jobs.

In addition to the members of the executive committee, the chief of staff also needs the help of the administrator if he is to carry out the duties of his position. The administrator is the real professional in the area of hospital administration. Cooperation between the chief of the medical staff and the administrator is vital because, without it, divisive fragmentation occurs. Such a dichotomy between medical staff and administration has been somewhat eased by the integration of the medical staff and the governing board. In many hospitals, at least one member of the hospital board is now a physician.

This kind of integration is highly desirable because the chief of the medical staff needs the action and informed help of the governing board. This board is normally composed of capable and sincere citizens who are legally responsible for the total operation and activity of the hospital. However, many members of governing boards come to their tasks with little background and little understanding, if any, of what is expected and desired of them. Continuing education of board members is necessary if they are to be able to contribute effectively to the operation of the hospital and to the medical staff as an important element of the hospital structure.

In order to make the administration of medical staff activities more efficient, it is advisable to combine certain traditional staff functions into three main categories or "councils." These three councils cover the broad areas of patient care, continuing medical education, and care evaluation.

PATIENT CARE

The council on patient care comprises a group of interrelated functions including pharmacy and therapeutics, infection control, emergency room, outpatient department, special care, and disaster. Each of these functions is oriented toward the care of the patient and each requires the cooperation of and support from administration and/or nursing. A doctor should be assigned responsibility for each of these functions and should work with his counterparts from administration and nursing in coordinating the particular function for which he is responsible with other hospital activities.

All the physicians assigned responsibility for the various functions that comprise the council on patient care constitute the members of that council. They should meet regularly in an attempt to familiarize each other with their views about each of the particular functions of patient care. In so doing, they should seek to coordinate these functions so as to achieve better patient care.

The chief of the medical staff should chair the council on patient care for various reasons: He is closely associated with the administrator and with the nursing director, both of whom are vital to any consideration of patient care. In addition, his position as chief of staff and head of the executive committee enables him to help resolve problems concerning patient care as quickly as possible.

PATIENT CARE COUNCIL

Pharmacy-Therapeutic

1. Advise the medical staff and hospital pharmacist on matters pertaining to the choice of drugs.
2. Recommend drugs available under emergency conditions.
3. Evaluate clinical data and report to the medical staff on new drugs suggested for use in the hospital.
4. Authorize the use of experimental drugs under well-defined rules.
5. Maintain a registry of adverse reactions.

Infection Control

1. Make recommendations regarding the control of all patient infections within the hospital.

2. Make recommendations regarding the hospital's isolation techniques.
3. Conduct epidemiological surveys of infections occurring in the hospital.

Emergency Room/Outpatient

1. Recommend policies regarding the care of patients in the emergency room and outpatient clinics and, after approval, supervise the implementation of these policies.
2. Make certain that the emergency room and the outpatient clinics are always ready to take part in mass casualty situations.
3. Supervise the proper record-keeping in the emergency room and outpatient clinics.
4. Aid in integrating the emergency room and outpatient clinics into the teaching program.

Special Care

1. Assume responsibility for the development of the medical policy for proper and efficient management of the intensive care unit, the pediatric intensive care unit, the coronary care unit, and such other special care units as recommended by the staff executive committee.
2. Develop policies for the admission, duration of stay, and discharge of patients in the special care units.
3. Serve in an advisory capacity for the nursing service in joint problems involving the special care units.

Disaster

1. Assess constantly the hospital's preparedness for any disaster which might strike the community at large or the hospital itself.
2. Re-evaluate the hospital's disaster plan periodically to eliminate defects, improve the plan, recommend improvements, and supervise practice sessions.

CONTINUING MEDICAL EDUCATION COUNCIL

Education

1. Develop a broad program for continuing education within the hospital, and, after approval, be responsible for its implementation.
2. Make recommendations for improving the program.
3. Assume responsibility for recruiting and appointing house staff.
4. Assume responsibility for recruiting outside speakers and integrating their presentations into the general continuing education programs.

Library-Publications

1. Recommend the purchase of books, periodicals, tapes, and visual aids.
2. Make recommendations regarding the operation of the medical library.
3. Make plans and recommendations regarding staff publications and, after approval, implement these policies.
4. Offer assistance to members of the staff who may wish to submit an article for publication.

Oncology

1. Offer a consultation service in the diagnosis and treatment of malignancies.
2. Provide leadership in the cancer teaching program.
3. Establish regular conferences for discussing cases of hospital patients with malignancies.
4. Supervise the operation of the tumor registry.

Research

1. Stimulate and guide critical investigation or experimentation that has for its aim the discovery and correct interpretation of new facts.
2. Aid or improve existing techniques or skills for patient care within the hospital.

Program

1. Develop programs for general staff meetings within the broad policies of continuing medical education.
2. Coordinate departmental and interdepartmental programs.
3. Integrate reports of the various committees and departments into the educational program.

CARE EVALUATION COUNCIL

Tissue Evaluation

1. Review and evaluate all surgery performed in the hospital on the basis of agreement or non-agreement with the pre- and post-operative and pathological tissue diagnoses, and on the basis of acceptability of the procedure undertaken.

Utilization Review

1. Offer assurance that the hospital stays and inpatient services are medically necessary.
2. Analyze and identify factors that may contribute to unnecessary or ineffective hospital stays or ineffective use of inpatient services and facilities.

Medical Records

1. Assure satisfactory completion of medical records within the time allotted.
2. Advise and recommend policies for maintaining medical records.
3. Supervise medical records to insure that details are recorded in the proper manner and that sufficient data are present to evaluate the care of the patient.
4. Advise and develop policies, with the aid of legal counsel, to guide the medical record librarian, the medical staff, and the administration insofar as matters of privileged communication and legal release of information are concerned.

Medical Audit

1. Evaluate the quality of patient care as reflected in the clinical record.
2. Audit complications that occur in the hospital.
3. Evaluate the efficacy, value, or harm of treatments and procedures used in the management of patients.
4. Audit all deaths occurring in the hospital.

CONTINUING MEDICAL EDUCATION

The council on continuing medical education also includes a number of interrelated functions. Education; library; publications; oncology; research; and various educational programs.

Post-graduate medical education is almost unbelievably complicated and competitive. The amount of printed material and the number of meetings every week, month, and year that vie for the physician's attention staggers the imagination. Almost everything that is offered is worth considering, and much is actually worth studying or attending. However, since time will not permit the individual physician to take advantage of everything that is offered, compromise is inevitable. Articles in special interest journals, meetings of selected organizations, and attendance at informal discussions on a regular basis must suffice.

Reading and attendance at outside meetings prevent parochialism. Assimilation and perspective are gained through small group discussions, and it is in this area that the hospital has a definite role. By providing physicians with an opportunity to discuss topics of current interest, the hospital enables them to keep informed.

The council on continuing medical education should be organized in much the same manner as the council on patient care, with a specific physician being assigned responsibility for each specific function. The director of medical education for the hospital should chair this council, and the council itself should provide direction and coordination for the hospital's entire educational program. Hopefully the director of medical education would also be a member of the medical staff executive committee, so that the educational function of the medical staff would be directly represented in this administrative body.

The hospital that has a house staff will find that the council on continuing medical education will have a larger role to play than it does in the hospital without a house staff. Interns and residents provide a source of stimuli for all physicians on the staff so that, in planning for their education, the hospital also plans for the education of all its medical staff members.

However, in another sense, the hospital without a house staff perhaps has an even greater need of a continuing education program, since the physicians in such a hospital do not benefit from the stimulus provided by the influx of interns and residents. At any rate, quality patient care cannot be achieved without an adequate continuing medical education program.

CARE EVALUATION

The council on care evaluation includes such functions as tissue evaluation, utilization review, medical records, and the medical audit.

This council is not designed primarily to seek out the incompetent and unskilled, but rather to pinpoint areas where patient care can be improved through continuing education. Education is the proper solution to the problem of lack of skill and/or judgment. If situations arise in which there is an uneducable lack of skill and/or judgment, they should be documented in the deliberations of the council. For this reason, the chairman of the medical staff's credentials committee should also chair the council on care evaluation.

The need for the council on care evaluation points logically to another need, that of discipline. Disciplinary rules and procedures should be written into the medical staff by-laws. They should be delineated in detail and checked thoroughly by legal council. The section on discipline should, of course, be publicized to the entire medical staff.

QUESTIONING CURRENT PRACTICES

Aside from the traditional medical staff functions of patient care, continuing medical education, and care evaluation, two additional functions must be added in order to meet the demands of modern health care. The first of these additional responsibilities is that of questioning the effectiveness of current programs and practices. No traditional practice should be allowed to continue without examination. The medical staff must ask itself if the practice is necessary, if it is being performed in the most effective and efficient manner, if it is worth the effort being expended, and if it contributes to quality care. Medical staff leaders must seek the answers to these and similar questions, hopefully with consultation and cooperation of the administration and the governing board.

AWARENESS OF NEW TRENDS

The second additional responsibility of today's medical staff is to be aware of national trends and developments and to plan local implementation of them.

Health Care Delivery. For over 50 years, the major focus in the delivery of health care has been the hospital. However, at the present time, there are not enough physicians and, at the current rate of production, there will not be enough in the foreseeable future. Vast numbers of people in the United States do not have ready access to quality health care. Yet, how many hospitals have seriously considered alternate ways of delivering health care? Is it enough for hospitals to boast that they will provide care for those who seek it at their doors? Or, must they become more actively involved in deciding how to decentralize health care delivery in order to be able to make their "product" more accessible to the public?

Planning. Another development currently receiving much attention is that of area planning. How many hospitals participate in inter-hospital cooperative programs? How many medical staffs have seriously considered the advisability of establishing a committee or council to coordinate the medical education programs of the various hospitals in the community, of centralizing the medical records and medical audit activities of the community hospitals; of establishing an acute care bed registry, common storage, common purchasing, and common food services? How many hospitals and medical staffs are willing to close their obstetrics service, pediatrics service, or newborn service in the interests of economy, efficiency, and quality care?

Allied Health Manpower. Good medical care is care provided by an initially well-trained and continually retrained physician. However, every patient condition does not require care at this level; some conditions can be cared for by a person at a different level of knowledge and skill. How many hospitals and medical staffs have seriously considered the possibilities which such an innovation presents? Efforts to make this innovation standard procedure are being made throughout the country.

Those involved in the delivery of health care should ask themselves whether the use of allied health manpower is possible in the outpatient department, the emergency room, the physician's office, the neighborhood health center. They should discuss this concept with legal counsel, insurance carriers, legislators. It is too exciting a possibility to be ignored and too promising to be disregarded.

Liability Insurance. One continuing development in which members of medical staffs should be particularly interested is that of liability insurance. Most claims arise as a result of hospital care. Is the answer to preventing or decreasing liability claims really so simple as peer review, a bigger and better tissue committee, audit committee, etc.? Medical staffs must begin seeking answers to the problem of rising medical care costs; they must not be satisfied with naive and oversimplified solutions, such as the creation of better utilization committees. Can the problem be solved merely by reducing a hospital stay to four days rather than five? Does the challenge to solve this problem lie only at the doorstep of medicine and nowhere else?

Political Influence. Responsible statesmanship seems to have given way to political opportunism, and health care has become the politician's golden opportunity. The issues and problems associated with health care and its delivery seem to mean a quick ticket to Washington, or a front-page story, or television coverage.

The national trends and developments listed above are some of the problems that face the health care system in general and the physician in particular in the 70's. They require serious consideration from every medical staff, every administrator, and every governing board. For those involved in the delivery of health care to say that everything about medicine is right and pure and innocent is just as ridiculous as to say that all detractors of the system are wrong, evil, and dishonest.

SYSTEM NEEDS LEADERSHIP

The present decade demands that the health care system provide more and better care for more people. To fulfill this demand, the system needs more doctors, nurses, and allied health personnel who are trained in such a way that they can provide more care, more efficiently and effectively at a lower unit cost. The system needs more hospitals in more locations providing care to more people at a lower unit cost. To achieve such goals, the system must encourage innovation and experimentation.

Physicians and hospitals must remember that they will have to work together if the demands of the public are to be met. If fragmentation ever existed, it must go. Medical staffs, administrators, and governing boards must find new ways of working more closely together. Physicians must not regard hospitals as their private workshops. Board members must not convince themselves that attending one meeting a month fulfills their obligations. Administrators must accept their roles as catalysts between the board and the medical staff. The key to all these requirements is the chief of the medical staff. His leadership is a single most important aspect of effective staff functioning.

How Changing Times are Changing Staffs

C. WESLEY EISELE, M.D.

C. Wesley Eisele, M.D., is a Professor of Medicine at the University of Colorado.

Changing concepts of the hospital medical staff organization are not so much a matter of new concepts as of changes in understanding and in emphasis of basic principles. The hospital itself is changing, and the community hospital increasingly is assuming the role of a community medical center. Education at all levels and laboratory research are augmenting the traditional role of patient care. The community hospital thus approaches the character of the university hospital. Regionalization of hospitals and cooperative arrangements among hospitals will proceed at an accelerated pace under the Regional Medical Programs of Public Law 89-239.

Even more important to the staff physician is the fact that more and more functions previously performed in the physician's office are now becoming functions of the hospital. To mention but a few, there is the exploding emergency service, the ever expanding outpatient department, and the many highly technical diagnostic and treatment procedures which require specialized facilities, equipment and personnel, with costs of such magnitude that it becomes totally impractical to perform them in the physician's office. For example, a decade or so ago, a patient could have a complete cardiac work-up in a physician's office. This examination now might involve a quarter of a million dollars worth of hardware weighing 10 tons.

Along with these changes, the image of the hospital has changed. Almost imperceptibly, patients are beginning to shift their identification from the solo physician to the hospital center.

Many of these changes have been brought about by the medical profession itself, with the hospital merely serving to fill the voids in medical care which individual physicians are unable or unwilling to fill. Whatever the cause, physicians feel threatened. They want to cling to the control of the hospital which they think they once had. Fragmentation may occur and a totally untenable situation may arise in which physicians hold the obsolete notion that the hospital is a twofold organization – a self-governing and more or less autonomous medical staff that renders medical care, and a separate, loosely related business and administrative organization that provides facilities and personnel to assist the doctors in the care of their patients, with a governing board around merely to raise money. The hospital is looked upon as the doctor's workshop. There is a gauze curtain between the medical staff and the administration, but, fortunately, most of the gauze used today is of the disposable variety.

The hospital is a single organization. This is the first basic principle to be emphasized. The primary purpose of all concerned is the same — to provide high-quality patient care. When this principle is firmly established, the hospital is no longer merely the doctor's workshop, and it is recognized that the physician's responsibility extends beyond the care of his own patients. The one-to-one physician-patient relationship can remain inviolate only so long as the one doctor provides good care for the one patient.

The entire medical staff, the board of trustees, and the administration share moral and legal responsibilities to take whatever steps are necessary to insist on high standards of care for all patients. On one legal theory or another, the courts have been saying for some time that a hospital is responsible to the patient for knowing what is going on professionally within its walls and for demanding high standards of care.

This leads to another basic principle. The medical staff must establish high standards of practice and it must effectively enforce and maintain them through its bylaws and its staff organization. This implies the necessity for a conscientious, continuous and systematic review of the clinical practice in the institution.

There are many approaches to this problem, but in all of them, whether they like it or not, physicians must express their critical judgment of the work performed by their colleagues. Happily, effective computer systems are available to assist the physicians in the more tedious aspects of the task and to ensure an objective and impartial selection of cases for critical review. More significantly, computers can now give any hospital staff, regardless of size, anonymous statistical comparisons of many facets of its work with that in hundreds of similar hospitals across the nation.

Traditionally, the hospital staff has elected its own leaders from among its membership with the chief of staff and other responsible positions often rotating on an annual basis. Not infrequently, elections have been decided not on merit but on considerations far removed from ability to provide able and impartial leadership. These situations are no longer tenable under any circumstances. At times, it may be expecting too much to hope for effective leadership from a busy physician who must continue to earn his living in practice, and who is untrained and inexperienced in management processes.

The problems are compounded when the tenure in office is but a year or two. All too often, the chief of staff has not even seen the bylaws, and seldom does he fully understand the table of organization of the institution or the structure and function of standing committees. Unless he is willing to accept guidance and support from an able administrator, medical staff functions may deteriorate and become stagnant and ineffective. The staff may find itself at a serious disadvantage in relationship to the trained management personnel usually found in the administration and the governing board of modern hospitals, and finally it may become adept only at blocking actions, without any positive program of its own. The medical staff is too important a cog in the complexity of the modern hospital for its vital function to be left to happenstance or to well-meaning but haphazard leadership.

As an antidote, a trend is emerging for the hospital staff affairs to be guided by a salaried medical director. In essence, he is a full-time chief of staff. Ideally, he is a clinician who is mature but still in his prime, who has stature, and who has been trained in administration. Not the least of his responsibilities is to provide leadership and expert knowledge to the staff in their continuing self-evaluation of clinical practice. He leads and coordinates staff activities, but by no means does he assume the staff's functions or responsibilities.

Many of the larger hospitals have found it desirable to employ additional salaried physicians to serve as chief of major clinical services, especially when there is an active house staff program. This further increases the effectiveness of staff function and improves the educational programs for house staff and attending staff alike.

The chief of staff is responsible to the governing board of the hospital, and to it alone, whatever his title, whether or not he is salaried, and whether or not he is elected by the staff. This is another frequently misunderstood basic principle. It is especially confusing when the chief is elected by the staff and he mistakenly believes that he is primarily beholden to his electorate. For this and other reasons, it is well for the governing body to appoint the chief of staff directly. Obviously the appointment should be made in consultation and in collaboration with the medical staff, but the responsibility and the prerogative rest with the board. It is appropriate for the staff to elect additional officers, including its own president, who serves as the voice of the staff.

Finally, the importance of an adequate and up-to-date set of medical staff bylaws deserves strong emphasis. The bylaws should be drafted to meet the specific needs of the individual staff; they must be explicit, and they must cover all staff functions. Further, they must be reviewed and revised frequently to meet the changing needs of a growing staff. As in all other hospital affairs, the medical staff bylaws are the final responsibility of the governing board. The bylaws must be approved by the boards before they become valid, and it is important that they be made a part of the hospital's own bylaws.

In summary, certain basic principles of medical staff function are becoming better understood and are receiving deserved emphasis. The hospital is a single organization, not separate ones for the medical staff and for the administration. The governing board is legally and morally responsible for all that takes place in the hospital, including the professional standards and the quality of patient care.

The medical staff must conscientiously and systematically review its clinical practice to assure the maintenance of high standards of practice. The chief of staff, whether salaried or not, is responsible to the governing board and to it alone. The appointment of a full-time salaried medical director to lead, coordinate and stimulate medical staff functions is a salutary trend. In some institutions, his leadership is supplemented by full-time chiefs of major clinical services. Finally, a precise, detailed, inclusive and up-to-date set of medical staff bylaws is an essential document, and it must be approved and adopted by the governing board as well as by the medical staff.

The Hospital Medical Director:
An Administrator's View

JAMES D. HARVEY

James D. Harvey is Administrator of Hillcrest Medical Center in Tulsa, Oklahoma.

The whole health care system is "under the gun" because of its inability to cope with the needs and demands of the public at a fair price. The press, television, periodicals, and non-fiction magazines chronicle the extent of the public's disillusionment with the current system.

The concept of effectiveness gained high public visibility when the Barr Report, the popular name for the Secretary's Advisory Committee on Hospital Effectiveness, was published in 1968. In this context, effectiveness means an optimal combination of efficiency, appropriateness of service, accessibility to the service, acceptability of the service from the public's point of view, and the quality of the service as measured by professionals working in the health care system. This definition of effectiveness suggest that proposed solutions to the health care delivery problem must include a solution to the problem of poor organization. In attempting to solve the organizational problem, the system should examine its existing resources and facilities to see if they can be more effictively used or arranged before spending more money, recruiting more people, or looking elsewhere for an answer.

Paradoxically, although hospital attending staff physicians direct the use of a majority of hospital resources, they are not usually organized in a way that promotes optimal use of their power. This situation exists as a result of the organization of early-day hospitals in which a doctor and nurse constituted the entire patient care team and in which either the doctor or nurse organized and managed the institution.

However, as medical research and skill have increased, hospital operation has become more complex but hospitals' organizational patterns—particularly those of the medical staff—have not changed significantly. This is not to say that management techniques and modern organizational trends have not developed in hospitals. For example, the increasing complexity of hospital operation has created the need for a hospital administrator whose work requires him to apply modern management techniques.

However, the application of such techniques has developed much more slowly within the medical staff. Hospital medical staffs are not organized to cope with the responsibilities which have been thrust upon them. The use of multiple physicians, as well as teams of supportive personnel, in the treatment of a single patient indicates a need for better organization of the medical staff. In addition, the general accountability of medical staffs for the practices of individual members has increased greatly because of legal precedents and decisions. Also, physicians are being faced with conflicting demands. They are becoming busier and busier, taking care of more and more patients, and consequently giving each one less and less time. At the same time, the demands of medical staff activities are mushrooming to the point where "something's gotta give."

Most medical staffs have what might be described as "sometime"—or "overtime"—leaders. Although physicians should be commended for giving their time to various elected or appointed staff offices, it is, indeed, an overtime job for them to undertake such responsibilities.

Ironically, the hospital administrator is often the first person to recognize the need for medical staff reorganization, probably because it is his job to think about hospital affairs on a full-time basis. Usually, after a series of fruitless attempts to coordinate activities with designated medical staff leaders, the administrator concludes that what is needed is a full-time, appointed medical staff "leader." Often, key doctors are not present at key meetings where important decisions are to be made. Those doctors who do give appreciable time and energy to their medical staff responsibilities do so at great personal sacrifice. Even though administrators appreciate such dedication they realize that such physicians "burn out."

Many doctors feel that full-time medical staff leaders represent a threat to the "clinical freedom" now enjoyed by attending medical staff members; many hospital administrators also consider the medical director as a personal threat. Such fears are unfounded.

One reason for apprehension on the part of both doctors and administrators is that the accountabilities of neither the administrator nor the medical director are understood—either by themselves or others. An examination of these accountabilities reveals the specific roles of those involved. The medical director must be recognized as a member of the institution's top management team. The medical staff does not exist in a vacuum; rather, it influences and is influenced by other activities within and outside the institution. Consequently, the medical staff's leaders must operate at the top management level so that these relationships can be dealt with effectively.

ADMINISTRATOR'S ACCOUNTABILITIES

In dealing with the positions of administrator and medical director, it is much more pertinent to ask, "What do we expect?" rather than, "What do they do?" In other words, their output should be of more interest than their input. By first asking what is expected, it is easier to identify the activities necessary to produce the desired end results.

"Accountabilities" is another word for end results. An examination of the administrator's accountabilities shows the relationship between them and the accountabilities of the medical director. His most basic and essential accountability is to make certain that his institution achieves and maintains full accreditation by the Joint Commission on Accreditation of Hospitals. This accreditation accountability is linked closely to medical staff activities.

Second, he must assure that an environment exists in which doctors can and do practice at optimum effectiveness. This accountability is one reason why the administrator should want a medical director with whom he can work. Another important accountability is to see to it that the institution maintains a viable financial condition. He must also make certain that the governing board of the institution receives enough information to enable it to make sound policy decisions. These are his primary accountabilities.

Other accountabilities which support those listed above include establishing and interpreting the goals of the institution and representing its interests and activities to the public. Changes within the institution may change the administrator's primary accountabilities to some extent; for example, the priority placed in research, education, rehabilitation, etc., may cause or be caused by some change in the institution itself.

MEDICAL DIRECTOR'S ACCOUNTABILITIES

Several of the medical director's accountabilities help an administrator fulfill his accountabilities. For one thing, the medical director must assure that the quality of medical care is appraised and maintained. Second, the medical director must attempt to improve communications between the medical staff and the institution, including the administration, the governing board, and the other operating departments of the institution. As a top management person and leader of the most important hospital department, the medical director has a significant impact on all hospital departments. Third, he must make certain that there are enough physicians on the medical staff to fulfill the philosophy and objectives of the institution.

Fourth, the medical director must strengthen the medical education program of the institution. The priority· of this accountability depends, of course, upon the philosophy and objectives of the institution and the extent to which education plays a role.

An administrator would expect a medical director to institute new patient care programs if there is a demonstrated need for them and if the resources of the institution can sustain them. He would also expect the medical director to be proficient in management and administrative skills.

These accountabilities are admittedly stated in broad terms. However, they represent end results, not activities.

ACCOUNTABILITY MEASUREMENT

Such broad statements are not meaningful unless the administrator and the medical director can agree on certain measurements by which they can determine whether the end results are being accomplished. For example, in appraising the quality of medical care, the medical director and the administrator should ask questions which lead to specific answers, such as "What would indicate that good quality appraisal be carried out?" They should search for several percentage or quantum figures that indicate the degree of quality of medical care. Regardless of what statistical measure is used, it is essential that the administrator and medical director agree on what the indicators should be. In mutually establishing measures or indicators to the medical director's accountabilities, the administrator and medical director are really establishing the standards of performance which the medical director should meet.

Such standards are met by performing "minding the store" activities; that is, those things which the medical director must do daily in order to fulfill his accountabilities. He should periodically raise his standards on the assumption that improvement is always desirable. Such improvement is acomplished through the establishment and achievement of goals. The achievement of such goals constantly changes the situation. Thus, an accountability standard is one thing, while a goal may be to improve the standard by some quantifiable measure. For example, if the administrator and the medical director agree that this year "X" number of single unit transfusions is acceptable, but that next year "X minus Y" is their aim, they will have come up with a combination of a "minding the store" standard and a goal. This is a true system of results-centered management—or management by objectives.

It is essential that the medical director's accountabilities have high visibility, so that the staff clearly understands what they are. Obviously, it is necessary for the medical staff to be involved in accomplishing results if the medical director is to "measure up." Thus, his talent for planning, organizing, implementing, and evaluating becomes of paramount importance. The medical director's job description should be amplified by an inclusion of his accountabilities. If the results expected of the medical director are attached to his job description, he will have a working document and can proceed to achieve the results for which he was hired.

If a medical director is going to achieve specific end results, he must work with other doctors, administrators, and governing board members. There can be no place for authoritarianism in his methods. Admittedly, he must have authority and top management prerogatives in order to get things done. However, he will not last long if he imploys high-handed tactics in appraising the quality of medical care, or if he uses terse communiques containing cold, calculated statements concerning activities of the staff. The results desired simply will not be achieved by using despotic techniques.

One of the medical director's first undertakings should be to eliminate unnecessary work previously required of medical staff members. He and his office staff should be able to prepare meetings and limit discussions only to those topics on which doctors must act. In addition, a full-time medical director should be able to communicate clearly with the medical staff about various hospital activities. This is important since his accountabilities require him to improve medical staff understanding and cooperation. As a result of his efforts, staff participation should gradually become much more meaningful and important to the institution. When this happens, attendance at meetings will increase and doctors' involvement in the issues that the institution faces will become more valuable. Measures of the medical director's accountabilities will be measures of the medical staff's progress. Because performance criteria will be well-established, goals will become self-evident and much easier to achieve.

NO ROOM FOR ONE-YEAR LEADERS

The medical director's incumbency should last over an extended period of time rather than rotate from year to year. An institution's fortunes do not change drastically in a year's time, yet far too many staff leaders are in office only for that period. The long-range implications of institutional stewardship are so profound as to nullify the notion that effective medical staff operations can be achieved when leadership responsibilities are passed around on a a yearly basis. Physicians should demand a change in this system.

A NATURAL CHANGE

Doctors practice in a results-centered profession: Their task is to make patients well, to make them more comfortable, to increase their longevity. It should follow, then, that in the organization and management of the medical staff, physicians should demand a results-centered management. However, this can be achieved only by a full-time, top-level medical executive skilled enough and on the job long enough to use the same results-centered approach to staff affairs as his colleagues use in their private practices. This kind of management has proved its effectiveness in industry, and physicians should be not only willing to accept it, but should demand that it be introduced in their institutions.

It is regrettable that many hospital administrators do not yet employ this kind of leadership. A medical director would certainly be hampered if he tried to introduce this kind of management when the administrator did not operate in the same way. However, the medical staff is so important to the institution's success that the medical director, as a member of top management, could initiate a results-centered approach and try to bring his administrator along with him into a full management by objectives program.

CONCLUSION

It is much better for the medical staff to voluntarily undertake this change to management by objectives than to be forced into it. When such a system is imposed, it will not work well, because it is much more difficult to achieve someone else's goals.

To those who are worried about socialism in medicine, what has been described in this article is capitalism in its most precious form. In this system, the rewards go to the people who produce the results and achieve goals. If the hospital system can be operated and managed in the way described above there will be nothing to worry about. In addition, physicians will be fulfilling their role in society—they will be marshalling resources and producing service at an optimal level and doing it in the most efficient way possible. Moreover, they will have maintained their freedom to act. However, they can keep this perrogative only so long as the results they produce are higher than those which can be reasonably expected from any other system.

Hospital Systems

This section presents the hospital organization from a systems point of view. Being a complex organization, material, financial, facility, and human resources must be drawn together and allocated in some manner to form an operational whole. The systems approach is a means of viewing the interrelated and interdependent activities of the organization. In addition to assisting in the identification of the relationship between component parts, the systems approach is a realistic managerial tool that can be effectively used in the decision making process.

In *SYSTEMS CONCEPTS FOR HOSPITALS,* the need for an integrated philosophy in hospital administration is made. The systems concept is presented as a tool for providing the opportunity for the administrator to look at the hospital as a whole. That is, a means of converting the diverse functions and resources into an effective institution.

In *HOSPITAL ADMINISTRATION AND SYSTEMS CONCEPTS,* the hospital organization is presented as one which does not fit the traditional bureaucratic or administrative management models. It is advocated that the traditional models do not solve the power conflicts between the various professionals in the organization and the administration. The systems concept with a structural and human—social orientation provides a more effective means of understanding and dealing with the activity relationships.

Systems Concepts for Hospitals

LEO B. OSTERHAUS, PH.D.

Leo B. Osterhaus, Ph.D., is the Director of the Center of Business Administration at St. Edwards University in Austin, Texas.

During the past few years, there have been many different approaches toward improving the management of organizations, e.g., organization theory, decision theory, planning theory, and the behavioral theory of the institution. Each of these philosophies has helped to sharpen administrative skills; however, there remains a need for a theory which provides a conceptual framework for better design and operation of the hospital.

The need for integrative philosophy in hospital administration has been dramatized by the rising costs, the increasing complexity, the emphasis on research and development, and the uncertainty associated with Medicare. Further, the conflict between the specialists and the generalists has not been resolved, i.e., the paradox of requiring more skills in special areas in the hospital in contrast to the more general and integrative knowledge needed by the administrator. The administrator of a hospital may solve many of its problems and improve its efficiency by operating the hospital as a system.

The systems concept is not new; it has been used by the natural sciences for many years, and it is also being applied to businesses, e.g., construction projects and military programs where specification and time requirements are critical.

The systems concept does not replace progressive management or leadership. It provides the opportunity for the ambitious and creative administrator to look at the whole or complete hospital. First, management decides on a specific job to be accomplished and facilities and manpower needed, and then technical assistance is provided to design a system.

The systems concept of organization can be defined as "an array of components designed to accomplish a particular objective according to plan."[1]

[1] Johnson, Richard A., Fremont E. Kast, & James E. Rosenzweig, *The Theory and Management of Systems,* (2nd edition) New York: McGraw-Hill Book Co., p. 113.

Figure 1 presents the general concept of the systems approach and the location of the administrator. The administrator and his various committees interrelate and coordinate the information in the communication network and decision system. He also tries to maintain equilibrium within the system. The more mature systems will have homeostasis built in the system.

Figure 1
GENERAL SYSTEMS CONCEPT

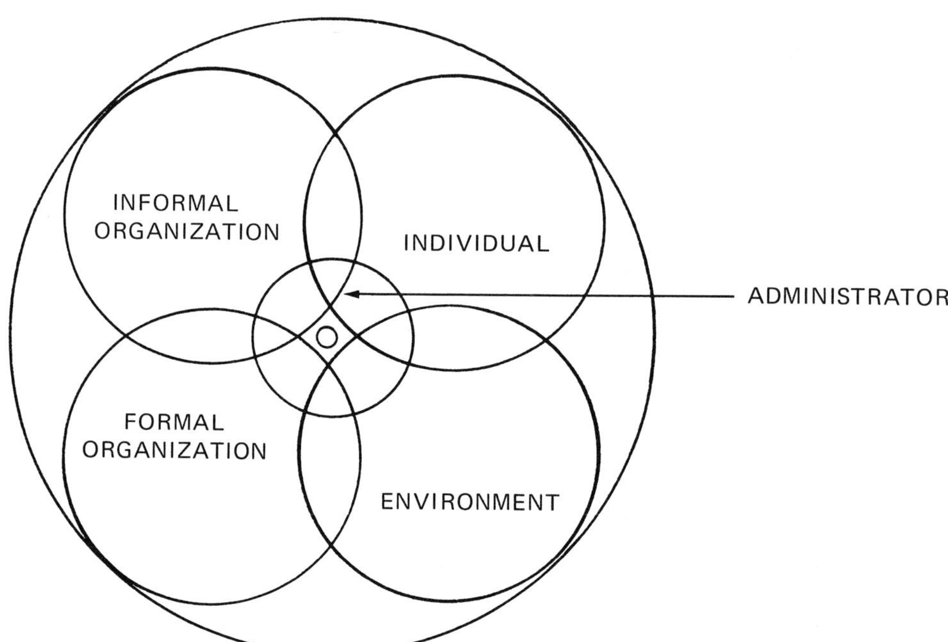

This model can be further developed into a flow process diagram which will show the causes of information, matter, and energy. A process in the system concept is defined as the transformation of matter, energy, and/or information over time in a system. In the model there are two critical processes—the decision process which transforms information through search into alternatives, and selection of a course of action. The decision process also uses energy to get others to implement the decision. The second process is the action process which transforms matter from one state to another or moves it from one point to another, for example, physical goods, orders, money, or personnel flows.

In terms of this systems design the information and energy flow into the decision center as inputs, and decision centers output flows to the action center to indicate the power relationship. It is necessary under this system of organization to supply the decision maker with the ability to use sanctions—this means delegation of authority in the formal organization. In the hospital the professional status of some managers gives them significant power to make decisions, e.g., the medical doctor. The manager's personality, skills, and general demeanor are also important elements.

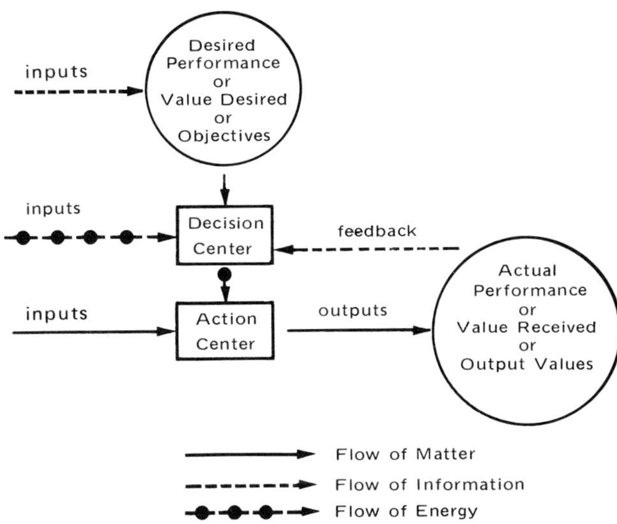

The information inputs to the circle labeled "desired performance or desired values or objectives" in Figure 2 are messages from environmental and internal forces, and they determine the objectives. After a working relationship has been established, the agreed-upon goals become the ends toward which organizational processes are directed. The goals are then arranged in a hierarchy with ". . . each level to be considered as an end relative to the levels below it and as a means relative to the levels above it. Through the hierarchical structure of ends, behavior attains integration and consistency. . . ."[3]

The actual performance or output of the system is the result of the action process. The decision maker implements action through the "action center" and regulates the flow through the system. Because of entropy (noise, bias, and delays) actual performance often differs from desired performance or objectives. It is therefore necessary to design the system so that the decision maker can monitor the performance and institute corrective action when necessary. The communication channel labeled "feedback" records, measures and reports the performance deviations to the "decision center."

Traditionally hospitals have not been structured to utilize the systems concept. In adjusting the typical hospital to fit within the framework of the systems concept, certain organizational changes may be required. It is quite obvious that no one organizational structure can meet the operational requirements for every hospital. Each institution must design its own unique system. However, a model can be developed as a starting point for the medium or large hospitals which have a number of major functions and provide several services, e.g., the general hospital.

[2] Carzo, Rocco, and John N. Yanouzas, *Formal Organization: A Systems Approach,* Homewood, Ill.: Richard D. Irwin, Inc. & The Dorsey Press, pp. 336.

[3] Simon, Herbert A., *Administrative Behavior,* New York: The Macmillan Company, 1959, p. 63.

HOW THE FUNCTIONS OPERATE

The primary purpose of the top management model is to illustrate the application of the systems concept to the hospital and to show how the various functions of planning, organizing, control, and communications operate. The master planning committee should relate the hospital to its environmental system, and make decisions concerning the service of the hospital. The master planning committee should establish the limits of the operating programs, decide general policy matters relative to the design of operating systems, and select the directors for each new project (see Figure 3). Members of this committee would be selected from key resources and operating agencies in the hospital.

Once the decision has been made by the master planning committee, the resources allocation committee would provide the facilities and manpower for the new system, and supply technical assistance for systems design. After the system has been designed, it would be furnished to the operating committee as a major project system, or as a facilitating system.

Figure 3
TOP MANAGEMENT MODEL[4]

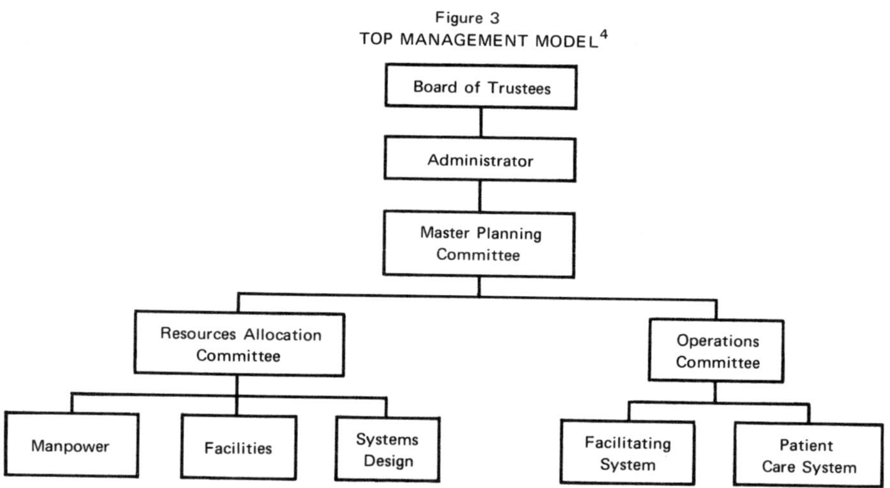

A facilitating system would include those systems organized to produce a service other than patient service. Each project system would be designed toward self-sufficiency. A facilitating system would be designed, therefore, to produce operating service for the major project systems. The outputs of the facilitating system would be material input for the project system and a fee should be charged for this input, just as if the input has been purchased from an outside source.

In order to illustrate the general systems design Figure 2, the (personnel subsystem) has been shown in Figure 4.

The flow of personnel includes recruiting, hiring, training, assigning to job, and leaving the organization for reason of retirement, sickness, dismissal, or resignation. In

[4] Johnson, *op. cit.,* p. 119.

the model it is assumed the personnel director has the authority to recruit, hire, train, and assign. The training director is the only action center shown for simplicity. The personnel director, as the decision maker, determines how fast employees will be processed on their way to the job assignments. He regulates the flow of personnel up to the point where the employee joins the department and enters a new subsystem. Thereafter, the decision on the flow of personnel is regulated by the subsystem where the employee is assigned (exceptions may be made for retirement, sickness, or resignations). When the feedback from the subsystem about actual and desired performance is fed into the personnel director, he takes the necessary corrective action, if any is required.

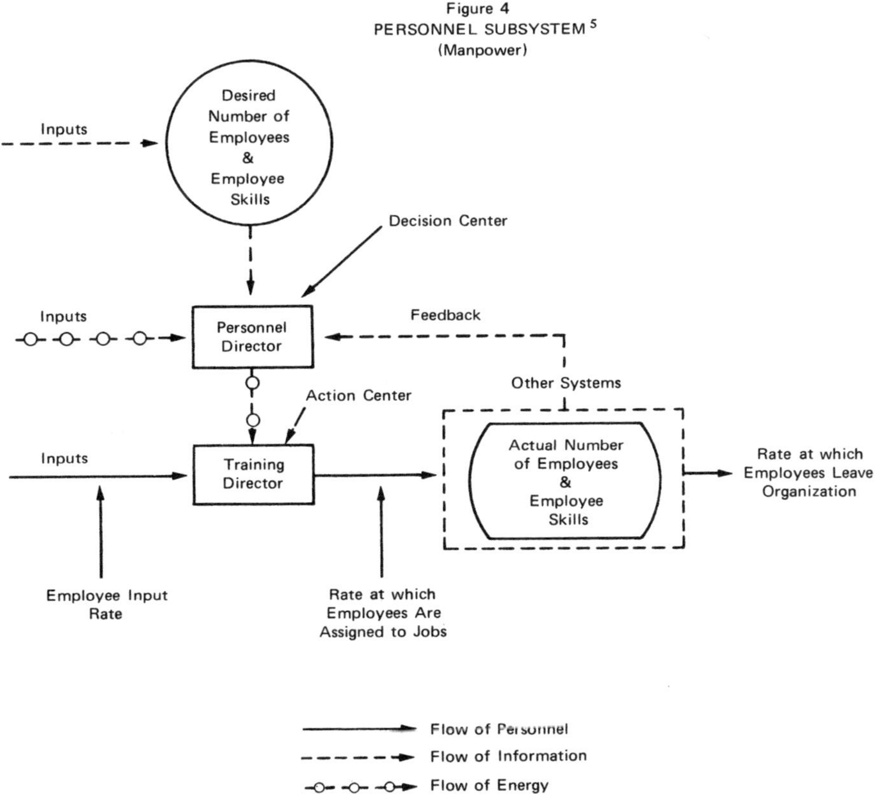

Figure 4
PERSONNEL SUBSYSTEM [5]
(Manpower)

The action process is completed by the training director who transfers an unskilled or semiskilled employee into a fully qualified employee. This training may be completed before the employee enters his assigned subsystem (vestibule training) or after he enters his permanent assignment through on-the-job training.

[5] Carzo & Yanouzas, *op. cit.,* p. 346.

In order to be more specific about the general framework for hospital organization, we can draw upon the work of Donald J. Clough (Donald J. Clough, *Concepts of Management Science,* Englewood Cliffs, N.J., Prentice Hall, Inc., 1963). A modified simple model is shown as Figure 5.

Patient information is obtained and fed to the decision center which represents the doctor who makes the diagnosis. He in turn orders certain supplies and services. These supplies and services are checked by the doctor or his representative, the nurse. The patient undergoes treatment and feedback is furnished to the decision center (doctor).

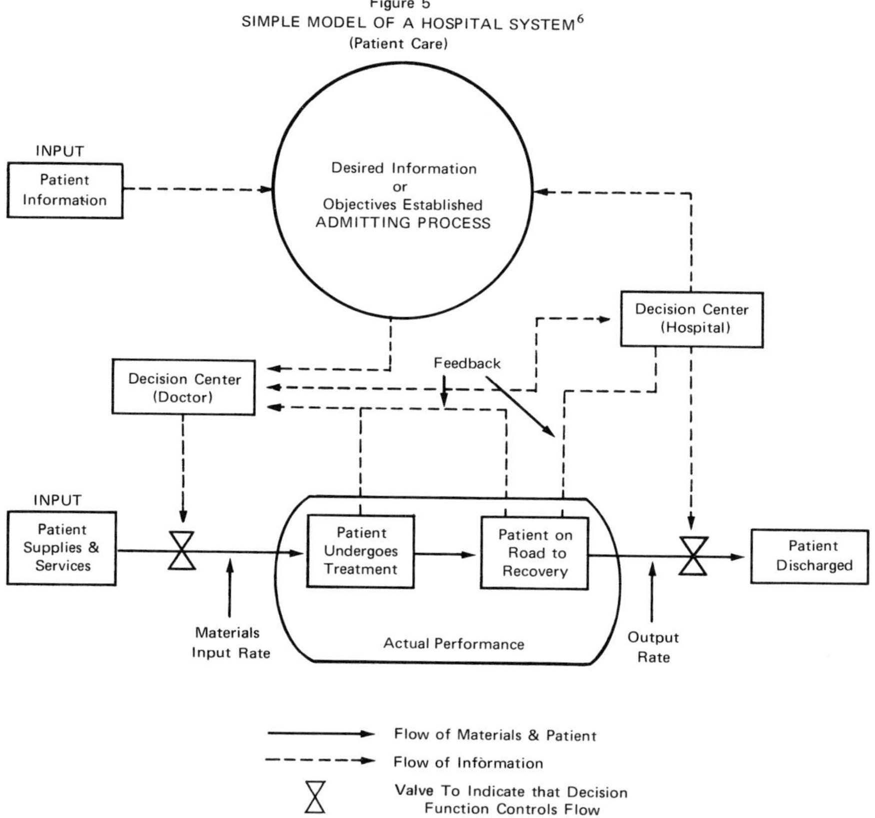

Action centers have not been identified in the diagram for simplicity, but their existence is apparent by the fact that there is a recovery or output rate. The second decision center (hospital personnel) as well as the first decision center regulates the flow of the patients and discharge. The valve is the symbol regulating the flow of patients, materials, and services during the patient's stay in the hospital. The regulatory function is accomplished by decision centers through their control over action centers.

[6] *Ibid,* p. 349.

To bring all the various subsystems together, a matrix organization which has been designed for project management might provide a clearer picture of the whole hospital and how the subsystems fit into the matrix.

Note that the left side of the chart shows some of the operating agencies which are often designated as projects in the business matrix. These agencies are controlled by the operating committee or coordinator. The right side of the chart depicts the support agencies for the care of the patient, which are under the supervision of the facilitating system committee. Both of these committees carry out the plans of the master planning committee. Horizontally across are shown the line service departments which support the operating departments. These departments provide the functional service, information, materials, and specialized manpower. The personnel may be "housed" for administrative purposes in the line service departments and assigned to duty with the operating units on the left on a permanent basis or temporarily for short term projects (i.e., emergency or disaster situations).

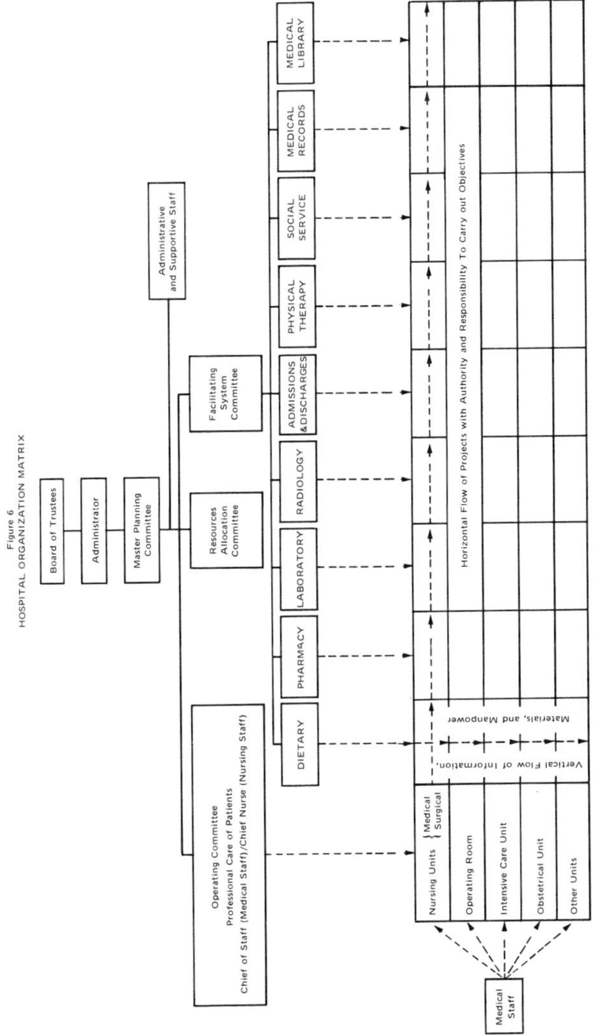

On the left the operating departments are arranged vertically with some major breakdowns. Each department would have a designed project manager. The operating departments control the horizontal flow of projects and have the authority and responsibility to carry out the mission. The people the manager needs to operationalize his project are drawn from specialists out of their respective administrative line service departments. When the project is complete, the project manager may return these people to their administrative "pool" for reassignment.

The resources allocation committee evaluates the need for manpower, facilities, and systems design. It will probably include representatives from the staff, (e.g., personnel director, business manager, etc.) the operating committee, and the facilitating system committee.

Similarity between the matrix organization and the usual functional organization can be seen. However, some differences occur; the unity of command principle is violated. The specialists have two bosses: the line or administrative head and the operating project manager. Another difference is noted in the scalar principle; there is an absence of the hierarchy in the organization. The project or operating managers and the administrative and line service departments stand on about the same level. They are laterally related in a way that accentuates forms of behavioral accommodation and tends to minimize conventional conflict. Some bargaining and compromises are common in resolving conflict over allocation of personnel and performance.

THE POTENTIALS OF SYSTEMS

The "modern organization theory" or "systems concept" is only a tool which the administrator can use to convert the disorganized resources of men, machines, and money into a useful and effective institution. Management is the process whereby those unrelated resources are integrated into a total system of objective accomplishment. The administrator gets things accomplished by working with people and physical resources in order to accomplish the goals of the hospital. He coordinates and integrates the activities of others rather than performing the job himself.

Under the systems concept everything revolves around the total system and its objective and the functions of planning, organizing, controlling, and communicating are carried out only as a service to this end. Its potential is great because it offers the opportunity of uniting what is valuable in the classical and neo-classical theories into a systematic and integrated conception of hospital organization.

Hospital Administration and System Concepts

FREMONT E. KAST, PH.D. AND JAMES E. ROSENZWEIG, PH.D.

Fremont E. Kast, Ph.D., and James E. Rosenzweig, Ph.D., are both Professors of Management and Organization at the University of Washington.

An omnipresent phenomenon of modern society has been the growth and development of large-scale, complex organizations. In most human activities there has been an evolution from small-scale, informally organized groups toward large, highly-structured, formal organizations. Hospitals, business enterprises, governmental units, educational institutions, labor unions, charitable activities, and even social and recreational endeavors have tended to become larger and more complex. These large-scale organizations have been primarily devices for rationalization of human effort and for the more effective accomplishment of many objectives. They provide a means for coping with the increased complexities and challenges of modern societies.

In spite of their prevalence, development of a general model or theory of large-scale, complex organizations has been extremely slow. Although a great deal has been written about large organizations in recent years, most of the models presented have been restricted or partial, rather than general models.[1] It is our view that at this stage, systems concepts provide the most useful general model for the study of complex organizations such as hospitals. In this article we will review general systems theory, show some broad applications of systems concepts outside the field of hospital administration, and then discuss more specifically the application of systems concepts in hospital administration.

DEFINITION OF A SYSTEM

A system is "an organized or complex whole: an assemblage or combination of things or parts forming a complex or unitary whole." The term system covers an extremely broad spectrum of concepts. The biologist Ludwig von Bertalanffy set forth

---

[1] Among the most significant of these are: James G. March and Herbert A. Simon, *Organizations* (New York: John Wiley & Sons, Inc., 1958); Amitai Etzioni, *A Comparative Analysis of Complex Organization* (New York: Free Press of Glencoe, Inc., 1961); and Peter M. Blau and W. Richard Scott, *Formal Organizations* (San Francisco: Chandler Publishing Co., 1962).

---

a model which he called open systems.[2] The basis of his concept is that a living organism is not a conglomeration of separate elements but a definite system, possessing organization and wholeness. An organization is an open system which maintains a constant state while matter and energy which enter it keep changing (so-called dynamic equilibrium). The organism is influenced by, and influences, its environment and reaches a state of dynamic equilibrium in this environment. Such a description fits complex organizations such as hospitals. The hospital is a man-made social system which has a dynamic interplay with its environment—the community, patients, medical practitioners, governments and many other elements. Furthermore, the hospital is a system of interrelated parts working in conjunction with each other in order to accomplish a number of goals, those of the organization *and* individual participants.

The systems concept is a useful way of thinking about the function of management and administration of large-scale, complex organizations. It provides a framework for visualizing internal and external environment factors as an integrated whole. It allows recognition of the proper place and function of subsystems. But, above all, it emphasizes the importance of the integration of these subsystems into an operational whole.[3]

GENERAL SYSTEMS THEORY

General systems theory is concerned with developing a systematic, theoretical framework for describing general relationships of the empirical world. One of the most important reasons pointing to the need for a general systems theory is the problem of communication between the various disciplines. Although there is some similarity between general methods of approach—the scientific method—the results of research are not often communicated across discipline boundaries. Increasingly, there has been a development of interdisciplinary studies. Areas such as social psychology, bio-chemistry, astrophysics, social anthropology, economic psychology, and economic sociology have developed to integrate various disciplines. Recently, areas of study and research have developed which utilize knowledge from various fields. For example, sybernetics calls on electrical engineering, neurophysiology, physics, biology, and other fields. Operations research is often pointed to as a multidisciplinary approach to problem solving. Organization theory embraces economics, sociology, engineering, psychology, physiology, and anthropology. Problem solving and decision making are becoming focal points for study and research, drawing on numerous disciplines.

With these examples of interdisciplinary approaches, it is easy to recognize a surge of interest in larger-scale, systematic bodies of knowledge. However, this trend calls for the development of an overall framework within which the various subparts can be integrated. General systems theory may help to provide this framework.

[2] Ludwig von Bertalanffy, "General Systems Theory: A New Approach to Unity of Science," *Human Biology,* December, 1951, pp. 303-61.

[3] For a more comprehensive discussion of these concepts see R. A. Johnson, F. E. Kast, and J. E. Rosenzweig, *The Theory and Management of Systems* (New York: McGraw-Hill Book Co., Inc., 1963).

THE HIERARCHY OF LEVELS

Kenneth Boulding has provided a useful classification of systems which sets forth a hierarchy of levels as follows:[4]

1. The first level is that of static structure. It might be called the level of *framework;* for example, the anatomy of the universe.
2. The next level is that of the simple dynamic system with predetermined, necessary motions. This might be called the level of *clockworks.*
3. The control mechanism or cybernetic system, which might be nicknamed the level of the *thermostat.* The system is self-regulating in maintaining equilibrium.
4. The fourth level is that of the "open system," or self-maintaining structure. This is the level at which life begins to differentiate from not-life; it might be called the level of the *cell.*
5. The next level might be called the genetic-societal level; it is typified by the *plant,* and it dominates the empirical world of the botanist.
6. The *animal* system level is characterized by increased mobility, teleological behavior, and self-awareness.
7. The next level is the *human* level, that is, of the individual human being considered as a system with self-awareness and the ability to utilize language and symbolism.
8. The *social system* or systems of human organization constitute the next level, with the consideration of the content and meaning of messages, the nature and dimensions of value systems, the transcription of images into historical record, the subtle symbolizations of art, music and poetry, and the complex gamut of human emotion.
9. *Transcendental systems* complete the classification of levels. These are the ultimates and absolutes and the inescapables and unknowables, and they also exhibit systematic structure and relationship.

Obviously, the first level is most pervasive. Descriptions of static structures are widespread. This descriptive cataloguing is helpful in providing a framework for additional analysis and synthesis. Dynamic "clockwork" systems, where prediction is a strong element, are evident in the classical natural sciences such as physics and astronomy; yet even here there are important gaps. Adequate theoretical models are not apparent at higher levels. However, in recent years closed-loop cybernetics, or "thermostat," systems have received increasing attention. At the same time, work is progressing on open-loop systems with self-maintaining structures and reproduction facilities. Beyond the fourth level we hardly have a beginning of theory. It is obvious that the social sciences are operating in the last four levels of this systems hierarchy.

RELATIONSHIP TO FUNCTIONALISM

There is a close relationship between general systems theory and the development of functionalism in the social sciences. This relationship is apparent in the following statement of Don Martindale:

In the period since World War II, as Western society readjusted to the radical change in milieu that followed, with the attempt to return to something that looked like "normalcy," but in a permanently transformed world, the essential unity of the social sciences has been revealed through the flooding of the functionalistic voint of view across the boundaries of the special disciplines. This point of view has had both theoretical and methodological dimensions. Theoretically, it consists in the analysis of social and cultural life from the standpoint of wholes or systems. Epistemologically, it involves analysis of social events by methods thought peculiarly adapted to the integration of social events into systems.

4Kenneth Boulding, "General Systems Theory: The Skeleton of Science," *Management Science,* April, 1956, pp. 197-208.

The functionalistic point of view has been manifest in all the social sciences from psychology through sociology, political science, economics, and anthropology to geography, jurisprudence and linguistics. Most primary theoretical and methodological debates in postwar social science have centered on functionalism and alternatives to it.[5]

Although there are several meanings of the word "functionalism," its most important aspect is the emphasis upon systems of relationship and the integration of parts and subsystems into a whole.[6] General systems theory and the functionalistic point of view (including dynamic equilibrium concepts from economics) offer a theoretical framework for the study of complex organizations.

SYSTEMS CONCEPTS FOR MANAGEMENT OF COMPLEX ORGANIZATIONS

Traditional organization theory, based upon Max Weber's bureaucratic model and the administrative management model, placed emphasis upon organizational structure, hierarchical relationships, specialization, span of control, and line and staff relationships. The traditional theory did not give sufficient emphasis to the problems of interrelationships or integration of activities. Nor did the neoclassical, or human relations, approach move in this direction. Its approach was aimed at interjecting back into the mechanistic, traditional models human motivations, aspirations, and limitations. Neither of these approaches provided a basis for an integrated, systematic organizational model.

Increasing attention is being given to the notion that the most useful way to study organizations is to consider them as systems. This view tends to treat them as systems of mutually dependent parts and variables, and the complex organization is thought of as a social system within the broader, more inclusive system of society. Sociologist Talcott Parsons expresses this view:

It seems appropriate to define an organization as a social system which is organized for the attainment of a particular type of goal; the attainment of that goal is at the same time a performance of a type of function on behalf of a more inclusive system, the society.[7]

Modern organization theory and general systems theory are closely related, with organization theory a special element of general systems theory. Systems theory and organization theory are both concerned with the investigation and performance of the organization as an integrated whole. However, general systems theory is concerned with all nine levels of systems whereas organization theory focuses primarily upon level eight, human social organizations.

Under the systems concept, the complex organization is viewed as a *conglomerate of subsystems* which include the individual, the informal work groups, the formal organization, and, finally, the environmental systems which have a direct impact upon it. Furthermore, under the systems concept, consideration must be given to the means

<hr>

[5]Don Martindale, *Functionalism in the Social Sciences* (American Academy of Political and Social Science Monograph 5, February, 1965), pp. viii-ix.

[6]Robert K. Merton discusses various connotations of the word "function" in *Social Theory and Social Structure* (Glencoe, Ill.: Free Press, 1957), pp. 20-22.

[7]Talcott Parsons, "Suggestions for a Sociological Approach to the Theory of Organizations," *Administrative Science Quarterly*. September, 1956, p. 238.

for *interrelating and coordinating* these various subsystems. These parts are integrated through various processes such as the information and communications network, the decision system, and built-in equilibrium mechanisms which exist in every organization.

APPLICATIONS OF SYSTEMS CONCEPTS

Actually, practical applications of many of the concepts stemming from the systems approach have preceded the development of adequate models or theories of complex organizations. Several of these applications are:

1. The weapon-system management approach has been used extensively in the development of the nation's advanced weapon and space systems. This approach calls for the systematic organization of a vast complex of strategies, technologies, industries, human and material resources, and other subsystems into an integrated whole toward the accomplishment of objectives.
2. Program management has been utilized in many of the advanced technology industries. It is essentially a managerial approach for adapting to the systems concept. Program management calls for integration of the activities related to particular projects into explicit organizational systems.
3. Automation represents an important application of the systems concept in industry. It requires the integration of many of the operations of the business firm into a formal man-machine system.
4. Systems concepts have been applied extensively in data processing; indeed the term data processing system has widespread usage. The most sophisticated data-processing systems are represented by real-time, or on-line, systems. In these cases, the computer is an integral part of the information-decision system and it is used to provide information during the actual decision process.
5. Many of the newer approaches in management science—operations research, industrial dynamics and simulation—are based upon the systems concept. These approaches structure the operation under analysis as an integrated system tied together by a series of equations. The use of computers in symbolic system simulation allows treatment of large-scale, complex systems. Thus an analyst can develop a model of a group of subsystems, their interrelationships, and the total system.
6. PERT, SCANS, RAMPS, and other techniques of network analysis are examples of more detailed applications of systems concepts. They can be used to recognize and identify all the interconnecting links in a single system or in a series or network of systems.
7. In considering human behavior in formal organizations there is a tendency to think in terms of systems concepts. For example, Rensis Likert suggests the interaction-influence system as the means for integrating and coordinating the efforts of participants in organizations.[8]

SYSTEMS CONCEPTS IN HOSPITAL ADMINISTRATION

Anyone familiar with hospitals as organizations realizes that many of the models and generalizations taken from other organizations are not directly applicable nor appropriate. Indeed, there are many reasons for questioning the usefulness of the traditional models for any large-scale, complex organization. Essentially, the traditional approach is based upon Max Weber's ideal bureaucratic model with modifications from scientific management and the administrative management approaches of Luther Gulick, Lyndall Urwick, James Mooney and Alan Reiley, and others. The basic dimensions of the bureaucratic model are:[9]

[8] Rensis Likert, *New Patterns of Management* (New York: McGraw-Hill Book Co., 1961).

[9] Richard H. Hall, "The Concept of Bureaucracy: An Empirical Assessment," *American Journal of Sociology,* July, 1963, p. 33.

1. A division of labor based upon functional specialization.
2. A well-defined hierarchy of authority.
3. A system of rules covering the rights and duties of positional incumbents.
4. A system of procedures for dealing with work situations.
5. Impersonality of interpersonal relations.
6. Promotion and selection for employment based upon technical competence.

Although these characteristics of the bureaucratic form may be applicable to large hospitals in certain instances, there are many factors which limit their value. Shortcomings are also apparent in the application of scientific management principles and generalizations from the administrative management approaches. Some of the key deficiencies in applying the traditional organization model of hospitals are discussed below.

WHY HOSPITALS DO NOT FIT THE TRADITIONAL MODEL

The traditional model calls for a definite hierarchy of authority with clear-cut superior-subordinate relationships. This may be appropriate where the administrator has superiority of knowledge and information, but it is not feasible where there is specialization of skills and knowledge on the part of participants at different levels in the organization. Particularly, there is often conflict between hierarchical authority and professional values of organizational members. This is true in organizations other than hospitals. William Kornhauser found that there was substantial conflict between the professional values of scientists in industry and the organizational requirements imposed by the administrative hierarchy.[10] Amitai Etzioni sees this as a major problem in many complex organizations.

Probably the most important structural dilemma is the inevitable strain imposed on the organization by the use of knowledge. All social units use knowledge, but organizations use more knowledge more systematically than do other social units. . . .Students of the professions have pointed out that the autonomy granted to professionals who are basically responsible to their consciences (though they may be censured by their peers and in extreme cases by the courts) is necessary for effective professional work. It is this highly individualized principle which is diametrically opposed to the very essence of the organizational principle of control and coordination by superiors—i.e., the principle of administrative authority.[11]

THE CONTINUAL POWER CONFLICT

While this conflict between the knowledge and values of the professional and hierarchical administrative authority is apparent in many organizations, it appears most critical in hospitals. A large hospital requires effective performance by many professional and semi-professional participants who have highly specialized knowledge and skills. Yet, their functions are not performed in a vacuum; they must be integrated into an over-all operation. It is understandable that there is a continual power conflict

[10]William Kornhauser, *Scientists in Industry: Conflict and Accommodation* (Berkeley: University of California Press, 1963).

[11]Amitai Etzioni, *Modern Organizations* (Englewood Cliffs, N.J.: Prentice-Hall, Inc., 1964), pp. 75-76.

between the various professionals and the hospital administration.[12] But, traditional management models provide no answers to these problems—they do not even recognize their existence. The systems model provides a more effective means for understanding and dealing with these relationships.

Another characteristic of the traditional model which is not completely appropriate for the hospital is the emphasis upon routinization and standardization of activities. To be sure, there are a number of hospital activities which fall within this category, but there are many others which cannot be standardized and made uniform. This is particularly true for activities which require interactions between the various participants in the hospital.

Eugene Litwak suggests an interesting distinction between different models for large-scale organizations:

> Weber's model is most efficient when the organization deals primarily with uniform events and with occupations stressing traditional areas of knowledge rather than social skills. The human-relations model will be most efficient for dealing with events which are not uniform (research, medical treatment, graduate training, designing) and with occupations emphasizing social skills as well as technical aspects of the job. . . .
>
> There are several models of organization with differential efficiencies depending on the nature of the work and the types of tasks to be performed. In this regard, at least three types have been suggested: Weber's, that found in "human relations" and what may be called the "professional bureaucracy." This third model is characterized by the degree to which the organization must deal with events both uniform and not uniform, or by the need to have jobs requiring great social skills as well as jobs requiring traditional areas of knowledge. Perhaps the outstanding illustrations of the third type would be a large hospital, a graduate school, or a research organization.
>
> The chief distinguishing characteristic of the professional model is its inclusion of contradictory forms of social relations. This model is particularly relevant to contemporary society where most large-scale organizations have to deal with uniform and non-uniform tasks or with occupations that demand traditional knowledge as well as social skills.[13]

MULTIPLE OBJECTIVES OF COMPLEX ORGANIZATIONS

Other studies suggest that the traditional bureaucratic model is not appropriate when applied to non-routine, "creative" decisions and activities. They show that departments or units whose tasks are nonroutine or difficult to standardize are significantly less bureaucratic.[14] Many aspects of hospital operations are also non-programmable and require freedom from the restriction of bureaucratic mechanisms. Interestingly, the same problem is evident in many complex organizations. Universities generally have been ill-adapted to the traditional bureaucratic model because of the need for freedom, creativity, and self-expression. Increasingly, in

[12]Many articles in *Hospital Administration* have dealt with these problems. Two of the more directly related are George Bugbee, "Administration and the Professional in the Hospital." Winter, 1961, pp. 26-33, and Harold L. Wilensky, "The Dynamics of Professionalism: The Case of Hospital Administration," Spring, 1962, pp. 6-24.

[13]Eugene Litwak, "Models of Bureaucracy Which Permit Conflict," *American Journal of Sociology,* September, 1961, pp. 177-81.

[14]Andre L. Delbecq has conducted an interesting study concerning the relationship between the bureaucratic model, types of decision-making problems, and various leadership styles in "Bureaucracy, Leadership Style, and Decision-making," *Proceedings of the 1963 Annual Meeting of the Academy of Management, Boston, Massachusetts, December 1963,* pp. 14-38.

business organizations and even in such formally structured activities as military units and governmental agencies, we find that the bureaucratic model must be modified to cope with non-programmed decision problems.

Traditional administrative models assumed well-defined, clear-cut objectives, toward which all organizational participants would strive. In the business organization the prime objective was assumed to be maximization of profits; in government agencies, it was the most effective use of funds in providing a service to the public. Increasingly, the complex organization is being viewed as a viable coalition of many interest groups who may have different and even conflicting objectives. Rather than maximization of any one overriding accepted objective, many objectives must be achieved satisfactorily in order to retain the cooperation of participants.

The large hospital is a prime example of a complex organization faced with attaining many diverse objectives. To be sure, the major objective is to satisfy the needs of the patient for treatment and care. But each group of participants—patients, the medical staff, department heads, the administrator, the trustees, and others—interpret the means for meeting this objective in terms of their own value system and requirements. And there are additional objectives, such as medical and nursing education and research, which have to be integrated into the operation. The entire organization must operate within the constraints of economic factors, the need for continued survival and growth, and the maintenance of balance and equilibrium both internally and externally. Traditional management theory assumes distinct, clear-cut objective and provides little help in dealing with the multiple objectives of complex organizations. The systems concept provides a useful approach for doing so.

THE HOSPITAL AS A HUMAN-SOCIAL SYSTEM

Large-scale, complex organizations such as hospitals should not be analyzed in terms of the traditional bureaucratic model, nor from the frame of reference of administrative management models adapted from other organizations. Rather, it should be viewed as a unique human-social system. This concept is certainly not new. Basil Georgopoulos and Floyd Mann expressed a similar point of view as follows:

An organization like the hospital is not merely a technological arrangement wherein people work according to the demands of the work plan, or in accordance with existing rules, regulations, and procedures, or in accordance with formal communication and authority lines and commands from above. It is a human-social system as well. It is a system whose members, unlike pieces of machinery and equipment, have (and use) the power to reason, to feel, to engage in informational relationships, and to make decisions—decisions which may be rational or nonrational, correct or incorrect, organizationally desirable or undesirable. . . .

Under the impact of recent experience and research, many hospital administrators, trustees, and others are becoming convinced that a hospital is basically, fundamentally, and above all, a man-system. It is complex, human-social system: its raw material is human; its product is human; its work is mainly done by human hands; and its objective is human—direct service to people, service that is individualized and personalized.[15]

THE FUNCTION OF THE HOSPITAL ADMINISTRATOR

The function of the hospital administrator in today's hospital is to coordinate the activities of the numerous operational units and to facilitate achievement of the goals

[15]Basil S. Georgopoulos and Floyd Mann, "Hospital Organization and Administration: Prospects and Perspective," *Hospital Administration,* Summer, 1964, pp. 25-26.

of the organization and its various participants. The administrator must understand the hospital, not as a number of isolated parts, but as a system; he must have knowledge of the relationships between the parts and be aware of their interaction. He must bring these individual, often diverse, functions together into an integrated, organized *system* with all the parts working toward common organizational goals. With growing size, specialization, and complexities of hospitals, this problem of integration has become increasingly difficult. In adapting the systems concept to hospitals the following aspects should be considered.

SUBSYSTEMS AND INTEGRATION

To illustrate the use of systems concepts, we will outline several approaches to organizational analysis based on subsystems. The age-old process of analysis and synthesis (subdivision and integration) has long been useful in theory building. It is also a useful approach for practitioners who want to understand any situation or environment in which they must operate. Any one or a combination of these approaches should be a useful frame of reference for administrators.

Strategic parts—It seems logical to focus attention on those parts of an over-all system which are strategic or crucial for its effective operation. Pfiffner and Sherwood describe substantive and adjective functions of organizations.[16] Substantive functions are those that must be done and done well in order for an organization to achieve its goals. Adjective functions, on the other hand, are those which facilitate the carrying out of substantive functions. Scott emphasizes systems concepts and strategic parts as follows:

> The distinctive qualities of modern organization theory are its conceptual-analytical base, its reliance upon empirical research data, and, above all, its synthesizing, integrating nature. These qualities are framed in a philosophy which accepts the premise that the only meaningful way to study organization is as a system.
>
> System analysis has its own peculiar point of view. Modern organization theory accepts system analysis as a starting point. It asks a range of interrelated questions which are not seriously considered by the classical and neo-classical theories of organization. Key among these questions are:
> 1. What are the strategic parts of the system?
> 2. What is the nature of their mutual interdependency?
> 3. What are the main processes in the system which link the parts and facilitate their adjustment to each other?
> 4. What are the goals sought by the system?[17]

Each administrator can identify the strategic parts of whatever system he is involved in. The strategic parts for a hospital administrator may be quite different from those of a plant manager in the metal fabricating industry. An administrator should understand the nature of subsystems and how they relate to one another. He should be able to identify the goals of individuals, informal groups, departments, and the organization as a whole. And he should understand the processes which integrate these various subsystems into a meaningful whole.

[16]John N. Pfiffner and Frank P. Sherwood, *Administrative Organization* (Englewood Cliffs, N.J.: Prentice-Hall, Inc., 1960), p. 171.

[17]William G. Scott, *Human Relations in Management* (Homewood, Ill.: Richard D. Irwin, Inc., 1962), p. 138.

Flow concepts–One general approach in systems design involves identification of material, energy, and information flow. These three elements are strategic parts of every system and subsystem. Consideration of them facilitates thinking about systems and subsystems. The material aspects of any system include the facilities involved and the raw material, if any, which flows through the process. A system must be designed to ensure the acquisition of raw material and/or components necessary for processing into finished products. Whenever the operation in question involves the flow and processing of material, appropriate systems can be identified. In a sense, patients represent material flow for hospitals. For operations such as insurance companies or other commercial institutions, there may be no material flow *per se*. Rather, the material in these systems is represented by the facilities, equipment, and supplies involved. Regardless of whether there is any material flow, all business operations, whether producing a product or service, contain elements of energy and information flow.

OBVIOUS SOURCE OF ENERGY: PEOPLE

Some source of energy is present in any operating system. It may be electricity obtained from available sources or generated by the firm's own power plant. The process may require natural gas, petroleum, coal or other fuel for production purposes. A business usually requires electrical energy for operating facilitating systems, if not for the main processing operation itself. Another obvious source of energy is people. Both physical and mental energy are required to operate organizations such as hospitals. People represent a renewable source of energy, at least for the short run. And, as an energy source, people are quite variable as individuals. However, in total, the group represents a reasonably stable source of energy for the system. An organization maintains a flow of worker energy throughout its life—on a day-to-day basis and from the standpoint of a long-range cycle which includes recruiting, hiring, orientation stages, and employment until retirement.Thus, all energy can be considered as a flow process both in and of itself and as part of other systems.

Another basic element in any system is information. It facilitates inter-relationships among subsystems and provides the linkage necessary to develop systems of systems. Information flow may be developed to flow along with the routing of material to be processed, for example, production control (or patient workups). For many systems where manufacturing and material flow are not present—service, commercial, and many governmental organizations—the flow of information is the critical element. Information must flow through key decision points where action is taken with regard to a service to be performed by the organization in question. In such cases, the system can be defined primarily on the basis of the flow of information to appropriate decision points. Subsystems can be identified on this basis, and they in turn can be interrelated to define the total system.

SIX MAJOR SUBSYSTEMS

Key subsystems–There are certain key subsystems and/or functions essential in every business organization which make up the total information-decision system, and which operate in a dynamic environmental system subject to rapid change. The subsystems include:

1. A sensor subsystem designed to measure changes within the system and within the environment.
2. An information processing subsystem such as an accounting, or data processing system.
3. A decision-making subsystem which receives information inputs and outputs planning messages.
4. A processing subsystem which utilizes information, energy, and materials to accomplish certain tasks.
5. A control component which ensures that processing is in accordance with planning. Typically this provides feedback control.
6. A memory or information storage subsystem which may take forms such as records, manuals, procedures, computer programs, or human experience.

The goal-setting function will establish the long-range objectives of the organization, and the performance will be measured in terms of factors such as sales, profits, and employment, or cost reduction—relative to the total environmental system. As described, these key subsystems seem vague and impersonal. Each statement outlines a function, one which will be performed in some fashion regardless of the size and/or type of organization. Often, technical and mechanical elements are involved—automated equipment, computers, paper work forms—which are coupled with human effort to close the loop. The specific approach for a subsystem can be tailor-made even though standard "hardware" items are utilized. Customizing can be accomplished via the "software" (sometimes referred to as "brainware") elements of the system. It is particularly important that attention be devoted to the people aspects of key subsystems.

PFIFFNER'S AND SHERWOOD'S "OVERLAYS"

Individuals interact with other individuals in both large and small groups to comprise the social system that is an organization. Both formal and informal organizations are involved. The organization chart depicts a system of interdependent roles in a job-task hierarchy. This basic job-task hierarchy is modified by a number of other systems which have been called "overlays" by Pfiffner and Sherwood.[18]

These modifying subsystems include:

1. The sociometric network
2. The decision network
3. The communication-feedback grid
4. The network of functional relationships
5. The power center network
6. The network of individual personalities
7. The network of personal and institutional values

Some of these overlays parallel key subsystems as set forth above. Others identify additional, confounding elements in a typical large-scale, complex organization. Pervasive value systems should be recognized as important factors in decision making. Personalities and sociometric networks, with their attendant systems of power and influence, alter the formal system of authority based on the job-task hierarchy. These "people aspects" should be considered in any analysis of key subsystems in an organization.

Each of the subsystems has interactions within its own framework. In addition, they interact with some or all of the other systems. The complexity involved is evident. Thus managers would be well advised not to succumb to the temptation to adopt

[18]Pfiffner and Sherwood, *op. cit.*, p. 207.

over-simplified views of organizations or "ten steps to managerial success" which are guaranteed in any situation. The administrator is better advised to attempt to understand the complexity and why straightforward, simple-minded approaches do not seem to work out in the real world.

CONCLUSIONS

Models based on systems concepts have not been designed to simplify the task of administration. On the contrary, this approach is a way of recognizing the complexity of the real world. And it facilitates anticipation of problems. By identifying the parts of a complex whole and the means of integrating such subsystems into a meaningful endeavor, approaches to solutions may become evident. As an old adage suggests: "A problem well stated is half solved."

To assume the real world conforms to the simplified, traditional models set forth decades ago is folly. Another adage states, "Ignorance is bliss!" However, such bliss is usually short lived as managers wonder why their perfectly straightforward, well--thought-out plans and programs evoke unanticipated responses. It is our contention that there is no set recipe for managerial success—cookbook approaches will not suffice in the long run. If there are ten steps to success, there are usually eleven or more critical problems in today's large-scale, complex organizations. Thus, rather than developing a list of "do's" and "don'ts," it seems more appropriate to develop a frame of mind which will help cope with current problems. Rather than trying to simplify the real world, it will be more fruitful to develop an understanding of its complexity and the concomitant need for flexibility in coping with problems as they arise. Systems concepts facilitate such understanding.

Part II

THE MANAGEMENT OF PERSONNEL IN HOSPITALS

This part of the book presents the management of personnel in the hospital organization. Employee motivation, supervision, leadership, and communication are important elements characteristic of the direction function. In order for the organization to operate effectively, attention must be given to its personnel and the management of them.

The first section, EMPLOYEE MOTIVATION, presents people as the catalyst that enables the technical processes of the hospital to function. A framework for understanding the needs of employees and the factors that motivate them is described.

The second section, SUPERVISION AND LEADERSHIP, provides a description of the various supervisory and leadership styles characteristic of those who direct others in the hospital setting. Leadership is presented as obtaining voluntary cooperation from subordinates while supervision is presented as the coordination of activities. Both, along with the motivation of subordinates, are necessary elements for the effective operation of the complex hospital organization.

Employee Motivation

This section is devoted to the subject of hospital employee motivation. People enable the structural organization to function toward the accomplishment of some objective. Since activities characteristic of the hospital require extensive coordination and cooperation, it is necessary to have an adequate understanding of why employees behave as they do. Those in supervisory positions not only have to be technically equipped, but must also be aware of the human relations requirements of their job.

In *THE ORGANIZATION AS A SOCIAL SYSTEM,* the point is made that people are the catalyst that enables the technical processes of the hospital to function. In addition, it is stipulated that the work of the administrator will be fruitless unless the members of the organization cooperate. Employee cooperation and effectiveness, being a function of the individual's attitudes toward his work, employer, and supervisor, are two elements which must be examined from the motivational point of view.

A framework for understanding human behavior in the hospital setting is presented in *HUMAN RELATIONS IN THE HOSPITAL.* By understanding the value system of employees it is possible to understand and anticipate employee behavior. An examination is made of the different motivations, attitudes, and behavior of various occupational groups such as the medical staff, nurses, nurses aides, and housekeeping employees within the hospital.

In *THE GROWING NEED FOR MOTIVATED NURSES,* leadership and the motivation of subordinates are presented as the primary functions of the professional hospital administrator. In addition to a treatment of motivational theory and presentation of nurses and patient's needs, the domino aspect of motivation theory is presented. The domino description depicts the filtering of motivation downward from the supervisor to the nurse and finally to the patient.

The Organization as a Social System

TED R. BRANNEN, PH.D.

Ted R. Brannen, Ph.D., is Dean of the School of Business at the University of Southern California, Los Angeles.

One of the most outstanding characteristics of modern society is the number and variety of tools in use. These tools fit into patterns that are combinations of interrelated parts devoted to common objectives. To operate this technological process, people are needed. Since each individual uses only a few of the tools included in the technological process, various individuals are responsible for the functioning of different parts of the process. These people must be formed into functional patterns consistent with effective co-ordination of the parts of the tool process. Patterns of technical relations between men grow out of the patterns of relations between the workers and their tools. In these patterns of relations some men must be given responsibility to co-ordinate the efforts of others.

The welfare of society, therefore, is a function not only of the availability of technology but of the efficiency with which it is used and the purposes to which it is applied. For the most part, society has delegated responsibility for the efficient use of the technological process to private and government administrators. These administrators are responsible for directing the tool complex in a manner that will achieve desired objectives.

The job of administrators is a most difficult one because, instead of performing the technical operations themselves, they must induce others to carry them out according to previously determined plans. The work of administrators will be fruitless unless the various members of their organizations are willing to contribute their efforts to the achievement of common objectives. Therefore, the primary function of administrators is to induce voluntary co-operation on the part of their subordinates and associates. It follows from this that the most important qualifications of administrators are (1) an understanding of why persons are willing to contribute their efforts and (2) skill in obtaining co-operation from the members of an organization in working toward planned objectives.

Reprinted by permission from *Hospital Administration: Quarterly Journal of the American College of Hospital Administrators,* Chicago, Vol. 4 (Spring, 1959), 19-25. Copyright 1959 by the American College of Hospital Administrators. All rights reserved.

The performance of every man falls within a range of effort and efficiency. The upper limit of this range is determined by his aptitude and ability. The lower limit is determined by superiors who establish the minimum level of performance that will be accepted without provoking punishment. Men who offer conscientious voluntary co-operation perform near the upper limit of their range of productivity. Other men may do no more than is necessary to avoid punishment. The level of productivity of the individual is determined by his own desire to co-operate. In short, the attitudes of the worker toward his work, his employer, and his supervisor determine his effectiveness in the organization.

ELIMINATE PROBLEMATIC SITUATIONS

Developments in the field of psychology indicate the life-process of man is a perpetual attempt to eliminate problematic situations, that is, to satisfy needs. Each person is continually making decisions he believes will help to satisfy his needs. Employees work, follow directions, and co-operate spontaneously when doing so appears to offer a means of satisfying their needs.

Unfortunately, many administrators do not recognize the fact that the eagerness of employees to absorb training, to perform their jobs well, and to co-operate with other members of the organization can be sustained or destroyed by their relations within the organization. Administrators often interpret the energy and co-operativeness of employees as being a reflection of the inherent worthiness of the individuals. Productive employees are given credit for accepting their responsibilities because they are honorable men. Unproductive employees are often discredited as being naturally lazy, stupid, or deceitful.

Every formal organizational structure (i.e., the hierarchy of supervisors and employees) tends to be permeated with a basic attitude toward the workers in the organization. The organizational attitude toward employees is determined by the highest level of administration, and it seeps down through the entire structure. There is a causal relation between this organizational attitude and the attitudes of employees toward the organization. In turn, the attitudes of employees toward the organization strongly affect the degree of employee cooperation obtained by the organization. Employees co-operate with those from whom they receive co-operation.

THESE ARE COMMON NEEDS

Administrators must be willing to help employees satisfy their needs, and they must know what needs employees expect to satisfy through their association with the organization. There are a few needs that appear to be held in common by all employees. Although it is not always consciously recognized, the basic desire probably is for recognition of the right of every man to human dignity equal to that of every other man. All employees desire respect for their abilities, appreciation for their efforts, a sense of sharing in the control of their own destinies, and a feeling of security, that is, the absence of frightening uncertainties.

However, while we know some of the basic needs employees expect to satisfy in the organization, we know far less about what is required to satisfy these needs. What one employee thinks satisfies his needs, another employee may resent. Each man interprets the situations he encounters from his own particular point of view. The individual's perception of his environment is a conditioned reaction. It is conditioned by his own background and beliefs. Thus one employee may need careful supervision, while another may function best with a minimum of supervision. When a supervisor stops by the desk of the first worker, this may be interpreted as an expression of interest on the part of the supervisor. But the same act may be perceived by the second employee as unwarranted investigation or an expression of insufficient confidence in the ability of the worker to control his own performance.

Administrators must anticipate the reaction of employees to situations that arise. Only by an understanding of the individual, his habits, expectations, and beliefs, can the administrator know what is needed to induce his spontaneous co-operation for the benefit of the organization. The administrator must recognize the elements of satisfaction and dissatisfaction in the life of each member of the organization with whom he has direct relations. There is no short cut to sound human relations. The problems involved in meeting the needs of each employee are somewhat different from the problems presented by every other employee. Each man is unique; his situation differs in some respect from all others. Administrators must seek to understand the individual—his problems, his ambitions, the way he thinks and feels, and why he has the attitudes he has. Patience and interest are required in order to determine the peculiarities of each member of the organization.

INDUCING CO-OPERATION

It also must be recognized that expectations and interpretations are subject to change. They may be altered as a result of changes in other factors. As an employee becomes older, he may become more interested in job security and retirement benefits. He may become somewhat less concerned with opportunities for advancement.

But the problem of inducing co-operation with the formal organization is even more complex. Administrators who are familiar with the sentiments, expectations, and interpretations of individual employees may still fail to understand some of their behavior because of the influence of the "informal organization."

Most formal organizational structures are comprised of smaller groups of employees who are in frequent contact with one another. Each individual will have frequent contacts with a relatively small number of people. These individuals often form identifiable groups. Their relations become standardized into certain patterns of acceptable behavior; each person knows what is expected of him and what he can expect of others. These groups make effective technical cooperation possible. They increase stability, provide channels of communication, and routinize many relations. Individuals derive satisfaction and a sense of security from identifying themselves with groups of this informal type. In addition, these groups have leadership positions that will be filled by one employee or another. They have certain relations with other groups, with supervisors, and with the organization as a whole. The pattern of relations and the hierarchy of status positions that grow out of these natural groupings of people are called the "informal organization."

The informal organization influences the perception of the members of a formal organization. We are all influenced by social pressures. We try to meet the expectations of people with whom we are in frequent contact. We want their good will. As members of various groups and social organizations, we encounter group values, attitudes, and sentiments that determine what is expected of the members of the group. We are subjected to considerable social pressure to conform to the group concept of acceptable behavior.

THE SYMBOLS OF RANK

The status hierarchy of the informal social organization is important to employees and is exemplified in every way possible. Each status position has associated with it certain customary symbols of rank. Everything in the work situation takes on a special meaning in terms of the social organization. Who gives directions to whom, the relation of one employee's wages to those of other employees, the size of one's desk in relation to the desks of others, and every other variable becomes associated with certain positions in the informal social organization. Administrators who do not recognize this fact and treat objects and relations solely in terms of concepts of efficiency are likely to encounter difficulty in obtaining employee co-operation.

The informal social organizations of some employee groups serve to induce co-operation with administrators, but other informal groups serve to limit co-operation. Therefore, the administrator must understand not only the individuals with whom he is in contact; he must also understand the informal groups into which they are organized. He must observe the attitudes and sentiments of these groups in order to be able to anticipate their reactions to various situations.

Once an informal pattern of relations and a hierarchy of status positions becomes established, it tends to resist change. A change resulting from action taken by administrators may be interpreted as a threat to the stability or the continuation of the informal social organization. If it is, the change will be resisted, and the members of the group will refuse to co-operate with their administrators.

ORGANIZATIONAL TREASON

Changes in methods, organization, or physical facilities that should produce substantial improvements in efficiency may result in drastically reduced efficiency if employees are suspicious or resentful of the change. The best systems cannot function properly if employees do not desire to see them succeed. This type of resistance, sometimes referred to as organizational treason, must be expected unless support is obtained from employees in advance of any change.

The most effective way to obtain prior acceptance of a change is to discuss with employees the problem that makes the change necessary. If employees are encouraged to participate in developing a solution, they will have an interest in seeing that the solution is effective. Under these conditions they will accept their responsibility to cooperate with others, and they will strive to perform their assigned tasks in order to avoid a breakdown in the chain of interrelated functions. For example, employees are always interested in receiving recognition as valuable members of an organization. If they are asked to participate in developing a cost-reduction program—and their suggestions are seriously considered—they will support the final program of action. In this way the efficiency of the organization may be substantially increased.

Unco-operative attitudes develop among employees who feel they can obtain support for their objectives only by forcing the formal organization to recognize their importance. Co-operative behavior cannot be maintained unless administrators seek to understand and satisfy the needs and expectations of individuals and informal groups of individuals.

In order to administer an organization in a manner designed to induce effective co-operation, the administrator must have a sincere interest in the needs of others. However, trying to meet needs and expectations will not produce co-operative behavior unless the administrator understands the sentiments of the individuals and groups with whom he works. The administrator must try to anticipate the reactions of others to his own actions. His directives, plans, and expressed attitudes must be viewed from the perspective of the people he is trying to influence. He must attempt to evaluate his own actions in terms of the beliefs, anxieties, and attitudes that will determine the behavior of others. To do this, he must understand the individuals and informal organizations with which he is in contact. This understanding can be gained only by observing the individuals and groups. However, it is important to remember that what the administrator sees when he tries to observe and understand the sentiments of the formal and informal organizations will be a product of his own attitudes, values, and sentiments unless he is aware of the problem and deliberately tries to view the situation from the point of view of the people and groups being observed.

Human Relations in the Hospital

THOMAS R. O'DONOVAN, PH.D.

Thomas R. O'Donovan, Ph.D., is Administrator of Mount Carmel Mercy Hospital in Detroit, Michigan.

The analysis to be presented here will focus on certain areas within the broad field of human relations in the hospital industry. The purpose is to provide an analytical framework for understanding human behavior in a hospital setting.

It is almost axiomatic that in order to predict, understand, and explain human behavior, we must have a willingness to attempt to do so, combined with a fairly firm knowledge of each person's or group of persons' frame of reference and system of beliefs and values.

VALUE SYSTEM ANALYSIS

Supervisors are more effective if they are able to predict, understand, and explain human behavior. Unless the supervisor has some skills in predicting certain behavior patterns of his subordinates, he is operating on a hit-and-miss basis. Explaining behavior is the most difficult of these areas and, while important, is the least necessary attribute of the supervisor.

Upon what bases can a supervisor predict the reactions and actions of his subordinates? What strategies might he adopt? What does the supervisor need to know about his people in order to narrow the range of error in behavior-prediction? The full ramifications of this subject are beyond the scope of this paper. However, we will examine restricted areas in some detail.

One of the most important bases of prediction is the value system of a subordinate.[1] Values are part of the belief structure of an individual. He holds certain things as more important than others. He reacts to various stimuli in certain ways. As these beliefs are interrelated one to another, they form a system—a value system. For example, if a supervisor knows that George resists change drastically, he should not be *surprised* at George's reaction to a proposed job transfer or a change in certain of his job duties.

Some values and beliefs stem from the individual himself as a particular and unique personality. Others stem from cultural heritage and family acclimation. For example, the son of the executive rarely desires a career in bricklaying. Such a person may seem restless in a management development program if he is assigned routine assignments. So little research has been done in the area[2] that full elaboration becomes difficult.

[1] "While investigations of social stratification universally conclude that people in different social strata vary in attitudes and values, the implications of these variations have seldom been studied. A few recent writings, however, indicate that such variations have profound consequences for social life as well as for individual behavior. It has been suggested, for example, that social rewards and 'life chances' are related not only to social background and personal capacity but also to the attitudes and value orientations possessed by persons of different social classes, socioeconomic levels, and occupations. Other studies have concluded that persons from different social levels have unlike occupational goals and conceptions of the function and meaning of work. It is likely that additional studies which seek to identify variations in attitudes and values and to analyze their consequences will provide insight into a variety of core problems in current research.

"In the study of administration, a core problem is that involving the values, beliefs, and motivations of men. The pressing problems of 'good morale' and efficiency in industrial, business, and governmental bureaucracies have in recent years caused administrators to become interested in the opinions, desires, and philosophies of persons holding positions in a variety of occupational levels. It is quite probable that the total ideology of the individual has profound effects upon his behavior on the job and, indeed, upon his career pattern and prospects. Yet few empirical studies have demonstrated the precise manner in which such ideologies differ or, for that matter, the consequences of these differences." Roland F. Pellegrin and Charles H. Coates, "Executives and Supervisors: Contrasting Definitions of Career Success," *Administrative Science Quarterly,* Vol. 1, No. 4, March 1957.

[2] Herbert H. Hyman, "The Value Systems of Different Classes: A Social Psychological Contribution to the Analysis of Stratification," in R. Bendix and S. Lipset, *Class, Status and Power,* Glencoe, Illinois: The Free Press, 1953. pp. 426-27: "The existence of stratification in American society is well known. The corollary fact—that individuals from lower strata are not likely to climb far up the economic ladder is also known. However, what requires additional analysis are the factors that account for this lack of mobility. Many of these factors of an objective nature have been studied. Opportunity in the society is differential; higher education or specialized training, which might provide access to a high position, must be bought with money—the very commodity which the lower classes lack. Such objective factors help maintain the existing structure. But there are other factors of a more subtle psychological nature which have not been illuminated and which may also work to perpetuate the existing order. It is our assumption that an intervening variable mediating the relationship between low position and lack of upward mobility is a system of beliefs and values within the lower classes which in turn reduces the very voluntary actions which would ameliorate their low position.

"To put it simply, the lower class individual doesn't want as much success, knows he couldn't get it even if he wanted to, and doesn't want what might help him get success. Of course, an individual's value system is only one among many factors on which his position in the social hierachy depends. Some of these factors may be external and arbitrary, quite beyond the control of even a highly motivated individual. However, within the bounds of the freedom available to individuals, this value system would create a self-imposed barrier to an improved position.

Since a person's value system determines his behavior, it is therefore possible for the supervisor to predict the behavior of his subordinates if he understands their value system. There are limits to this prediction, of course. However, in the hospital industry as in any other industry, there have been very few attempts made to discover on an organized basis why man works, why he behaves in certain ways, why one man attains high productivity as other employees produce at a relatively low level. We can reduce conflict, increase output, promote intra-group cohesiveness, maintain or increase morale, develop top flight subordinates, increase profits . . . providing we can obtain willful cooperation from subordinates!

Within an "occupational" frame of reference, how does a person's value system determine or condition his behavior? We shall answer this question[3] by citing examples and presenting bibliographic references that will enable the reader to dig out an extensive analysis of the interplay between value and behavior.

One major example is the role of education and achievement. High status occupations in the United States are increasingly being earned by individuals with a university degree. The motivation for advanced education is stronger among the offspring of middle and upper class families than among the working class. There are exceptions, but this tendency does exist. The source of the motivation for advanced education is the value placed on education. Thus, the cultural heritage of an individual conditions values which create motivation to increase education which in turn can result in upper class occupational attainment.

The literature has demonstrated with countless research studies that occupational level of attainment is highly related to such factors as the individual's level of aspiration, education, education of father, and occupational level of father.[4]

"Presumably, this value system arises out of a realistic appraisal of reality and in turn softens for the individual the impact of low status. Unfortunately, we have at the moment little information on its genesis."

[3]Herbert H. Hyman, "The Value Systems of Different Classes: A Social Psychological Contribution to the Analysis of Stratification," in Reinhard Bendix and Seymour M. Lipset, eds., *Class, Status and Power* 1953, pp. 426-42; Genevieve Knupfer, "Portrait of the Underdog," in *Ibid.*, pp. 255-63; and Bernard C. Rose, "The Achievement Syndrome: A Psycho-cultural Dimension of Social Stratification," *American Sociological Review*, 21 (1956), pp. 203-11. Elizabeth C. Lyman, "Occupational Differences in the Value Attached to Work," *American Journal of Sociology*, 61 (1955), pp. 138-44; and Nancy C. Morse and Robert S. Weiss, "The Function and Meaning of Work and the Job," *American Sociological Review*, 20 (1955), pp. 191-98. Delbert C. Miller and William H. Form, *Industrial Sociology, The Sociology of Work Organizations,* 2nd edition, New York: Harper and Row, 1964. Robert K. Merton, "Social Structure and Anomie," in his *Social Theory and Social Structure*, pp. 132. Hyman, *op. cit.*, pp. 427. Leonard Reissman, "Levels of Aspiration and Social Class," *American Sociological Review*, 18 (1953). A. H. Maslow, *Motivation and Personality*, New York: Harper and Row, 1954. Richard Centers, "Motivational Aspects of Occupational Stratification," *Journal of Social Psychology*, 28 (1948), pp. 214-15; Thomas R. O'Donovan, "Differential Extent of Opportunity Among Executives and Lower Managers," *Journal of the Academy of Management*, Vol. 5, No. 2, August, 1962, pp. 139-49. A. Etzioni, "Authority Structure and Organizational Effectiveness," *Administrative Science Quarterly*, June, 1959. L. E. Rogers, "Measurement of Status Relations in a Hospital," Bulletin 175, Columbus, Ohio State University, Engineering Expt. Stn., 1959. O. Hall, "Motivation and Morale," *Hospital Administration*, Summer, 1959. C. Argyris, "Diagnosing Human Relations in Organization—A Case Study of a Hospital," New Haven, Labor and Management Center, Yale University, 1956.

[4]W. Lloyd Warner, and James C. Agegglen, *Occupational Mobility in American Business and Industry*, 1928-1952, Minneapolis: University of Minnesota Press, 1955. Necomber, Mable, *The Big*

Even though the research evidence is so well documented, we still read and hear of people who fail in their prediction of behavior because they do not see the connection between value systems and behavior or because they misinterpreted a person's value system. As one example, the following statements appeared recently: "In America, only girls of minority groups are strongly motivated to seek the highest education possible, according to Mrs. Charles U. Culmer, past president of the Girl Scouts, who addressed Detroit's annual council meeting last night at Ford Auditorium.

"Mrs. Culmer is also a member of the World Committee of the World Association of Girl Guides and Girl Scouts.

" 'I am increasingly concerned over this general lack of motivation in this country,' she said. 'In the '20's women coming of age were eager for accomplishment, but now only minority groups encourage their girls to do the best that's in them. Women in other countries are extending themselves and setting up standards of excellence, but not here.' "[5]

These are emotional statements that are totally incorrect. The tendency is exactly the opposite.[6]

How do "values" condition aspiration level? Pellegrin and Coates describe it this way: "Logically the experienced worker, in realistically appraising his career chances, will set a high level of aspiration for himself only if he possesses the advantages of a middle-class or higher social background. Without such a background, he typically lacks not only the technical qualifications for high-level positions, but, as Bernard C. Rosen has remarked, he has not been thoroughly exposed during his childhood to those values which encourage behavior leading to vertical mobility."[7]

ROLE CONFLICT

Before examining the value systems of certain occupational groups, we will discuss the concept of role conflict. "Resolving conflict" is the most important, most difficult, and most time-consuming function of the majority of supervisors and executives. In many cases, the classic managerial functions of planning, organizing, and controlling simply do not apply. The latter approach has limited usefulness.

Business Executive, New York: Columbia University Press, 1955. Roger V. Clements, *Managers: A Study of Their Careers in Industry,* London: George Allen and Unwin, 1958. Delbert C. Miller and William H. Form, *Industrial Sociology,* New York: Harper and Bros., 1951. Suzanne I. Keller, "Social Origins and Career Lines of Three Generations of American Business Leaders," Ph.D. thesis, New York: Columbia University, 1954, Microfilm. Natalie Rogoff, *Recent Trends in Occupational Mobility,* Glencoe: Free Press, 1953. Roland J. Pellegrin and Charles H. Coates, "Executives and Supervisors: Contrasting Definitions of Career Success," *Administrative Science Quarterly,* March 1957, pp. 506-17.

[5] *The Detroit News,* Thursday, May 14, 1964, p. 1c.

[6] Thomas R. O'Donovan, "Intergenerational Educational Mobility," *Sociology and Social Research,* Vol. 47, No. 1, October, 1962, p. 58: "A person will tend not to go to college unless he has (1) the motivation, and (2) a certain amount of economic means in order to pay the cost. Both of these factors are closely related to the cultural and economic position of the family. The enumeration of social problems connected with disproportionate opportunities for advanced education is a crucial research area in our society."

[7] Pellegrin and Coates, pp. 513, *op. cit.*

What is meant by conflict? What is role conflict and how does it differ from personality conflict? Conflict will be defined here as any form of antagonism (felt inwardly or expressed overtly) between employees, supervisors, or in any superior-subordinate relationship. Conflict can be quite a problem in any organization because it conditions our thinking and the way we react to interaction by setting up negativism. It can create the tendency for a supervisor or any individual to jump to conclusions without adequate evidence. In most instances, conflict is unfortunate and preventable because the original source of the conflict is usually rooted in miscommunication, or perhaps because we do not look at a situation from the other person's standpoint.

PERSONALITY CONFLICT

Any two individuals can experience conflict in their daily interactions based upon personality or related reasons. For example, two secretaries may argue among themselves and end up not on speaking terms for several weeks. One maid may be against one of her fellow workers because she works "too hard" or evades work too often. These are the usual antagonisms and conflicts that arise and the effective supervisor largely overlooks them unless he expects the situation to affect the general morale and productivity.

Role conflict is generally more difficult for the supervisor to cope with. Role conflict can exist totally independent of the personalities of the people involved. For example, the role of the time study man in the factory is different from the role of the assembly line worker. It is not unusual for conflict to arise here.

The taxpayer may experience conflict in his interaction with an income tax investigator. Other examples include: prosecuting attorney and defense attorney; doctor-nurse; student-teacher; nursing floor supervisor-maintenance department head; policeman-fugitive.

There is another form of role conflict that we should mention. When a particular individual occupies more than one role himself, he may find that there could be a conflict among these roles. For example, an individual could be a husband, father, and executive at the same time. Any of these three roles could conflict with one another. Thus, the term "role conflict" can have two different meanings. In any event, analysis of role variations is important. People with differential occupational roles:

1. are motivated differently;
2. have different attitudes;
3. behave differently;
4. look to administration for different things.

Not all of the occupational groups that exist within a hospital will be described here. It is important to keep in mind that we are talking about tendencies in each of these cases. Not every characteristic will be valid in the case of every employee in all hospitals.

THE MEDICAL STAFF

Physicians are not employees of the hospital. They are paid by the patient directly or through the patient's insurance company. Potential role conflict can arise between attending doctors and hospital administration because of this arrangement. The value system of the physician centers around his desire to advance the medical profession and his own stature within the profession. He is greatly interested in the well-being of the patient. The hospital is viewed by him as a vehicle of service to carry out his professional needs. He may appear conservative and to resist change because he seeks stability in the hospital since, of necessity, his time is devoted to the pursuit of other professional interests. The physician will tend to value independence and resent interference and restriction. A sharp head nurse can save herself a good deal of frustration if she attempts to know and understand the value structure of the doctor. This applies to other groups too.

Their norms have been assimilated in medical school. Doctors are judged by their colleagues and they tend to resist bureaucratic interferences. The doctor's primary loyalty is to the patient, the hospital employee's primary loyalty is to the hospital with a direct focus on patient care. Thus he may miss many hospital meetings that he probably should have attended. He may not always be the most efficient committee chairman either.

THE REGISTERED NURSE

The value system of the staff nurse centers around the professional care of the patient and an entrenched dedication to the service of sick and diseased people. Most nurses retain the role of performing general nursing care while others move into other areas such as supervisory positions, anesthesia, medical doctor. Her first concern is the well-being of the patient.

The shortage of nurses coupled with the increased utilization of hospitals to near full capacity has resulted in a vast increase in the dynamic activities on hospital floors. This often results in tensions and strained human relationships. Many nurses have felt a good deal of frustration because they find themselves not being able to extend the kind of patient care they want to due to the shortage of nurses. Entire floors often end up with one nurse and a few aides and perhaps a practical nurse.

Nurses often have to work part time because they are married with a family. This gives them a role conflict within themselves: the working wife and mother. Sometimes supervisors see her as *only* having one role: employee. Therefore, conflict can arise between the nurse and the supervisor. Afternoon and midnight shifts of hospitals tend to have a greater percent of part time nurses; this creates hospital identification problems. Group cohesiveness among the nurses becomes less strong. In addition, they tend to feel that their hospital has a greater shortage of nurses than of any other occupational group.

Most nurses resist promotion. There is a tendency among the majority of nurses to resist promotions into positions of head nurse, assistant head nurse, or floor supervisor. A good deal of research is necessary in this area. Aspiration levels of the typical nurse do not include promotion into supervisory duties. They resent and resist unreasonable "assembly line" techniques that prevent them from treating the needs of the whole patient. Nurses want to be considered partners with the doctors on the medical team rather than "handmaidens."

Burling, Lentz and Wilson have identified six areas that showed differences in the point of view of nurses and doctors toward the hospital:

The nurse's world is the hospital. The doctor's world on the other hand is only partly the hospital, for much of his professional time is spent in the community or his office. The doctor uses the institution as a facility while the nurse is employed by it and subject to its administration. The doctor prescribes and thus initiates many of the nurse's activities. She assists him and does those things for the patient for which she is qualified. The nurse has had to struggle to attain a respected position in the hospital and in society at large, while the doctor's prestige is legendary. The tradition that the nurse is a helpmate to the doctor in a differential, quasi-servant capacity is still in the background of the doctor-nurse relationship, although the situation is changing, and a more nearly equal relationship than existed in the past is developing. Furthermore, nurses band together as a group more readily than the medical staff. Any doctor soon acquires a hospital-wide reputation and nurses have been known to shrewdly "gang up" on a doctor who has offended one of them.[8]

In the past, the typical hospital patient was often a charity case and was therefore in no position to rebuke his nurse or resist her authority. Such is not the case today, however. With hospitalization insurance, the patient has become much more independent and is likely to challenge his nurse in a vigorous fashion about anything that he does not care about in the hospital situation.

KEEPING UP TO DATE

The role of the nurse as a first line supervisor is quite different from the first line supervisor in corporate industry. A head nurse must be technically competent in nursing in order to retain the respect of the staff nurses and other nursing personnel on her floor. She must also have the skills in organizing activities and in planning and control. If she becomes out of touch with modern techniques in nursing while she becomes very proficient as a "manager," she will tend to lose her general effectiveness because it is essential that technical competence be maintained. Burling, Lentz and Wilson have stated it this way:

The theory that a supervisor should stick to supervising may make more sense in business than in hospitals. Where techniques change rapidly, a nurse who doesn't keep in practice may become out of date in a short time. As a result her staff loses confidence in her as a craftsman.[9]

WHITE COLLAR EMPLOYEES, NON-SUPERVISORY CLERICAL

As hospitals grow in size and complexity, the variety of skills that must be utilized increases; this results in the need for increased clerical help with high competency. The following discussions will describe some of the sociological areas that affect white collar employees in a hospital. In many cases, the value systems of people in this group can be deducted from an analysis of these points.

The white collar job is one of the few hospital jobs that is directly comparable with jobs in other industries. However, even though in the past clerical skills were interchangeable with those in the commercial world, there are indications that hospital clerical work is beginning to be a specialty. A certain amount of professionalization is occurring among clerical workers in the hospital industry. One of the reasons for this is the increased significance of the contribution that is being made by the white collar employee in the hospital industry.

[8]Temple Burling, Edith Lentz, and Robert Wilson, *The Give and Take in Hospitals,* New York: G. P. Putnam's Sons, 1956, pp. 87. The sociological value system analysis presented in this classic research study is one of the best in the literature.

[9]*Ibid.,* p. 145.

The major motivation of most white collar employees is to identify with members of the healing profession. The prestige of doctors and nurses tends to spread to less highly skilled clerical employees. Also, people who work in hospitals are often credited with health knowledge by their friends and relatives on the outside. They pick up vocabulary that lifts their "advice" above the level of gossip.

Both social and psychological security exists for the clerical employee in the hospital. In addition, a good deal of economic security is present. Very few lay-offs occur in the hospital industry. Variety of work can facilitate psychological security. Hospital jobs are said to be more varied and less routine than most industrial clerical jobs. A hospital deals daily in "crisis" situations; even the business office participates in daily hospital drama.

Some hospitals are less demanding employers than industrial concerns. The pace varies from moderate to quite high, but a general air of unchanging conservatism often prevails.

The hospital is sometimes at a disadvantage in regard to wages, hours and benefits, so that other advantages of employment need to exist in order to attract qualified personnel. These differences in the hospital industry and in commerical organizations are narrowing, however.

Blocked mobility tends to exist in white collar employment. There are few rungs on the clerical ladder. In fact, promotions tend to be blocked among *most* occupations in hospital industry. A nurse aide, for example, cannot become a nurse regardless of the amount of on-the-job experience she has. Professional education is the sole road to advanced status throughout most hospital employment. Few industries are characterized with as high a proportion of professional personnel as is the hospital industry. This is especially significant since it is the fifth largest industry in the United States.

INTER-DEPARTMENT CONFLICT

Internal conflict can be present in certain departments within the hospital. For example, the business office can be subject to a good deal of internal conflict because of the attempts that must be made to balance humanitarian ideals of service with financial solvency. Blue Cross and other prepayment insurances have helped the situation for both the business office employees and patients. However, there is still a general reluctance on the part of the public to pay for hospitalization costs, and the trustees of hospitals tend to insist that balanced budgets are a strong virtue. Therefore the business office employee can be caught between these two pressures.[10] Cashiers and other business office employees must be polite but firm. It is quite an art to achieve good patient relations while maintaining a watchdog vigilance. However, as with any white collar department, the better the organization of the department, the less the tendency for such conflicts to arise.

The clerical employees are employed throughout the hospital and therefore are not an identifiable and cohesive work group. Anytime a work group is geographically decentralized within an organization, they do not become highly cohesive. Values held by members of cohesive groups are different than values held by members in a noncohesive group.

[10]Arthur X. Deegan, II, "The Personal Touch in Hospital Relations," *Hospital Progress,* November, 1964, Vol. 45, No. 11, pp. 90-93, 108.

Medical staff and professional personnel directly concerned with medical care feel no competition from clerical employees. There can still be conflict however, because doctors and nurses may tend to feel that records are of secondary importance compared with the direct objective of patient care. They may, therefore, consider the clerical worker's insistence on consistently following stated procedures as unimportant. One example of this is the common practice of the doctor's delinquency in keeping up the medical record of each of his patients.

NURSE AIDE

There is a potential role conflict between the role of the nurse and the nurse aide that can exist at any time on any floor in any hospital. Knowing the value system of the nurse aide, as with all major hospital employment groups, is quite important to the supervisor who expects to be effective in his relations.

The first nurse aides in the hospital industry were amateur nurses who performed patient care services before professional nurses or the modern hospital came on the scene. After nursing took hold, very few nurse aides were employed. During the great shortage of nurses in World War II, the nurse aide began to reappear on the scene.

It is alleged that "white" is the highest status color in the hospital. This is certainly insignificant in many ways. Nevertheless, white is predominantly used by professional people such as doctors and nurses, while the nurse aide often wears a blue uniform and the dietary employees may wear yellow uniforms. In any event, the nurse aides generally are not allowed to wear white uniforms. There is a functional value in differentiating colors of uniforms of certain occupational groups. If everyone wore white, the patients and other people would not be able to tell the difference among certain of the employee groups. In some cases, it is important to tell the difference between a nurse and non-professional personnel. (Disagreements have been known to occur over the right to wear full length white lab coats).

Because of the drastic shortage of nurses in most hospitals, the function of the nurse aide has taken on phenomenal significance in recent years. Most hospitals have witnessed a relative increase of the ratio of nurse to nurse aides in the past 15 years. In addition, there tends to be a wide range of abilities among nurse aides; on the one hand you find nurse aides of great skill and ability, while on the other end of the scale, certain nurse aides are very lax in their work. The range of ability for most occupational groups, especially the professional groups, is generally not as wide as in the nurse aide groups.

Training of nurse aides is important because of the effect this can have on their efficiency. This can be accomplished in a variety of ways. Some hospitals hire only experienced aides. Other hospitals have a formal training program that lasts two to five weeks. Still others perform on-the-job training by turning the aides over to the head nurse to do it. However, she is very often too busy to do the job that she would like to do and, therefore, she may delegate the training function to experienced aides to "show them the ropes." This has many advantages as well as disadvantages. Such differential systems result in different value systems.

JURISDICTIONAL CONFLICT

Jurisdictional disputes may often arise. For example, they may arise in the daily work interaction among nurse aides, practical nurses, and staff nurses. The problem arises when the person with the lower level of responsibility attempts to perform functions that are characteristically performed by the next higher level of responsibility. When this happens, such an individual is usually rebuffed because she allegedly does not have appropriate training. Of course in most cases they do not have this training. However, when you have a great shortage of personnel such as nurses, you may find in emergencies that a nurse aide or practical will be called upon to help out in a higher level of work on a temporary basis. She becomes trained during the emergency rather than in a formal classroom. Sometimes she would not receive any coaching from the nurses at all but would attempt to perform such an activity based upon her own judgment and experience observing the nurse. However, when the crisis passes, the nurse expects the practical nurse or nurse aide to go back to their former level of responsibility. The nurse aide or practical nurse may be reluctant to do so even though she is required to do so by the nurse.

The greater the shortage of registered nurses in a particular hospital, the more the existing nurses will "accept" lesser skilled personnel in working with nursing activities. Thus, practical nurses and nurse aides tend to be accepted more when there is a shortage of registered nurses than where there is not.

DEALING WITH TRANSFERS

The job of nurse aide carries more status than the job of maid but in only rare cases does a nurse aide receive higher pay. This suggests that pay is not necessarily related to status in our society. It certainly is not true in many hospital jobs. Very often we see that the more promising maids who work in patient room areas tend to do little things for patients and often wind up requesting a transfer to the job of nurse aide. In most hospitals when a maid approaches her supervisor in the housekeeping department and requests a transfer to the department of nursing services in order to become a nurse aide, the housekeeping supervisor tends to feel that the department of nursing services is raiding them of their best maids. Obviously the housekeeping department needs high quality maids in order to perform the housekeeping function on a high level basis. It becomes difficult for them to do this if their best maids are taken from them. However, what happens if the transfers are declined? The maid may leave the hospital and become a nurse aide at *another* hospital. In any event lowered morale will result if such transfers are automatically restricted.

Sometimes a nurse aide will request a transfer from the department of nursing services to the physical therapy department. The reason behind such a request may be because the physical therapy department is open Monday through Friday, 8:00 a.m. to 4:30 p.m. Thus the nurse aide will transfer and obtain a more desirable set of working hours for herself. Again it is not a good policy to restrict such transfers. However, most hospitals have found it advantageous to require two weeks' notice before any employee can be transferred. In this way some training time for replacements is provided for.

NON-PROFESSIONAL MALES IN HOSPITALS

Non-professional male positions in hospitals are, in most instances, "dead end" jobs. Because promotional opportunities are scarce, their turnover tends to be high. Even when hospitals adhere to a "promotion-from-within" policy, such promotions are a function of educational attainment rather than of length of service. The orderly cannot become an inhalation therapist without training; on-the-job experience does not prepare an orderly for higher paying professional positions.

Since hospital wages are often lower than industrial wages, when a hospital does begin to become modern, i.e., installing a computer, etc., certain job holders that it did not have previously become difficult to recruit. Most jobs are priced on an internal basis, which means that a job title is priced in relation to jobs of similar responsibility within the hospital. When attempts to employ key punch operators are made, difficulties arise. Supply and demand account for this difficulty. Jobs of similar responsibility to key punch operators which are paid equally are easier to fill; however, the job of key punch operator is in higher demand. If the hospital pays market rates, they upset their internal job relationships; if they do not, they either obtain no key punch operators or low quality operators.

These problems do not arise as often in hospitals that utilize the traditional jobs, but if hospitals are to become dynamic they must modernize their approaches. When this happens, the problem as described above can occur.

This is not the only problem in hospital wage and salary administration. An interesting question to ask is whether or not males get more money than females when performing the same job. This has been a long standing social and legislative fight in the United States. The answer is generally that in the hospital the males and females performing the same job *do* receive the same pay. However, when two jobs are of equal responsibility, and would probably belong in the same pay grade, but are different jobs—one being performed only by females and the other by males—we often find that the male job will be placed in a higher pay grade than the female job.

For example, in most hospitals, the relative value to the hospital of the nurse aide and orderly is fairly similar. This means that both of these jobs could receive the same pay and would not result in any unfair pay structure. However, the vast majority of hospitals in the United States pay the orderly more than the nurse aide *solely* because the orderly job is a male job and the nurse aide job is a female job. Certain other hospitals have argued that the jobs are significantly different even in responsibility. As a justification for paying the orderly more, they use the physical effort of the orderly involved in lifting patients, stating that this gives the floor more flexibility in patient care than if they only had nurse aides. This problem is prevalent in wage and salary programs throughout the United States and not just in the hospital industry.

HIGHER PAY PROBLEMS

It is harder to change attitudes than policies. Most communities feel that hospital employment is in part charitable work and that it should be low paid. However, raising pay rates creates two problems. It increases problems in morale because existing older and long service people expect to receive the raise also. But from a productive standpoint, they may not meet the standard and lack the specifications of the job that has been upgraded. Thus, while the new people being hired may be doing the same type of work as the old timers, their relative efficiency may be much higher. Newly hired, supposedly efficient, workers may learn bad habits from the old guard employees or they may become discouraged and quit. It creates certain problems if a hospital terminates people who cannot meet the new standard.

The male job holder in the hospital industry tends to have a high regard for the autonomy of his position. He seeks the opportunity to "figure things out" without close supervision or pressure for speed. If supervisors attempt to provide close supervision over male employees, they may meet severe resistance. The successful supervisor will attempt to recognize these different needs and will attempt to fulfill them whenever possible. For example, the supervisor can recommend and provide training, job transfers, and/or counseling.

LAUNDRY AND HOUSEKEEPING EMPLOYEES

Many research studies have pointed out that technical factors relating to work and work organization can affect human relations.[11] For example, if the nature of the job is such that the workers performing the task do not work together in the same area, this has an effect on group cohesiveness in the informal organization. In such cases, their group cohesiveness would be less and morale would tend to be lower among such workers.

In contrast, if the employees work together as a team on projects, there is an opportunity for greater cohesiveness, a strengthening of the informal organization, and potentially greater morale. In the hospital, we find that housekeeping workers tend to be geographically dispersed through the hospital in their work assignments. Thus, the maids do not have a close-knit, informal organization among themselves. However, laundry workers tend to have their working area centralized and therefore their cohesiveness is greater and high ties of acquaintanceship develop. Thus, we see among female laundry workers a greater homogeneity among the workers, higher morale, lower rate of turnover, and a higher average job tenure.

In the supervision of non-professional workers, it is sometimes necessary to use a *closer* type of supervision than would be necessary in the supervision of professional employees. However, if we supervise too closely, this can result in negativism on the part of the workers being supervised. When workers are centralized in the same working area, it is possible to extend more *general* supervision than if the workers are geographically decentralized in their work schedule. Therefore, maids generally need to be more closely supervised than female laundry workers *because* of the spatial considerations. It is quite likely that the supervisor who is effective in supervising laundry workers would be ineffective as a supervisor of maids. The supervisory role tends to change somewhat because the role of the supervisor in supervising maids is that he must follow them carefully and provide inspection for their work. Whereas, among laundry workers, the groups themselves can police each other. It is much easier to spot a shirker in the laundry department than it is in the housekeeping department. If the group of laundry workers has high cohesiveness and high morale, they will tend to look askance at a member who is not doing his share of the work.

Upward communication is somewhat restricted by spacial considerations. When the workers are performing their functions in the same room with supervision, it is much

---

[11]William Foote Whyte, *Human Relations in the Restaurant Industry,* New York: McGraw-Hill Book Company, Inc. 1946, and also Temple Burling, Edith Lentz, and Robert N. Wilson, *The Give and Take in Hospitals,* New York: G. P. Putnam's Sons, 1956. Robert N. Wilson, "The Social Structure of a General Hospital," *The Annals of the American Academy of Political and Social Science,* Volume 346, March, 1963, pp. 67-76.

easier to communicate than when the work is dispersed throughout several floors and you may not see your supervisor more than once or twice per day.

It should also be noted that maids in the hospital industry are surrounded by professional personnel as they perform their daily tasks. Thus, they are constantly reminded of their relative status, whereas the laundry employees may not think of their status at all while they are performing their work tasks. Maids with long service tend to be better adjusted to their jobs than maids with a short amount of tenure. They tend to make a special effort to work with others. Thus, while there are built-in problems in the job of supervising maids, there is certainly a good deal that the supervisor can do to improve himself as a good supervisor. Understanding the value system of the maids and porters plays a very important role.

CONCLUSION

The more we know about people and the more we understand and seek to understand them, the more effective we are as supervisors. Knowledge of supervisory behavior is built on the foundations of the behavioral sciences—in particular, sociology, psychology and cultural anthropology. These sciences provide an empirical basis for predicting, explaining, and understanding human behavior. Without this knowledge the supervisor is less able to effectively "influence" or "control" the behavior of his subordinates.

Throughout this paper we have centered on human relations. By integrating findings from research studies from the behavioral sciences into supervisory behavior, we increase our knowledge of how to obtain *willful* cooperation from subordinates.

Our major focal point has been value system analysis. In examining this concept we have shown some of the dynamics of human complexities that exist within the hospital environment. Because man is complex, we dare not make simple assumptions in predicting his behavior! Also, it should be noted that acquiring knowledge of the value system of an occupational group does not mean that each *member* of that group will hold the same value system. The tendency will be there, but exceptions will occur.

In addition, knowledge of value system analysis helps identify areas of potential breakdowns in human relationships. When the total picture is brought together, patterns begin to develop. Unfortunately, this process is not automatic. The major part of the job must still rest with the supervisor. Working with subordinates in the most effective way is the challenge and responsibility of every supervisor.

The Growing Need for Motivated Nurses

FRANCIS G. EDWARDS

Francis G. Edwards is a Vice President of Louis A. Allen Associates, Inc. in Palo Alto, California.

The nineteenth century angel of mercy has today been replaced by a seemingly less angelic and considerably more mercenary counterpart. With increased technical skill has come an apparent lessening of sensitivity to the sufferings of the patient. With demands for higher wages and better working conditions, the modern Florence Nightingale is undoubtedly more efficient, but somehow less comforting.

SENSITIVITY TO THE NEEDS OF THE USER

While this may seem a matter of minor moment to the hospital administrator, his management counterpart in other fields is showing growing concern with problems in motivation. He has already observed that with increased technical sophistication the product or service produced tends to become more important to the technician than the people using it. Pardonable pride in his technical accomplishments lessens his sensitivity to the needs of the user. This is particularly true when the product or service caters mainly to physical needs. Too often more subtle but equally real psychological needs are ignored or rationalized away.

In the admittedly difficult area of providing adequate nursing care for physically damaged and psychologically impaired patients, modern motivation theory gives rise to some interesting speculations and offers a strong possibility for marked improvement if seriously applied. To bring the topic into focus for the hospital administrator, he must first be aware that one of his primary functions as a professional manager is the leadership and motivation of his subordinates. Its importance, expressed in economic terms, is most readily apparent in "strained" relationships with the patients, his customers. Time-consuming, unreasonable demands and embarrassing complaints—all adding to operating costs—can be avoided if patients are properly motivated by the nursing staff. The nursing staff in turn must be motivated by their supervisors, and

Reprinted by permission from *Hospital Administration: Quarterly Journal of the American College of Hospital Administrators,* Chicago, Vol. 16 (Winter, 1971), 44-53. Copyright 1971 by the American College of Hospital Administrators. All rights reserved.

they in turn by their managers. To understand this fully, we must first determine exactly what motivation is and then examine the types of problems which arise when people are not motivated. Once this has been done, the experience of management in other fields can be examined to see if there are direct areas of application to hospital administration.

WHAT IS MOTIVATION?

Motivation, to behavioral scientists, is a satisfactory pattern of behavior which reaches an objective corresponding to the individual's need or needs. Since purposeful human behavior is instigated by need and directed toward objectives, reaching these objectives produces a feeling of satisfaction and a temporary disappearance of the need. This we call motivation. A motivated individual is one who accomplishes worth-while objectives related to his personal needs. In a social situation this satisfaction is greatly increased if recognition and esteem on the part of other members of the group accompanies the achievement of the objective.

Based largely on the work of Frederick Herzberg, modern motivational theory distinguishes between motivating and maintenance needs. This is particularly important in a socially structured situation such as working for a company or as part of a hospital staff. The contractual implications of employment are such that the employee feels he has a right to certain considerations. Among these considerations typically are fair policies or administration, effective supervision, adequate salary, reasonable interpersonal relations, and adequate working conditions. While precise descriptions of these conditions will vary from one type of work to another, the individual has certain standards which he feels should be met. As long as these standards are met, the individual has no reason to be dissatisfied. However, these factors, in and of themselves, do not motivate or satisfy him. For this reason they are sometimes referred to as maintenance factors, sometimes as the dissatisfiers or hygiene factors.

On the other hand, there are certain considerations to which the individual has no right in virtue of his employment contract. However, he needs them if he is going to be a completely satisified human being. These, known as motivating factors, include the work itself, achievement, recognition of this achievement, responsibility, and advancement or growth. These represent the challenge and pleasure people get out of work. They provide a basis for recognition from other members of the group and from one's supervisor. They produce a desire for advancement and a sense of continuing accomplishment.

Successful application of Herzberg's theories to various industrial situations has produced an additional observation. When people are not motivated—that is, when they are not receiving enough recognition, growth, sense of achievement, etc., they do not complain about lack of motivation or attack the motivation factors which are directly responsible. Instead, they pick on the dissatisfiers and complain about working conditions, management policies, inadequate supervision, wages, etc. Further, if the complaints are taken at their face value and salaries are increased, working conditions are improved, etc., the effect is relatively short-lived. Soon other objects or the same factors again become renewed sources of dissatisfaction and the cycle tends to repeat itself endlessly.

On the other hand, motivated workers, that is, those who are achieving a strong sense of growth, adequate recognition, a feeling of accomplishment, etc., not only do not complain about environmental factors, but tend to have a greater tolerance for substandard conditions and are quite unlikely to complain unless some major inequity develops.

IMPLICATIONS FOR MANAGEMENT

The implications of modern motivation theory for professional management are at the same time distressing and encouraging. The disquieting thought that the mini-welfare states, created by some companies, were both unnecessary and largely ineffective is in the former category. (The interesting speculation as to how many union demands might have been averted if workers had been adequately motivated must remain forever unanswered. The suspicion, however, is strong today that giving in to demands without creating better motivation simply produces more demands and a basis for further dissatisfaction.)

On the encouraging side, however, is the thought that management understanding the importance of the motivating factors, can now begin to create a climate in which workers can find personal satisfaction in everything they do. Combined with modern emphasis on management objectives, it produces a realistic climate in which the worker's need for recognition, growth, achievement, etc., can be satisfied by enlightened management handling of superior/subordinate contacts.

WORTH-WHILE OBJECTIVES

In the basic management task of securing results through others, the professional can combine an ability to effectively predetermine their courses of action with a climate that inspires and encourages each individual worker and gives him a continuing sense of his own importance so necessary to produce a continuing feeling of satisfaction. To motivate his subordinates, the modern professional must create a climate in which the individual can select and work towards worth-while objectives. He must give him necessary recognition and a sense of achievement when he accomplishes them and hold out opportunities for continuous personal growth and development.

If the manager can do this, the motivated subordinate not only produces more effective results, but can also increase both his physical and psychological capacity for useful work. Attendance records show that well-motivated, satisfied employees have fewer days off, fewer physical complaints, whether real or imaginary, and can progressively take on more difficult objectives. Of even greater significance is the observation that motivated subordinates can, in turn, create a climate in which motivation of people with whom they come in contact becomes possible. This is particularly true if they are taught to understand the important implications of motivation and its practical value, both for themselves and the company or institution they represent.

MOTIVATION IN THE HOSPITAL

Since the primary reason for a hospital's existence is to provide care for its patients and to satisfy their needs, it may be well to first examine the modern patient's needs, both physical and psychological, then to draw implications for the primary interface between the hospital administration and the patient, namely, the nursing staff. From this, we can proceed through the supervisory to the upper management levels.

In the course of the last thirty years, the needs of the average American have changed considerably in emphasis. In the era during and immediately after the depression of the 1930's primary emphasis was placed on satisfying one's bodily needs and on survival. A lot of physical and emotional energy was spent getting a job, making ends meet, and adding to or replacing one's possessions. This sense of insecurity persisted for most Americans throughout World War II. It was only in the growing affluence of the postwar period that the emphasis slowly shifted from safety and survival to a broader acknowledgment of social values, the need for status, and more recently, a strong sense of individual potential which can be actualized to an ever-increasing degree.

PROTRACTED SURVIVAL

The economic, education, and technological forces which spawned this change have also produced an extended life expectancy, superior remedies, and more sophisticated surgical techniques which have generated in modern man a stronger hope of protracted personal survival. At the same time, a growing concern and heightened dissatisfaction with ailments and physical disabilities has become apparent.

Among the par values or maintenance factors of our society today must surely be included good health and long life. For this reason the potential dissatisfaction of the individual with anything that threatens these rights is correspondingly greater. Evidence of this can be found in increasing preoccupation with health, diet, exercise, and all matters affecting one's physical well being. This is understandably heightened by the mirror-affect of mass communications, presenting health problems in highly dramatic form.

EXPECTATIONS VS. REALITIES

Concomitantly, expectations of people regarding medical services and what these can and cannot accomplish are exaggerated, and the opportunity for potential dissatisfaction greatly increased. In contrast, attitudes of patients to hospital care in less highly developed societies than ours is less demanding and considerably more permissive. In many parts of the world patients cheerfully put up with conditions that would be regarded as intolerable in any U.S. or Canadian hospital.

Seen in this light, the cool, clinical detachment of many nurses does little to provide the climate of reassurance so necessary to offset the disappointment of the individual at being confined to hospital in the first place. The proliferation of equipment, the various clinical routines and procedures to which he is required to submit, the preoccupation of the nursing staff with the mechanics of running a ward, all tend to heighten the patient's feeling of dissatisfaction with his condition.

THROUGH THE PATIENT'S EYES

Whatever his physical condition, his psychological need immediately is for adequate orientation in the new routine, a strong sense of recognition on the part of the nursing staff of his problems and their importance to him, an encouraging attitude toward the progress he makes, and an ability on the part of the nurse to see the minor objectives which he achieves through *his* eyes rather than on an absolute scale of patient achievement.

To do this adequately, minor achievements, such as eating solid food, taking a first step, sleeping through a night, etc., should all be given recognition in proportion to the patient's sense of their importance. Clearly, a nurse who is unhappy or dissatisfied with her position and is not adequately motivated will find it very difficult to develop the necessary empathy to produce this type of reaction.

THE NURSE

During the extensive period of training the nurse is required to undergo, major emphasis is placed on procedures, both diagnostic and therapeutic, knowledge of pharmacology, and other technical areas. Minor emphasis is placed on clinical psychology, with some insight into largely abnormal working of the human mind. She receives little formal training in normal human behavior, and even less in correct attitudes toward various types of patients. Supposedly, good common sense and the right type of personality will help her to improvise in the various situations which she will confront in the course of her nursing life. Even when formal training is given in this area, it unfortunately tends to take the form of a "how to be nice to patients" session and rarely explains in sufficient detail the important connection between mental attitudes and physical recuperation.

Small wonder, then, that the hardened professional tends a few years after school to classify patients into two groups: "good" patients, meaning those who make no demands outside of regular routine, and "bad" patients, meaning those who externalize psychological needs that she is not ready or equipped to satisfy. If the demands of the latter become too oppressive, a nurse will typically refer the incident to her supervisor who, depending on her type of personality, either will seek to mollify the patient through some form of verbal therapy or will reinforce the rejection which the nurse has already exhibited.

LEARNING BY PRECEPT IS RARE

Nowhere in her training is the nurse told that the role of her supervisor is to lead and motivate her so that she, in turn, can lead and motivate the patient. She is not aware of the fact that avoidance of the conflict not only does not satisfy the patient's needs, but unfortunately lessens her ability to cope with more demanding situations. If she is fortunate enough to have a supervisor with natural leadership and motivation ability, she may learn by example, but rarely will she learn by precept. Were her supervisor adequately trained in the management side of her responsibilities, she could undoubtedly anticipate a lot of the problems that nurses—particularly younger nurses and trainees—run into, and through adequate training set up a program of preventative psychological maintenance that would solve problems before they occur.

That this is not just an idle speculation was amply demonstrated in a recent two-and-a-half year study at Yale–New Haven Hospital in Connecticut, as reported in the June 20, 1969, issue of *Time* magazine. The study, under the direction of a New York psychiatrist, attempted to determine changes in attitude on the part of the nursing staff toward terminal cancer patients.

TREATING PATIENTS IN A REALISTIC MANNER

In describing the attitudes of the nurses, the article notes, "As custodians of terminal cases, nurses bear particularly heavy burdens. The girls show a tough and cold exterior—an attitude quickly acquired in hospital service." Under the psychiatrist's direction, the nurses were convinced of the importance of their task, and were asked to treat the patients in a much more realistic manner.

The success of the experiment perhaps is best summed up in the concluding works of the article: "With life rapidly slipping from her, an old Italian woman called to a nurse one day. 'It is the end, isn't it?' she asked. The nurse nodded, sat next to the old woman and held her hand. 'I don't want die alone,' the old woman said. 'You won't be alone,' the nurse replied. Ten minutes later, the old woman's labored breathing stopped, with the nurse still holding her hand."

THE NURSING SUPERVISOR

As the lowest level of hospital management, the nursing supervisor must engage in certain technical activities and provide some management functions. Among the latter, elementary planning and control and a high degree of leading and motivating skill are undoubtedly required. While new systems and procedures have placed heavy emphasis on the former, unfortunately her responsibilities in the latter area are often neglected. In order to act as an effective leader, she must know how to make logical decisions, how to communicate them effectively to her subordinates, and how to motivate her subordinates so that they in turn may obtain both personal satisfaction from their work and at the same time create an effective climate of motivation and cooperation with their patients.

This can generally be accomplished by some form of supervisory training that would adequately convey to supervisors the notion that part of their responsibility includes getting results through others. If the experience of management outside the hospital field holds true, this can prove to be one of the most valuable training investments a company or a hospital could make.

However, applying the domino aspect of motivation theory, if the supervisor is not herself adequately motivated by her immediate superior, the chances of her being able to pass this on to her subordinates is somewhat remote. It is necessary to set up an adequate instructional program throughout all levels of hospital management, so that the importance of motivation cannot only be preached, but effectively practiced.

THE HOSPITAL ADMINISTRATOR

In the evolution of modern management, as described in *Management Today,* in the spring, 1969, issue of this journal, emphasis has shifted from the autocratic to the supportive role, or from a posture of reacting to problems as they occur to an ability to anticipate problems before they arise. The change is similar from one of fighting fires by whatever means to installing a sprinkler system, so that when the fire occurs, it will automatically be extinguished.

The modern hospital administrator is called on to combine two seemingly impossible tasks. On the one hand, he must create a climate within which people can achieve their own personal objectives and, at the same time, he must also seek through them to achieve the economic objectives of the institution he manages. To accomplish the latter he must carefully predetermine what people are going to do, and have them do it in the most efficient manner possible. To accomplish the former, he must permit them enough freedom in working toward their part of the economic objectives of the institution so that they can find personal satisfaction in their work. Fortunately modern management planning systems, such as those built around management objectives permit him to overcome the apparent incompatibility.

MUST DETERMINE COMMITMENTS

As a professional manager, the hospital administrator must determine the economic, functional, service, and patient commitments of the hospital. He must communicate them effectively to all levels of supervision, and, through them, to the nursing staff. At the same time, he must create the necessary motivational climate so that all levels, depending as they do on the level above, and ultimately on him, can find the necessary freedom and self-determination to obtain maximum satisfaction from the work that they perform.

If all employees understand the intimate connection between profitability and patient satisfaction, the hospital will not only survive, but will have an opportunity to grow and expand its services to satisfy both the needs of patients today and the more demanding and complex needs of patients tomorrow.

FURTHER READINGS SUGGESTED BY THE AUTHOR

Argyris, Chris. *Personality and Organization.* (New York: Harper & Rowe, 1957).

Gellerman, Saul W. *Motivation and Productivity.* (New York: American Management Association, 1963).

Herzberg, Frederick, Bernard Mauser, and Barbara Synderman. *The Motivation to Work.* (New York: John Wiley & Sons, Inc., 1960).

Katz, Daniel. "The Motivational Basis of Organizational Behavior," *Behavioral Science,* April, 1964

Supervision and Leadership

The topics of supervision and leadership are presented in this section. Supervision and leadership are two essential elements inherent within the directing of personnel. Along with motivation and communication, leadership is a method utilized in gaining the voluntary cooperation of employees. Supervision, on the other hand, consists of the specific supervisory actions related to allocating, delegating, and controlling work activities.

Leadership, in *EFFECTIVE SUPERVISION REQUIRES LEADERSHIP,* is presented as a process of obtaining voluntary cooperation from others. The Democratic, Mature Autocrat, and Bureaucratic leadership styles are presented along with the many supervisory styles.

One of the causes of ineffective supervision is presented in *WHY SUPERVISORS HAVE SPLIT PERSONALITIES.* Since various hospital jobs lack clear definition, supervisors are not sure of their duties. The case of upward promotion to a supervisory position is presented as one where the distinction in duties may not be clear. Various suggestions such as development are offered for improving the supervisor's skills.

Cooperation and coordination are presented as two indispensable managerial processes necessary for effective hospital management. In *VOLUNTARY COOPERA- TION AND COORDINATION: REQUISITES FOR EFFECTIVE HOSPITAL AD- MINISTRATION,* voluntary cooperation is presented as resulting from leadership and facilitated by two-way communication. Coordination is described as resulting from organization and yields the orderly arrangement of group effort. In addition, suggestions are made for enhancing both voluntary cooperation and coordination within the hospital organization.

Effective Supervision
Requires Leadership

THOMAS R. O'DONOVAN, Ph.D.

Thomas R. O'Donovan, Ph.D., is Administrator of Mount Carmel Mercy Hospital in Detroit, Michigan.

The concept of leadership refers to a process in which an individual is able to obtain voluntary cooperation in a goal or activity from another person or group of persons. Managers and supervisors who possess formal delegated authority in an organization become more effective when their style of leadership brings forth willful cooperation from their subordinates. This article will discuss some of the ways the supervisor can obtain the full support of his team. A major goal of any hospital is to provide a high level of patient care. Such care is administered by people. Therefore, supervision of these people is vitally important to the achievement of hospital goals. Without leadership, the supervisor's ability to obtain willful cooperation from his subordinates is impossible.

KINDS OF LEADERSHIP

The style of leadership that a supervisor should adopt depends upon a great many factors. His own personal goals and values, the character and goals of the organization, the type of subordinates involved, and the particular situation all will influence the choice of a particular leadership style. Each situation has to be considered on its own merit; however, some general statements can be made that are highly useful. Principles of leadership, like vitamins, are useful only when they are used correctly, and adaptation must be made to the individual situation. What is correct in one case may not be correct in another. A "correct" leadership style is important because of its effects on employe morale and productivity.

An improper leadership style may result in:

a. A lowering of employe morale and motivation because of oversupervision (sometimes referred to as "snoopervision"), overly strict or distant supervision, etc. Management is interested in employe morale not only because of a humanistic concern for the employe's wellbeing but also because of its effects on employe productivity.

b.   A lowering of employe productivity. This may be a decrease in either quantity or quality of employe work output per given unit of input. In a hospital for example, lower employe productivity would be reflected in a lower quality of patient care, increasing expenses, and waste.

c.   Increased employe absenteeism and turnover.

d.   Employe resistance to change.

e.   A decrease in the individual development of employes.

We shall identify six major question areas and give the implications for each area: 1. Shall I supervise my subordinates very closely by keeping tabs on every detail or shall I supervise them only in a general way? 2. As a supervisor, should I attempt to identify with my subordinates or with my superiors? 3. In the management of subordinates, should I tend to be distant toward them or friendly? 4. Should I be strict or lenient in supervision? 5. Should I tend to be "person-centered" in my leadership style or "work-centered?" 6. Which of the following specific leadership styles works best and under what conditions: the mature autocratic, the democratic, or the bureaucratic?

CLOSE VERSUS
GENERAL SUPERVISION

Whether or not we should supervise subordinates very closely or in a general way depends upon a large number of variables. Unskilled or clerical jobs tend to require closer supervision than professional or managerial jobs. For example, maids and porters generally need closer supervision than medical secretaries and nurses. Supervision of unskilled or clerical jobs is typically related to actual job performance while supervision of the professional or managerial employe is related more to the checking of results. If an employe has been trusted in the past to do a good job, a supervisor would be grossly unfair if he did not demonstrate his trust appropriately.

New employes may require closer supervision than employes who have been on the job for a long period of time. This point may seem self-evident, but we must be quite careful not to give the impression that this temporary closeness of supervision is merely a "taste" of what is to come.

Close supervision is important in emergency situations. In a highly critical situation, it may be neccessary to give very specific instructions and follow every detail very closely. For example, in our orbital flights, the top officials of the National Aeronautics and Space Administration watch details very closely because small errors can cause complete disaster. The surgeon-nurse supervisory relationship during an operation is another example.

In general, people who have an optimistic view of how well their subordinates will perform tend to supervise in a general way, while the more pessimistic supervisors who feel that they cannot trust their employes to do an honest or accurate job will tend to watch things in closer detail. Obviously, if supervision is *too* general, control over results is reduced and serious error may creep in before it is possible to determine the problem. In most organizations, however, there is a tendency to supervise too closely rather than not close enough. The problem for the supervisor is one of striking a happy medium.

Several studies are available in the research literature that provide useful information regarding the second question. The Prudential Insurance Company Study[1] of office employes examined the productivity of work groups under supervisors who had different patterns of identification. The first group of supervisors tended to identify more with subordinates than with higher management. The results of the study showed that productivity was higher in the group in which the supervisors tended to identify more with the subordinates than with upper management. A similar study of foremen was performed at General Electric Company.[2] Here the findings were quite similar. The foremen in high-producing areas tended to identify more with their subordinates than with upper management.

Certain people, in interpreting these findings, point out that it is not a question of *which* group one should identify with, but *how* much identification should be made with each group. In other words, it is important to identify with both groups. The workers who report to a superior must trust him and respect his willingness to support them. At the same time, management must depend upon the supervisor to carry out established policies. Obviously, this situation can create conflict in the supervisory role. The superior is literally the "man-in-the-middle." It is up to him to determine the best course of action for his particular situation. The most that can be said is that there is no firm answer as to which group should be identified with the most. It depends upon the individual situation.

Nonetheless, the supervisor must occupy a different role than the worker, although a lack of organizational resources may make this impossible in certain temporary situations. The supervisor who plays a different role does not perform the same functions as rank and file workers, but assumes more of the functions traditionally associated with leadership. Research studies of clerical workers, railroad workers, and workers in heavy industry point out that supervisors with the better production records gave a larger proportion of their time to supervisory functions, especially to the interpersonal aspect of their jobs. The supervisors of the lower producing sections were more likely to spend their time in tasks which the men themselves were performing or in the paperwork aspect of their jobs.

DISTANT SUPERVISION?
FRIENDLY SUPERVISION?

Whether or not a supervisor should be distant or friendly with his subordinates is another question which cannot be answered easily one way or the other. One should be distant enough to retain the respect of his subordinates, yet friendly enough so that he can work well with them as a team. In the military service, officers are instructed not to become too involved in the personal lives of their troops. This is especially true in war time. In corporate management a military type of organization is seldom needed, but there is much to be learned from the military experience. If one is too friendly with subordinates, it may prevent him from disciplining an employe when discipline is warranted, or from organizing and structuring work activity. On the other hand, a too distant attitude may be interpreted by the employe as a lack of interest in him as an individual, with resultant lower employe morale. The supervisor again has to draw a happy medium, depending upon the particular situation.

STRICT SUPERVISION?
LENIENT SUPERVISION?

Douglas McGregor[3] provides us with a solid analysis of the role of supervision with regard to strictness versus leniency. He suggests that there are two major parts in the leadership process. The supervisor must have a warm, genuine human concern for the well-being of his subordinates and at the *same* time, he must require and maintain a high standard of performance. He suggests that the supervisor must be fair with his subordinates but at the same time he must be firm. If the supervisor does not require a strict standard of performance, then both performance and respect will tend to degenerate. If the supervisor is too wishy-washy, he cannot command the respect that is needed. The important thing is that these two behavior patterns must co-exist. If we are firm but not fair, we tend to lose the cooperation of the group. If we are fair but not firm enough, we lose control of the group.

PERSON-CENTERED?
WORK-CENTERED?

The issue of being "person-centered" rather than being "work-centered" refers to the following: the "person-centered" supervisor tends to look toward the individual human being as the center of the productivity wheel. He interprets his job as one of increasing employe motivation. A supervisor who is "work-centered" tends to ignore the human factor and concentrates on the production and technical aspects of the job. The "work-centered" supervisor thinks of his employes as cogs in the wheel of production.

Many studies have shown that the "person-centered" supervisor is far more effective than the "work-centered" supervisor.[4] Employe productivity and morale tend to be much higher when the supervisor is "person-centered." Many supervisors are work-oriented because their experiences have been heavily weighted this way. They have been trained to make things or to perform things. They were trained to accomplish the work that they are now delegating. For this reason, when confronted with a work problem, some supervisors who have this tendency will look around the problem involved to the work itself in searching for the cause. If the problem is with the people involved, it may be completely overlooked.

Several years ago, the Survey Research Center of the University of Michigan[5] studied the leadership and production aspects of a large number of clerical departments of the Prudential Life Insurance Company. Many sections of this company had comparable working conditions. The clerical work output was measurable and it was possible to relate production records to various kinds of supervisory practices. One finding of the study was that approximately 85 per cent of the supervisors in the high-producing groups were "employe-centered" whereas only 30 per cent of the supervisors in the low-producing groups were "employe-centered."

This last section will describe three different leadership styles and discuss briefly their implications. These approaches were adapted from the writings of Eugene E. Jennings.[6]

THE DEMOCRATIC APPROACH

The democratic supervisor looks to the group for direction. He values the group above himself and above the organization. He caters to the group's wishes and desires. He tends to knit his group into a harmonious team, so that the resultant cohesion disguises who is actually running things. Rather than making himself indispensable, his primary goal is to develop subordinates so that he becomes almost unnecessary. The democratic supervisor seeks, therefore, to involve every member in determining group activities and objectives. He is more interested in group competency than in his individual competency.

In its extreme form, this is the description of the "democratic" supervisor. Perhaps no supervisor is this way all the time. Most will vary their pattern to fit the situation and they must do this to be effective. The majority of supervisors agree that they should be democratic and seek the participation of subordinates. What if time and circumstances do not permit? Some subordinates do not wish to share in many decisions. People change, both as supervisors and as subordinates.

One can appraise himself and fellow supervisors, but will be unable to classify each supervisor as democratic, mature autocratic, or bureaucratic. Most supervisors attempt to adjust their behavior pattern as needed. The better supervisors know how to adjust to the needs of their subordinates. However, we do tend to lean toward one model more than to any other and constant shifting of gears is no easy task.

THE MATURE AUTOCRAT

The mature autocrat is not the ruthless autocrat that existed in the "captains of industry" era. Reference is not had here to the complete "one-man show" style of leadership although this is one of the styles available to supervisors. The mature autocrat is the supervisor who wants to run with the ball but, at the same time, wants to make the team feel needed. The mature autocrat is a highly competent individual and an excellent decision-maker. He controls individually and uses personal influence. He is a decision-maker but he works through and with people. The mature autocrat is highly polished while the typical stereotype of the autocrat tends to be very crude.

The most important quality that the mature autocrat should possess is sincerity. This means that the mature autocrat makes up his mind and then works with the group in such a way that they come up with the same decision. Thus, when the decision is implemented, group members feel they have played a significant role. If, however, a supervisor attempted to use this leadership style and was insincere, then the entire model and perhaps the entire work group organization would likely split wide open. Mature autocracy and insincerity are incompatible. If at any time, the group does *not* come up with the same decision as the mature autocratic supervisor, he must either successfully show why the group's decision cannot be implemented (i.e., due to top management policy), or he must accept the group's decision. Thus, the mature autocrat doesn't "get his way" all the time and does not expect to. His major skill is in his ability to predict the group's reactions.

THE BUREAUCRAT

The bureaucrat does not recognize the individual or the group as much as the organization. He is a system-builder and places his faith in the ultimate perfectability of that system. This supervisor allows no violation of rules and procedures under any circumstances. If violation occurs, disciplinary action follows immediately. He wants every potential situation covered in a procedures manual so that individual judgment becomes unnecessary. This is a brief description of the bureaucratic model of leadership as viewed in its extreme form.

Managers today are tending more toward the bureaucratic leadership style than toward the mature autocratic or the democratic style. The aggressive attitude of the autocrat assures the enterprise of periodic rejuvenation and is largely the reason why our business system in the past has maintained its healthy vigor. As businesses increase in complexity, the importance of a bureaucratic structure becomes increasingly important. However, at the same time that bureaucrats replace autocrats, the essential creativity of our business system may be subjected to considerable dilution. The organization cannot become too engulfed in excessive rules and regulations. What the organization requires is a style of supervisory leadership that is a balance of the bureaucratic, the autocratic, and the democratic approaches—the *multicrat.*

CONCLUSION

As can be readily seen, most of the major areas discussed overlap closely.[7] A supervisor who is distant may also be strict. A supervisor who identifies with superiors may be somewhat distant. Each of these major subject areas that have been examined should be integrated with the others in order to establish the kind of leadership style that each supervisor would look forward to shaping for himself. These things have to follow in a natural way. A leadership role cannot be turned off and on like a faucet. The integration of a leadership style depends on individual philosophy and values, individual opinions, and individual attitudes toward people. A successful supervisor is a product of his team.

The choice of a leadership pattern is usually quite limited because of the factors listed at the beginning of this article. Certainly one limiting factor is the style of leadership exhibited by the supervisor's supervisor. The supervisor can, however, look ahead months or years to strategically determine at which point on the continuum he will act. This point will vary with the objectives he wishes to accomplish, his own personality and values, the characteristics of the situation.

There is no *one* leadership style correct for all supervisors at all times and in all places. This does not mean, however, that leadership cannot be scientifically examined. When the *total* situation has been carefully examined, a correct and satisfying pattern of leadership can be developed. Leadership is an art built upon scientific inquiry. We must be ourselves but at the same time, we must understand and watch ourselves. Supervision requires "super-vision."

REFERENCES

[1] Morse, Nancy C., *Satisfactions in White Collar Jobs.* Ann Arbor, Survey Research Centers, University of Michigan, 1953.

[2] Ponder, Quentin D., "The Effective Manufacturing Foreman," in *Proceedings of the Tenth Annual Meeting.* Madison, Wis., Industrial Relations Research Association, 1957, pp. 51-54; General Electric Company, Public and Employee Relations Research Service, *The Effective Manufacturing Foreman* (processed 1957).

[3] McGregor, Douglas, *The Human Side of Enterprise.* New York, McGraw-Hill Book Co., Inc., 1959.

[4] Cartwright, Dorwin and Zander, Alvin. eds., *Group Dynamics,* Evanston, Ill., Row, Peterson, 1953.

[5] Kahn, Robert L. and Katz, Daniel, "Leadership Practices in Relationship to Productivity and Morale," *Group Dynamics.* Dorwin Cartwright and Alvin Zander, eds., Evanston, Ill., Row, Peterson, 1953, pp. 612-628.

[6] Jennings, Eugene E., *The Executive.* New York, Harper, 1962.

[7] Jennings, Eugene E., *An Anatomy of Leadership,* New York, Harper, 1960.

Why Supervisors have Split Personalities

PAUL J. GORDON, PH.D.

Paul J. Gordon, Ph.D., is a Professor of Management at Indiana University.

How many readers can identify the existence of these situations in their own hospitals?

The executive housekeeper who goes about the hospital picking up after the maids.

The engineer who makes all the repairs himself while his employes hand him tools and run errands.

The head nurse who ignores the working relationships among the nurses, the aides and the maids to spend her time in arranging a meticulous linen closet.

The head dietitian who spends her time in ruling up blank forms, on which she records in longhand every menu and time schedules for all her employes, while employes work without adequate supervision.

The head laboratory technician who performs many routine tests herself because "employes cannot be relied upon to produce accurate results."

The laundry manager who spends most of his time on production records and machine maintenance, and frankly resents the efforts of employes to upset the "efficiency" that he has planned for all mechanical aspects of the laundry operation.

SURVEY SHOWS NEED

While many supervisors are able technicians, office workers or manual workers, a survey of three up-state New York hospitals recently completed by the New York State School of Industrial and Labor Relations in cooperation with the Central New York Regional Hospital Council, Inc., revealed that supervisory personnel in the hospitals studied wanted more information and a clearer definition of their own responsibilities concerning administrative and personnel matters. Some of these supervisors quite frankly raised such questions as:

"What is my job? Am I supposed to do the work, to supervise exclusively, or both? . . . I am trained to conduct highly technical research; (or I attended professional courses in dietetics, or library work); (or I can do more work, and tell better if work is done right than any member of my staff). . . . I know very little about personnel. . . . There isn't much planning here—we're busy—all the time—act as needed—don't have time for records."

Based on the evidence of the survey the conclusion can be drawn that the job of a supervisor in a hospital lacks definition. This does not mean that hospitals are unique in this regard. Many industries find difficulty in defining the extent and the limits of supervisory responsibility.

For the purpose of this article the term "supervisor" is used to include hospital supervisory personnel at all levels. Thus the term "supervisor" would include the administrator, the assistant administrator, department heads, supervising nurses, head nurses—any person in any department who directs the effort of other employes at work, especially if the supervisor is responsible for their work and responsible for administering personnel policies affecting other employes.

The conflicts in regard to understanding of their own responsibilities that now exist in the minds of supervisors who are trying their best to do a good job may be evident in these statements which are representative although not exact quotations:

The people in this department take up so much of my time with their personal problems, their personal disputes, and their requests for job instruction that little time is left for my own important work of making out records on their production.

My assistants just don't know how to supervise the employes. In addition to making out work schedules, time records, and all the other clerical work that I must do myself, I have to be out of the office supervising the work a good part of the day.

Training people in this department takes up so much of my time that I have to continue my own specialized work after hours. I can direct the others and I think I do a good job, but I am much happier working with a small group where I can work too.

These sentiments reveal a wish among some supervisors to withdraw from the difficult responsibility of supervising people, for which they may not be trained, and a wish to spend more time on the technical, manual or clerical work for which they are trained. If the supervisor is not trained in personnel work, he may derive more sense of personal security and tangible accomplishment in doing the work for which he has been especially trained.

THEY CAN'T DO BOTH

When supervisors try to spend a major portion of their own time performing work that they should assign to other people and should supervise, they operate below their proper level; effective supervision is stymied and the hospital pays more money to have work done.

This conflict, between the wish to perform work and the duty to supervise employes, can be strong and can result in unnecessary tension and fatigue among supervisors.

The supervisor's interest in continued exercise of the professional skills is, at times, entirely a personal pursuit influenced by a strong professional tradition in hospitals, striving for status through specialization of personal skills. Unfortunately, at other times the burden of dual responsibility, to supervise and to perform, may be imposed by the hospital as a make-shift arrangement awaiting relief.

If the department or section activities are such that its supervisor must perform as expert technician, and must also supervise, steps should be taken to assist the supervisor. A place to start might be with analysis of the supervisor's job. Eliminate from the job those items that do not require the supervisor's training or that cause him to operate at the worker level. This step can free time for supervision and can reduce hospital costs by having the work done at less money per hour. The hospital might also supply, or use more effectively, assistance for the supervisor on clerical work.

If the department is large and the work is sufficiently technical, two people at the supervisory level might be justified: one for the assignments that require technical training and one for administrative direction of the department.

As a result of thorough study of each supervisor's job, a new concept of the supervisor's job, or a better defined concept of the supervisor's job, should be developed. That concept should emphasize that supervisors get work done through other people; that the supervisor is a leader rather than a technician, and that leaders direct and develop followers.

FROM WORKER TO SUPERVISOR

Outside the professionally trained supervisor group, as well as within this group, both the individuals and the hospital have sometimes failed to appreciate the tremendous step, the learning process, and the emotional adjustment involved when a performer of work becomes a supervisor of people. The skilled operator ceases to perform and delegates with reluctance. The conscientious producer accepts responsibility for another's results, with inner turmoil, because the job may not be done just as thoroughly and accurately as he believes he would do it. The skilled craftsman, proud of his tools and his knowledge of what they can do, stores them away with some measure of regret to accept as his new tools subordinates, whose qualities, values and uses he has not tested.

The man who becomes a supervisor increases his capacity and makes a sacrifice to do it. The price he pays is to give up the pride and the dignity of his own craftsmanship in order to accept greater volume from others, even though the new results may contain flaws in his more critical view.

The attitudes, the knowledge and the skills required of the supervisor include a range quite different from those of the worker. The shift in emphasis is away from the professional and technical skills and toward the administrative and the social skills. The capacities of the supervisor in areas of personnel and human relations are not less important than his professional and technical qualifications.

In hospitals, the contrary view has often been expressed as a matter of tradition. According to hospital supervisors, the emphasis has been on training in the healing arts and training for a technical profession, not on training for administration and supervising subordinates.

Where the potential or present supervisor lacks training in the supervision of personnel, he needs help, needs development, needs training in order to master the new job. Where consistency of administrative philosophy and practice is desired throughout the hospital, the individual supervisor needs guidance on what constitutes a personnel area wherein consistency is desirable, and what remains as an area wherein the exercise of personal discretion might produce better results.

Guidance for the department head and the line supervisor in matters of personnel administration may be one of the most necessary and most rewarding personnel activities that hospitals can undertake in order to improve patient care through improved internal administration.

At the October 1951 conference on "Effective Utilization of Hospital Employes," held at Cornell, the concensus of a group of 30 administrators and department heads seemed to be that hospitals are aware of *what* they need in personnel administration, but that progress may be retarded because of insufficient knowledge on *where* and *how* to start. If the foregoing is true, then a recommendation for supervisory development on personnel matters will have relatively little value, unless some specific areas for development are outlined.

Records of the interviews in three hospitals with 44 supervisors have been analyzed and, based on these interviews, the supervisors appear to be concerned about or to want more information on the following matters:

1. Clarification of organization structure
2. Analysis and specification of job content at all levels
3. Definition of the supervisor's job
4. Better utilization of supervisory time
5. Better utilization of the services of hospital employes
6. Improved communication among and within departments
7. The importance of factors of tradition and status in the hospital field
8. Need for written personnel policies
9. Need for procedures to implement policies
10. Need for adequate records and systematic analysis of personnel practices
11. Analysis and reduction of turnover and absenteeism
12. Induction and orientation of new employes
13. Job instruction and on-the-job training
14. Improvement of work hours and work schedules
15. Wages and salaries for employes and supervisory personnel
16. Personal recognition and participation for employes and supervisors
17. Information on group leadership and discussion leadership
18. Information on interviewing and employe counseling

Any item which appears on the foregoing list has been mentioned by supervisors often enough and with sufficient force so that the list may provide a useful agenda in planning discussion for supervisory meetings or in planning for a program of supervisory development in hospitals beyond those surveyed.

Even though the listing of problem areas constitutes the judgment of supervisors themselves and not the judgment of the survey team, the list is substantiated by the school's experience in conducting programs for diverse groups of hospital people wherein the same problems were mentioned in conference discussions.

APPROACHES TO DEVELOPMENT

Approaches and methods can be as important as subject matter in deciding the reception and the success of such a program among supervisors.

Many industrial experts in the field of executive and supervisory development advise against the word "training" applied to a supervisory program. People who have held supervisory positions for some time resist "training" or "going to school" in order to learn a job that they have been doing for five, 10 or 20 years. They may resist the teacher-pupil or the lecturer-listener relationship.

Also, "training" seems to imply a formal program or classroom situation, whereas the approaches to supervisory development are many. Probably some of the best supervisory development takes place in the day-to-day work environment.

Some of many possible means and aids to supervisory development that might be practicable in the hospitals studied include:

1.   Involvement of supervisors in discussion of personnel problems, needs and the handling of specific personnel situations.

2.   Involvement of supervisors in personnel policy discussions and policy development.

3.   Supervisory conferences directed toward the production of a supervisor's policy manual.

4.   Preparation and distribution of printed personnel policies, if not developed by supervisors, then at least subject to their genuine criticism and acceptance before policies are established.

5.   Constant review and recommendation for improvement of personnel policies and personnel procedures on the part of supervisors.

6.   Periodic consultation among superior and subordinate supervisors on the administration of personnel policies and the current status or progress on specific personnel problems.

7.   Initiation of supervisory seminars for general education in approaches to personnel administration and personnel problems.

8.   Initiation of discussion clinics on the handling of day-to-day interdepartmental and intradepartmental relationships.

9.   Availability of a competent, professional full-time staff adviser and coordinator on personnel matters in the hospital whose principal duties in this specialized area are not lowered in priority by the assignment of other duties.

10.   Availability of such qualified person to serve in a consulting relationship to more than one hospital, through cooperation among hospitals, or through the offices of a regional hospital council.

These suggestions are offered to stimulate further thought on the need for supervisory development and some possible approaches, either along with or apart from a formal program as such.

Ideally, supervisory development should take place throughout the hospital from top to bottom and across all departments. During the experimental phases, meetings might be limited to a top management group or to particular departments until a workable approach is decided on. Later, the program may be extended and continuous follow-up and evaluation will be required to make the program worth while.

Voluntary Cooperation and Coordination: Requisites for Effective Hospital Administration

OWEN B. HARDY

Owen B. Hardy is Vice President of Gordon A. Friesen International, Inc. - health care consultants - in Washington, D. C.

The noted philosopher, Jacques Barzun, now at Columbia University, recently stated that the general hospital is one of man's most complex organized efforts to date.[1] This observation is undoubtedly true. The distinct and separate departments of most modern general hospitals number from ten to twenty, and additional services demanding the best in both technical and managerial skills are being added yearly.

All of these hospital departments have as their ultimate aim the successful attainment of the hospital's goals and objectives; these, too, are usually plural, embodying such aspects as care of the sick and injured; education of physicians, nurses, and other personnel; disease prevention; other public health functions; and research. Additionally, the hospital is a dynamic social institution, tied in a thousand ways to the community which supports it. Religious, political, economic, charitable, and personal interests are constantly influencing and sometimes impinging directly upon the operation of the hospital. Thus, the administrator is placed in the tediously exacting position of guiding and directing the efforts of the numerous departments toward the attainment of multiple goals in such a way as to satisfy the diverse interests which encompass him.

On the surface the task is a formidable one and, in truth, it is even more difficult than is readily apparent. For example, often the organization of the hospital will be structured in such a way as to put the medical staff beyond the pale of the administrator's power; auxiliary groups sometimes assume responsibility but desire to be loosely controlled; and independently contracting medical specialists sometimes

[1] Telephone interview with Jacques Barzun at Columbia University, New York City, November 3, 1965.

circumvent the administrator through direct negotiations with the governing board. There is also great likelihood that in some hospitals the de facto locus of power may not rest in the office of the administrator.

Considering these many factors, the statistical possibility of the administrator achieving maximum success (even if this tenuous term could be defined or measured) would seem to be well-nigh zero.

SUB-PROCESSES OF MANAGEMENT

In an enterprise of this complexity, where functions are both myriad and diverse and where the authority actually possessed by the administrator may not be commensurate with the duties and obligations ordinarily considered inherent in the position, the usual emphasis and balance accorded the various elements of management in industry and other organizational entities may not be the optimum. Without a doubt, the entire spectrum of managerial processes is both useful and necessary in the operation of hospitals; however, due to the unique role of these institutions and their singular organizational structure, two sub-processes of management which have been recognized as of great importance to all managers may be considered particularly indispensable for the use of the hospital administrator. These two sub-processes, the one usually identified as a function of leadership and the other a part of organization, are voluntary cooperation and voluntary coordination, respectively. Of course, those authorities who consider coordination as a separate process of management identify that coordination which occurs voluntarily as a sub-process of the broader term. These two sub-processes are sometimes confused, but a distinct difference exists between them; this difference is somewhat apparent from the terminology used for their identification.

Newman and Summer define voluntary cooperation as being predominantly an emotional response, wherein there takes place willing and enthusiastic participation in carrying out plans and striving toward organizational objectives.[2] These authors also maintain, as do most authorities, that the response is developed through effective leadership. It would seem, then, that voluntary cooperation should be dependent to a significant extent upon two-way vertical communication, and a search of the literature reveals that the weight of authoritative opinion is in concurrence with this view.

INTERPERSONAL, HORIZONTAL RELATIONSHIPS

On the other hand, in the words of Mooney, coordination deals with "the orderly arrangement of group effort to provide unity of action in the pursuit of a common purpose."[3] It follows, of course, that voluntary coordination would include those synchronizing and unifying actions which are not brought about through supervision or control, or even primarily by reason of the proper structuring of the organization,

---

[2] William H. Newman and Charles E. Summer, Jr., *The Process of Management* (Englewood Cliffs, N.J.: Prentice-Hall, Inc., 1964), p. 497.

[3] James D. Mooney, *The Principles of Organization* (New York: Harper and Bros., 1947), pp. 5-13.

but which are generated through interactions that are willingly and voluntarily undertaken. After reflection it can be seen that although voluntary cooperation and voluntary coordination differ in distinct respects, the former is undoubtedly the sine qua non for the latter. Most authorities, while recognizing the fact of coordination between superior and subordinate, are also in agreement with Mary Parker Follett's opinion that coordination, including voluntary coordination, is achieved in the main through interpersonal, horizontal relationships;[4] in short, it is achieved by means of horizontal communications.

Assuming that many hospital administrators might do well to employ these two sub-processes to the fullest advantage, an investigation of measures for consciously effecting them should prove beneficial.

If one accepts the thesis that appropriate leadership is the primary tool with which voluntary cooperation can be developed, the question arises as to the type of leadership most desirable for the purpose at hand. As regards eliciting a cooperative attitude among subordinates within an organizational hierarchy, Likert expresses a cogent view: "The leadership and other processes of the organization must be such as to ensure a maximum probability that in all interactions and all relationships with the organization each member will, in light of his background, values, and expectations, view the experience as supportive and one which builds and maintains his sense of personal worth and importance."[5] Autocratic leadership is thus rejected, and supportive leadership is cited as begetting the response most desired. Further, the connotation is explicit that for leadership to be perceived as supportive by the subordinate, the individual's need system must be satisfied to the extent that experiences build and maintain a sense of personal worth and importance. Inasmuch as the designation of a sense of personal worth and importance leaves unmentioned other needs, as identified by Maslow,[6] that may be possibly dominant to the individual Likert might well have added to his statement "as well as contributing to the satisfaction of other motivating needs."

LONG-RANGE BEHAVIORAL CHARACTERISTICS

In order to provide the supportive leadership to which Likert refers, the hospital administrator must develop within himself certain attitudes, and these attitudes must be reflected clearly in his interpersonal relations with his subordinates and in the behavioral image he presents within the role assigned to him. Although each subordinate with whom the administrator interacts regularly within the frame of the leader-subordinate relationship must be evaluated and dealt with on the basis of individual characteristics, to some extent, demands on the administrator's limited time usually preclude attempts to analyze the many facets of each individual's personality or to serve the numerous specific needs of all immediate subordinates. In fact, such

[4] H. C. Metcalf and Lyndall F. Urwick (eds.), *Dynamic Administration: The Collected Papers of Mary Parker Follett* (New York: Harper and Bros., 1941), pp. 297 ff.

[5] Rensis Likert, *New Patterns of Management* (New York: McGraw-Hill Book Co., 1961), p. 103.

[6] A. H. Maslow, Reading 2-1 in Timothy W. Costello and Sheldon S. Zalkind (eds.), *Pyschology in Administration* (Englewood Cliffs, N.J.: Prentice-Hall, Inc., 1963), p. 60.

attempts are considered undesirable from the standpoint of creating excessive dependency and delving unnecessarily into private lives.[7] Instead, the administrator in his efforts to evoke voluntary cooperation should display those behavioral characteristics which are not hastily designed for the expediency of the moment, but which will carry through periods of adversity and wear well over a period of years.

Among these characteristics are fairness, objectivity, dignified but genuine friendliness, empathy, trust, and a supportiveness which allows adherence to reasonable standards of performance.[8] The administrator must avoid being picayunish concerning matters of minor importance; he should encourage self-reliance and emphasize and give praise to correct behavior as well as point to deficiencies. The philosophy of the law of the situation can be used with particular effectiveness in hospitals, where the lives of many people are literally held in trust.

TWO-WAY COMMUNICATION ESSENTIAL

There are opinions that the only occasions in which participation in decision making is warranted are those when better decisions will be forthcoming.[9] In this modern age, however, when one considers that the physiological, safety, and social needs of almost all workers except the unskilled are largely met, other needs may well have to be employed as motivators. Most authorities agree that participation in decision making arouses egoistic needs which, in turn, function as motivators toward voluntary cooperation in the attainment of objectives. For example, the most successful work simplification programs in hospitals have been those where department heads were genuinely and responsibly involved in the establishment of the program's policies and in the implementation of its methodology.

Effective two-way communication is, of course, essential, and the art of listening has not been overemphasized. For voluntary cooperation to become a reality, the administrator's leadership must generate confidence and trust in the subordinate, and this result will not be possible where there is an absence of ample opportunity for feedback in the form of both positive and negative reactions.

The foregoing has focused only on winning voluntary cooperation from subordinates. However, as has been indicated, groups and individuals such as the medical staff, individuals under independent contract, auxiliary organizations, and others over whom the administrator possesses little or no authority must also cooperate willingly or his efforts will remain largely sterile. Where his office possesses a minimum of authority in relation to these elements, leadership arising solely from influence would appear to be the principal means whereby the administrator may elicit voluntary cooperation. Within this particular phase of the administrator's role, there are two factors which probably contribute more to the enhancement of influence reaching outside the direct chain of authority than any others. These are:

---

[7]Newman and Summer, *op. cit.,* p. 447.

[8]*Ibid.,* pp. 501-8.

[9]*Ibid.,* p. 509.

TWO IMPORTANT FACTORS

1.   The status accorded the administrator by the governing board: If the board regards the administrator as the chief executive officer of the hospital, and through word and act exhibits this regard in an unequivocal manner, the influence emanating from the office will be substantial, provided the incumbent possesses the conceptual skill required for its proper use. Conversely, if the board delegates minimally and treats the administrator as merely a tool of necessity, his influence will be diluted to a considerable degree.

2.   The respect and status accorded the administrator by his subordinates: It can be seen easily that leadership which is effective in arousing voluntary cooperation from the members of the organizational hierarchy will indirectly produce influence effecting similar cooperation in both those who are loosely bound to the hierarchy and those who operate in a close relationship with it.

Other factors augmenting the administrator's ability to project his influence beyond his delegated authority include his diligence and skill in communicating, his possession of current and pertinent facts, the adequacy of his educational background, and purposeful personality—all will assist in awakening interests which subsequently evolve into cooperation.

A word of caution should be noted concerning the administrator's relationship with those over whom he exercises no command function. Sociological research, in studying somewhat similar relationships among members of volunteer groups, has isolated definite indications that the pressure to produce or to participate effectively (by inference, to cooperate) must come from sources regarded as "acceptable."[10] The administrator must wisely refrain from attempts to usurp power that he does not and cannot possess.

HOW TO GAIN ADDED COORDINATION

In organizations less complex than the general hospital, it is quite possible that objectives can be satisfactorily accomplished with small regard for voluntary coordination, for coordination can be achieved by skillful execution of the various processes of management. As Terry states: "Fundamentally, coordination should result from the effective execution of the management process. When the managerial work of planning, organizing, activating, and controlling are performed properly and adequate consideration is given to interrelatedness, the results should be an integrated, well balanced composite of efforts exerted by an informal and satisfied work group."[11]

Certainly the intent of this paper is not to impart the idea that hospitals should sacrifice any effort to coordinate by the appropriate application of the management processes; to the contrary, it should be emphasized that no managerial tool or technique ought to remain unconsidered in the effort to achieve coordination at its

---

[10] Likert, *op. cit.,* p. 145.

[11] George R. Terry, *Principles of Management* (Homewood, Ill.: Richard D. Irwin, Inc., 1964), pp. 161, 163.

best. The thesis here is simply that coordination which the administrator is able to generate by these classical and formal means may not be sufficient to harmonize and adapt effectively the necessary efforts and actions of the many diverse categories of people found either within the organizational hierarchy or at its periphery.

What other measures or devices are available to the administrator, then, for his use in achieving the added coordination which accrues through voluntary actions?

Since coordination is a function of communications, primarily lateral, it follows that the best communication systems and devices which can be designed and provided are highly desirable. In fact, as a prerequisite to any coordination, including that which is voluntary, it is believed that good systems of communication should stand first. Also, most authorities are agreed that voluntary coordination is facilitated and encouraged by those same processes described by Terry above— processes which when properly executed usually bring about what might be called formal coordination.

FOUR HELPFUL SUGGESTIONS

Beyond these means, however, the administrator with expertise can set the stage so that those whose best work contributions are necessary or desirable will voluntarily synchronize and direct their combined efforts toward the objectives of the hospital. The administrator may:

1.   Imbue both those under his leadership and within its fringe with a profound psychological commitment toward the institution's objectives. Objectives should be unified to the extent possible and dominant objective established.[12] Hospitals, with the altruistic and noble purpose of alleviating the ills of man, have a motivating appeal stronger perhaps than possessed by any other human enterprise. Those who become generally absorbed with this high purpose will recognize that a subordination of departmental and individual group interests must occur and that a total team effort is necessitated for maximum achievement of the dominating objective. Some modern-day spokesmen decry the use of a strong leadership through emotional appeal; however, when that appeal is not made to stir motivations which substitute for rightful individual needs and is for the more successful achievement of the best there is in our culture, no harm is done, and much good can be gained.

2.   Arrange and encourage face to face contacts among the key people of groups whose actions must be coordinated. Fayol, in recommending weekly department head meetings, recognized that there was no substitute in this regard for the verbal give and take which will occur when people are placed in conference.[13] Hesitancy is sometimes shown by the insecure administrator to hold frequent group meetings due to imagined threats to ego or authority. However, the administrator who is bent on highest efficiency will boldly use this aid to gain not only voluntary coordination but many other benefits as well. Prudent use can be made of standing committees, meeting on a scheduled basis, as well as of ad hoc committees for the accomplishment of specific short range goals.

[12]William H. Newman, *Administrative Action* (Englewood Cliffs, N.J.: Prentice-Hall, Inc., 1951), p. 399.

[13]Henri Fayol, *General and Industrial Management* (London: Sir Isaac Pitman & Sons, Ltd., 1961), p. 205.

3. Encourage group decision making. In selected instances where face to face contacts are arranged to provide opportunity for the free interchange of ideas and proposals, one step further can be taken—group decision making can be encouraged. Not only will voluntary cooperation be enhanced thereby, as previously cited, but voluntary coordination can also be developed through the ego-involvement of those making the decision.

4. Nurture and utilize the informal organization. No hospital is lacking in informal organizations, many of which cut across departmental lines and reach outside the organizational hierarchy. Their presence may be recognized, encouraged, and utilized for several purposes, not the least of which is voluntary coordination. Barnard recognized their value in producing this response when he described the organization as being formal when the activities of two or more persons are consciously coordinated toward a given objective, and as being informal when interpersonal relationships are without conscious joint purpose, even though producing common or joint results.[14] Further, informal organization is born and sustained among friends, and certainly those who maintain friendly relations will coordinate their efforts without compulsion much more readily than those who are near strangers.

Although informal organizations are based on emotions and can be highly irrational (sometimes working directly against the administrator), they inevitably come into being and can be used successfully for constructive purposes, such as the subject under consideration.

Undoubtedly, the thoughtful hospital administrator, faced with the reality of his particular and often unique situation, will be able to modify and adapt for his use some of the aids to voluntary coordination enumerated here. They are employed successfully in various enterprises, either through design or intuition, and may provide the answer to some of the perplexing problems of hospitals.

To sum up, voluntary cooperation and voluntary coordination are elusive organizational qualities, much to be desired. To bring them into being, the administrator must possess knowledge and persistence. With these qualities, their attainment is possible, and thereby many of the difficulties stemming from the complex nature of the general hospital and its anomalous o.ganizational structure can be overcome.

[14]Chester I. Barnard, *Functions of the Executive* (Cambridge, Mass.: Harvard University Press, 1940), p. 122.

Part III

LABOR RELATIONS IN HOSPITALS

This part of the book presents the area of labor relations as it pertains to the hospital organization. The labor relations functional area of the hospital is charged with providing policy and carrying out activities related to employee collective bargaining. With an increasing trend in the unionization of hospital employees, the administrator should be aware of the labor law as it applies to his organization and the reasons why people frequently unionize. Since the hospital industry is labor intensive, unions can have a significant impact on hospital costs and administrative control. Thus, serious attention should be given to the hospital's stance vis-a-vis unions.

The first section, FEDERAL LEGISLATION, presents the major laws and their applicability to the hospital industry. The major piece of legislation is the Taft-Hartley Act which specifically excludes non-profit hospitals from the National Labor Relations Board's jurisdiction. The effect of that legislation is that non-profit hospitals are not required to recognize collective bargaining organization efforts unless state legislation applies. The legislation as related to for-profit hospitals, governmental hospitals, and nursing homes is also presented. In addition, two provocative points of view pertaining to Taft-Hartley exclusion are included.

The second section, HOSPITAL UNIONIZATION, presents the effects of unions on hospital management along with a discussion of the causes that frequently give rise to the desire for unionizing. The administration philosophy toward unions appears to be changing. Rather than resist unions as a matter of policy, liberal administrators are attempting to rectify the causes so that most employees will perceive no useful advantage to bargaining collectively.

Federal Legislation

This section presents Federal labor legislation as it pertains to the hospital industry. With an increasing trend in the unionization movement, the hospital administrator must evaluate his labor relations policies in light of the complex legal environment. This section presents the Wagner Act, Taft-Hartley Act, and the Landrum-Griffin Act as they apply to health care facilities.

The first reading, *THE LABOR LAW STATUS OF HEALTH CARE FACILITIES*, treats the topic of Federal labor legislation and court interpretation of that legislation in three parts. Part 1 discusses the Wagner Act. Even though the National Labor Relations Act of 1935 (Wagner Act) did not specifically exclude non-profit hospitals from its coverage, the main body of court interpretation considered the act as inapplicable. Part 2 presents the Taft-Hartley and Landrum-Griffin Acts. The former was enacted in 1947 to amend the Wagner Act. It specified for the exclusion of non-profit and governmental (Federal, state and municipal) hospitals from its coverage. However, it did not exclude for-profit institutions. The major effect of exclusion is that non-profit hospitals are not required by law to recognize formal organization drives unless state legislation applies. Part 3 deals with the labor law status of proprietary hospitals, nursing homes, and governmental hospitals. Under certain conditions the National Labor Relations Board will assert jurisdiction over proprietary hospitals and nursing homes. Federal hospital unionization is, in turn, permitted under presidential executive order.

The disadvantages resulting from the exclusion of non-profit hospitals from coverage by the Taft-Hartley Act are presented in *LABOR RELATIONS*. It is stipulated that the lack of federal legislative coverage has resulted in inconsistent state legislation, could cause the proliferation of bargaining units, and could possibly result in conflicts of interest. It is advocated that hospitals need federal legislative protection, similar to the Taft-Hartley Act, as much as industrial firms. A call is made for the institution of a lobby for the purpose of advocating federal legislative coverage of non-profit hospitals.

In *TAFT-HARTLEY EXEMPTION,* a different point of view is made which advocates the continuation of exclusion for non-profit hospitals from federal law coverage. The author rebuts the arguments raised in the previous writing. It is argued that the disadvantages of federal coverage would outweigh the advantages.

The Labor Law Status of Health Care Facilities

Part 1: The Wagner Act

DENNIS D. POINTER, PH.D.

Dennis D. Pointer, Ph.D., is an Assistant Professor in the Graduate Program in Health Administration and an Instructor of Administrative Medicine, The City University of New York.

Collective bargaining and unionization in health care facilities have only recently begun to attract widespread public and professional attention. The issues surrounding hospital "industrial relations" increased dramatically in 1959-1960 due to a series of extended strikes across the nation: A strike in New York lasted for 46 days, one in Seattle for 84 days, and one in Chicago for more than four months.

As a greater proportion of industrial workers have come under union agreements, the unions themselves have become increasingly interested in organizing the "fringe areas" of American labor. Some of the factors inhibiting union growth in health care facilities in the past have been: 1. The general lack of legal protection regarding organizational activities in hospitals; 2. the union's preoccupation with organizing more lucrative areas; 3. the low density of hospitals in a given area; 4. the relatively small number of employes per facility; 5. the unstable nature of the hospital labor pool; 6. the large number of women employes; 7. the multitude of professional and semi-professional employes; and 8. the great number and variety of skills operative in the hospital setting.

Union efforts at organizing clerical, professional, and hospital workers are illustrative of a relatively new trend. So long as the American labor force was essentially manual in nature, American unionism could consider itself the modern social mass movement. However, when one considers the proportional decline of the "blue-collar" worker in the labor force, it is clear that, unless the union movement increases its enrollment density in the expanding job categories such as the hospital industry, the union's social, economic, and political power in modern society could be substantially weakened.

Some indication of the increased penetration of unions in the health sector can be gained by examining data presented by Miller and Shortell.[1] They reported that between 1961 and 1967 the percentage of hospitals with collective bargaining contracts had more than doubled, from 3.2 per cent in 1961 to 6.8 per cent in 1967. In addition, they noted that in 1967, 370 hospitals, representing 5.2 per cent of the nation's 7,127 hospitals received requests for collective negotiation recognition.

COMPLEX LEGAL ENVIRONMENT

American society is becoming more legalistic in nature. This increased legalism is due both to the increasing complexity of group and interpersonal relations at all levels and to the accelerated pace of social change. Legislative enactments and court decisions establish the operational boundaries within which unions and hospital administrations must act and react. Developing and evaluating alternative administrative policy regarding personnel management and labor relations must be done within this increasingly complex legal-legislative environment. This series of articles will describe, analyze, and evaluate the federal labor law status of health care facilities. Present behavior and future policies must be based upon and guided by this legal foundation.

HOSPITALS AND THE WAGNER ACT

The National Labor Relations Act of 1935, more commonly known as the Wagner Act, was the United States' first piece of comprehensive labor legislation. Section 1 of the code noted that the purpose of the Act was "... to remove obstructions to commerce and restore equality of bargaining power arising out of employers' general denial to labor of the right to bargain collectively with them from which denial resulted a number of detrimental consequences. . . ."[2]

Section 8 of the Act prohibited management from: 1. Interfering with employes' rights to organize and bargain collectively; 2. dominating a labor organization with regard to organization or control; 3. discriminating against an employe for participating in union activity; 4. discriminating against an employe for filing charges under the Act; and 5. refusing to bargain in "good faith." In addition, the Act created the National Labor Relations Board (NLRB). The NLRB was given the responsibility to determine bargaining units, conduct elections to choose bargaining representatives, and hear cases dealing with unfair labor practices.

The Wagner Act did not specifically exempt charitable, religious, or educational institutions. Generally speaking, the courts in several cases also found no implied exemption. For example, *NLRB v. Polish National Alliance*[3] established that the mere fact that a fraternal benefit insurance plan was not organized for profit did not exempt

---

[1] Jon D. Miller and Stephen Shortell, "Hospital Unionization: A Study of the Trends," *Hospitals,* Aug. 16, 1969, p. 67.

[2] A. Howard Myers, *Labor Law and Legislation,* Cincinnati, Ohio, Southwestern Publishing Company, 1968, p. 1.

[3] *NLRB v. Polish National Alliance,* 332 U.S. 643.

the organization from coverage under the Wagner Act if, in fact, the activities of the organization had an impact on interstate commerce. The same conclusion was reached in *Christian Board of Publication v. NLRB,* [4] in which the court noted that the jurisdictional touch-stone of the Wagner Act was its impact on interstate commerce rather than whether or not the organization was formed for the purpose of making a profit. Both of these cases dealt with non-profit organizations *per se,* rather than those considered to be eleemosynary in character.

The question concerning the applicability of the Wagner Act to voluntary hospitals was raised for the first time in regard to the request of two unions to be recognized as the bargaining agent of workers employed at Central Dispensary and Emergency Hospital in Washington, D.C. In a hearing before the NLRB, the hospital moved to dismiss the proceedings on the grounds that: 1. The Wagner Act did not apply to hospitals because they were not engaged in "trade, traffic, or commerce" within the meaning of the Act; and 2. the hospital should be exempt from jurisdiction because it was a non-profit institution.

INTERSTATE TRADE

The NLRB found no merit in the contention that the jurisdictional words of the Act were inappropriate to describe a hospital's activities. It noted that the facility did import each month, from points outside the District of Columbia, material and supplies valued at $5,000. Thus, its dealings were deemed interstate in nature. Furthermore, the NLRB ruled that hospital activities could be considered "trade" based on a precedent established in *U.S. v. American Medical Association.*[5] In this case a federal court of appeals ruled that the AMA violated the Sherman Anti-Trust Act because it restrained trade among hospitals located in several states (by limiting hospital privileges). In the AMA decision, the court noted that the word "trade" had a developed meaning which covered any occupation in which men were engaged to earn a livelihood. Since workers employed by a hospital were engaged in earning a livelihood, the hospital itself was engaged in trade as defined in the Wagner Act.

The counsel for the hospital stressed the fact that the facility was not organized for profit as a reason for exemption from the Act. However, no cases were cited which held that the power conferred on Congress by the commerce clause of the U.S. Constitution was in any way limited to inter-state transactions entered into with a motive of financial gain. It was observed that the hospital was entering into contracts with firms whose activities were commercial in every sense. Observing that transactions with such organizations did not lose their commercial character even though the hospital had a motive other than profit, the NLRB said: "The commerce clause looks to the activities carried on, rather than to the motives. The jurisdiction conferring words of the National Labor Relations Act, 'trade, traffic, commerce, transportation, or communication' are words of activity, and when used together do not give a connotation of essential motive."[6] The precedent for this decision can be traced to

<hr>

[4] *Christian Board of Publication v. NLRB,* 113 F. 2d 753 (D.C. Cir., 1942).

[5] *U.S. v. American Medical Association,* App. D.C., 110 F. 2d 703.

[6] *Central Dispensary and Emergency Hospital,* cited in 44 NLRB at 540 (1942).

*Caminetti v. United States,*7 in which the U.S. Supreme Court held that the use of the word "traffic" in the title of the White Slave Traffic Act did not indicate that Congress intended the Act to apply only to white slaving undertaken with a motive for profit.

OTHER ATTEMPTS AT EXEMPTION

All else failing, the hospital attempted to gain exemption from the Wagner Act by stating that the facility was semi-public in nature and thereby excluded under Section 2(2) of the Act. This section states that ". . . the United States or any state or any political subdivision thereof . . ." is not considered to be an employer within the meaning of the legislation. Central Dispensary and Emergency Hospital argued that it received appropriations from Congress and thus should be considered as an integral part of the federal government. The NLRB ruled that the Congress had a contractual arrangement with the hospital for the provision of specifically delineated services; it observed that this was only a contractual relationship and not a statement of organizational integration.

The Central Dispensary and Emergency Hospital case was later appealed to a federal court, which enforced the NLRB decision to include the non-profit hospital under the jurisdiction of the Wagner Act. In its ruling, the federal court stated:

". . . the hospital argues that the spirit or policy of the Act is such that we should read into it an exemption of charitable hospitals. . . . We cannot understand what considerations of public policy deprive hospital employees of the privilege granted to the employees of other institutions. The opinions . . . , holding that charitable hospitals and their nonprofessional employees are subject to the labor relations acts of those states, present what seems to us the only tenable view. . . ."8

PUBLIC SENTIMENT

Since the Wagner Act neither specifically included nor excluded non-profit hospitals, interpretation of the legislative intent of the Act was left to the discretion of the courts. The Central Dispensary and Emergency Hospital case proved to be the exception to the majority of court rulings that dealt with the applicability of comprehensive labor legislation to non-profit hospitals.

Immediately preceding the passage of the Wagner Act, several states enacted labor legislation that incorporated provisions similar to those contained in the federal statute. Public sentiment toward the acceptability of hospital unionism can be perceived by examining several state court cases that considered whether or not non-profit hospitals should be treated like other business enterprises with regard to the regulation of labor-management relations.

A New York court ruled that a non-profit hospital, in caring for the indigent sick, is in fact, if not in name, a government agency performing a governmental function that would become a responsibility of the state if not successfully discharged by the

---

7*Caminetti v. U.S.,* 242 U.S. 470.

8*Central Dispensary and Emergency Hospital v. NLRB,* 145 F. 2d 852 (D.C. Cir., 1944), cert. denied 342 U.S. 847, 65 Sup. Ct. 684 (1945).

hospital. The court decided that the same doctrine that exempted the state and its political subdivisions from the statute required that a charitable institution such as a voluntary hospital also be excluded.[9]

COURTS ADJUST TO CONDITIONS

In considering whether non-profit hospitals could be included under the jurisdiction of a state labor law modeled after the Wagner Act, a Pennsylvania court noted that:

"... [the operation of such facilities] would be impossible should we hold the Labor Act applicable with all its attending ramifications, interruptions, and possible cessations of service due to labor disputes and attending financial inability to function. Surely the legislature had no such intention...."[10]

During this period, the great majority of court decisions followed the general line of reasoning developed in the preceding two cases. The courts concluded that: 1. The Wagner Act (and associated state labor laws modeled after it) was not intended to extend coverage to the workers of non-profit hospitals; 2. the delivery of health care was essentially a governmental function. Thus hospitals, like governments and their political subdivisions, were excluded from labor law coverage; and 3. making voluntary hospitals subject to the provisions of comprehensive labor statutes was not in the public interest. In addition, the rationale for excluding charitable institutions from labor legislation coverage centered on a distinction between those organizations created for gain and those whose goal was eleemosynary. A New York court stated that "... the character of such employers [non-profit charitable institutions] ... was sufficient assurance of fair dealing with their employees to render unnecessary the protection of the Labor Relations Act."[11] There also seemed to be some concern that if non-profit institutions were required to bargain collectively, much charitable contribution would be withdrawn.

Neil Chamberlain and James Kuhn state that "... labor law can best be understood if one thinks of the courts as an instrument of society adjusting to changed social conditions."[12] Courts base their rulings not only on precedent but also on the perceived mood of the public at any given time. The environment created by the preceding court decisions formed the foundation for a statutory enactment that embodied the prevailing mood of the public regarding the control of labor--management relations in health care facilities.

The next article in this series will examine the status of voluntary hospitals under the Labor-Management Relations (Taft-Hartley) Act of 1947 and the Labor--Management Reporting and Disclosure (Landrum-Griffin) Act of 1959.

[9] *Jewish Hospital of Brooklyn v. Doe,* 252 App. Div. 581 at 584 (1938).

[10] *Western Pennsylvania Hospital v. Lichliter,* 340 Pa. 382, 17A 2d 206 (1941). Cited in 6 LRRM at 1133.

[11] *Trustees of Columbia University v. Herzog,* 269 App. Div. 24 aff'd., 295 N.Y.S. 605 (1945). Subquoted from: Judith Vladeck, "Collective Bargaining in Voluntary Hospitals and Other Non-Profit Institutions," *Proceedings of New York 19th Annual Conference on Labor,* ed. Thomas G. S. Christensen, Washington, D.C., Bureau of National Affairs, Inc., 1965, p. 279.

[12] Neil W. Chamberlain and James W. Kuhn, *Collective Bargaining* 2nd ed., New York, McGraw-Hill Book Co., 1965, p. 223.

Part 2: The Taft-Hartley and Landrum-Griffin Acts

The expansion of union membership in the industrial sector, stimulated by the provisions of the Wagner Act, gave rise to new problems regarding the regulation of union-management relations. Jurisdictional strikes (disputes over which union should do what), abuses of the secondary boycott, the refusal of some unions to bargain in good faith, and the sharp increase in industrial conflict in the immediate post-war period created widespread public demand for remedial action. In this environment, Congress passed the Labor Management Relations (Taft-Hartley) Act of 1947. Today, this statute stands as the nation's major piece of labor legislation.

The Taft-Hartley Act amended the Wagner Act and maintained that it was unfair labor practice for a union to: 1. Coerce employes in the execution of their rights; 2. cause an employer to discriminate against his employes; 3. refuse to bargain in good faith with an employer; 4. engage in certain strikes and boycotts deemed unlawful in their objectives; 5. require the payment of excessive or discriminatory fees under a union security agreement; and 6. engage in "featherbedding" practices. In addition, the legislation expanded management's rights of free speech, excluded supervisors from the provisions of the Act, and gave the President the power to enjoin a strike if it would imperil the national health or safety.

Of particular interest regarding the status of health care facilities is Section 2(2) of the Act, which delineated those employers considered to be exempt from the legislation's provisions. This section states that the Act "... shall not include the United States or any wholly owned government corporation ... , or any state or political subdivision thereof, or any corporation or association operating a hospital, if no part of the net earnings inures to the benefit of any private shareholder or individual. . . ."[1]

This statutory directive reflected the climate of opinion created by the courts prior to 1947 regarding the regulation of labor-management relations in health care facilities. Under the Taft-Hartley Act, non-profit hospitals were specifically excluded from the provisions of the legislation. Federal, state, and municipal government hospitals were also exempt because they were operated by governments or recognized political subdivisions thereof. Proprietary hospitals and nursing homes were not specifically excluded from coverage and it appears that, if their operations had impact on interstate commerce, federal labor law would be applicable.

This article will examine the federal labor law status of voluntary non-profit hospitals under the Labor-Management Relations (Taft-Hartley) Act of 1947 and the Labor-Management Reporting and Disclosure (Landrum-Griffin) Act of 1959.

VOLUNTARY NON-PROFIT HOSPITALS

The original bill to amend the National Labor Relations (Wagner) Act was reported out of Congressman Hartley's Committee on Education and Labor, and Senator Taft's Committee on Labor and Public Welfare. The House Bill recommended exemption of all employers considered to be religious, charitable, scientific, or educational

---

[1] *National Labor Relations Act of 1947,* Public Law 101, 80th Congress, 1st Session, as amended by Public Law 188, 82nd Congress, 1st Session, Section 2(2).

institutions not organized for profit. The rationale governing the exemption focused on the fact that these facilities frequently assisted local government units in carrying out their essential functions and thus should be left to exclusive local jurisdiction.[2] The Senate bill mentioned no exemptions other than those that had been incorporated in the Wagner Act. However, when the proposed bill reached the Senate floor, Senator Tydings of Maryland offered an amendment exempting non-profit hospitals, which was eventually incorporated into Section 2(2) of the Taft-Hartley Act. In introducing the amendment, Sen. Tydings commented:

> ... this amendment is designed merely to help a great number of hospitals which are having very difficult times. They are eleemosynary institutions; no profit is involved in their operation; and I understand from the Hospital Association that this amendment would be very helpful in their efforts to serve those who have not the means to pay for hospital service, enable them to keep the doors open, and operate the hospitals.[3]

An examination of the record makes it obvious that the hospital exemption amendment was consciously considered and later enacted on the premise that *only* charitable non-profit hospitals should not be deemed as employers under the Act. Non-profit institutions that are not charitable in nature, as well as for-profit hospitals, were included in coverage. The exemption of non-profit hospitals hinged neither on their non-profit status nor on their functions as hospitals, but rather on their "charitable" character.

The implications of the exemption of non-profit hospitals from the provisions of the Taft-Hartley Act were clear. In the absence of any state statute which specifically included non-profit hospitals, such hospitals had no obligation under the law to recognize or deal with their employes on a collective basis. Additionally, hospital management could engage in direct action to halt or limit union activity (e.g., discharging union organizers or limiting promotions of those employes sympathetic to the union cause). Phillip Taft, in his widely acclaimed book on the history of American unionism, notes that when a particular employe group is denied the protection of labor legislation, union recognition and subsequent collective bargaining are essentially impossible to achieve.[4]

Before examining the status of voluntary hospitals under the Labor-Management Reporting and Disclosure Act of 1959, it would be helpful to investigate the effect of national labor legislation upon voluntary hospital shared service organizations and subcontracting activities. The shared service concept is an outgrowth of comprehensive health facility planning, in which several hospitals join together to operate a service needed by all. (Shared data processing, laundry, and pharmacy services are the most common.) With subcontracting, a hospital negotiates with an independent firm to assume a portion of the hospital's operation. (Contracting for the performance of food service and maintenance functions are the most common.)

VOLUNTARY HOSPITAL SHARED SERVICE OPERATIONS

The shared service venture of a group of non-profit hospitals, if properly organized, enjoys the same tax exempt status as its member hospitals. The question arises as to

[2] Comments of Congressman Hartley, H.R. No. 245, 93 *Congressional Record* at 3520 (1947).

[3] Comments of Senator Tydings, 93 *Congressional Record* May 12, 1947.

[4] Phillip Taft, *Organized Labor and American History,* New York, Harper & Row, Publishers, 1964, p. 579.

whether or not the shared service organization can also gain exemption from the provisions of the Taft-Hartley Act. Although this issue has not been addressed in the federal courts, several decisions of the National Labor Relations Board have dealt with it.

In *Southern Permanente Services, Inc.,*[5] the NLRB ruled that a for-profit shared service corporation, organized to provide services to a group of Kaiser Foundation (non-profit) hospitals, would fall under the jursidiction of the Act. The NLRB concluded that the functions of Southern Permanente Services were not intimately related to the operation or purposes of the non-profit hospitals to a sufficient degree to warrant withholding jurisdiction.

In *United Hospital Services, Inc.,*[6] the NLRB ruled that a non-profit corporation, organized to provide services only to member non-profit hospitals, was exempt from the provisions of the Taft-Hartley Act. The jurisdictional element in these two cases appears to be the non-profit status of the shared operation, on one hand, and its degree of integration with member non-profit hospitals, on the other. Hence, "properly organized" shared service corporations would probably be considered exempt from the federal labor law. The jurisdicational touchstone appears to be non-profit status rather than degree of integration.

VOLUNTARY HOSPITAL SUBCONTRACTING

The author is aware of only one decision regarding the question of whether or not independent subcontractors performing services for a non-profit hospital are bound by the provisions of the Taft-Hartley Act.

Prior to Jan. 1, 1962, New York Medical College Flower and Fifth Avenue Hospital operated its own food service (patient food preparation, employes' dining room, and coffee shop for hospital visitors). In January, 1962, the hospital entered into a 10-year contract with Horn and Hardart Company, a firm engaged in the preparation and retail sale of food, in which the latter undertook to operate all food service facilities for the hospital. On June 4, 1965, the NLRB received an election request from Local 1199, Drug and Hospital Employes Union, to represent dietary workers at the hospital. The hospital and Horn and Hardart Company filed a petition with NLRB asking that the election request be denied on the grounds that the hospital (and hence its subcontractor) was exempt from the Taft-Hartley Act and thus from NLRB jurisdiction. The union maintained that it was seeking recognition from Horn and Hardart Company, a profit-making, independent subcontractor that was under the jurisdiction of the Taft-Hartley Act, and not from the hospital.

In deciding the case, the NLRB ruled that the food service functions performed by the subcontractor were "intimately connected with the patient care and medical education purposes of the hospital."[7] It was further noted:

---

[5] *Southern Permanente Services, Inc.,* cited in 172 NLRB at 148 (1968).

[6] *United Hospital Services, Inc.,* cited in 172 NLRB at 188 (1968).

[7] *The Horn and Hardart Company,* cited in 154 NLRB at 129 (1965).

"In view of the close relationship found to exist between the employer's operation here involved and the activities of the hospital, and as the latter is exempted from the Board's jurisdiction, we find . . . that it will not effectuate the purposes of the Act to assert jurisdiction in this case."[8]

Thus it appears that properly executed subcontracting arrangements of non-profit hospitals are exempt from the provisions of the Taft-Hartley Act. However, a word of caution is warranted: The NLRB has always taken a more critical stance regarding organizational arrangements designed only and specifically to gain a jurisdictional or operational advantage under the labor laws.

THE LABOR MANAGEMENT REPORTING AND DISCLOSURE ACT OF 1959

The Labor-Management Reporting and Disclosure (Landrum-Griffin) Act of 1959 is the only federal statute that regulates the labor-management relations of non-profit hospitals. The statute places controls on the internal affairs of labor unions and on conduct of the union-management relationship. Specifically, the Act requires employers to report:

1. Promises to make or the making of payments on loans to officials or other representatives of labor organizations.

2. Payments to employes for the purpose of causing them to persuade other employes to exercise or not to exercise or as to the means of exercising their rights to organize and bargain collectively.

3. Payments to labor relations consultants under such circumstances to interfere with certain rights of employes.[9]

Reports of these actions must be filed with the Secretary of Labor. Penalities for failure to file such reports or for filing false reports include fines up to a maximum of $10,000 and/or imprisonment for one year.

The Taft-Hartley Act contained provisions for filing reports and affidavits, but did not require unions to comply unless they wanted to use the services of the NLRB. Since local unions dealing specifically with non-profit hospitals not covered under the Act were not susceptible to NLRB jurisdiction, they had no reason or duty to file such material. However, the Landrum-Griffin Act rescinded this 1947 provision and replaced it with a mandatory reporting requirement. Every labor union must now file a report with the Secretary of Labor containing information regarding: The names of union officials; fees and dues required of members; provisions of membership, ratification procedures, and participation in benefit plans; changes in union constitution, bylaws, or rules; and financial dealings and statements of the union.

In 1962, Arthur Goldberg, then secretary of labor, brought suit against the Public Building Service, Hospital, and Institutional Employes Union, Local 113. The union, which represented 2,500 non-professional employes in 20 Minneapolis area hospitals and nursing homes, was charged with failing to file copies of its constitution, bylaws, and yearly financial statements with the Department of Labor. The union contended

---

[8]*Ibid.* There have been several cases of this general nature, although not dealing specifically with non-profit hospitals. See: *University of Miami, Institute of Marine Sciences Division,* cited in 146 NLRB at 1448, 1450; and *The Prophet Company,* cited in 150 NLRB at 1559.

[9]*Labor-Management Reporting and Disclosure Act of 1959,* 79 Stat. 519, Section 203.

that it was involved in local activities only and that, as a result, it should not be covered by the Act. It also argued that reports were not filed because its members received no protection under either state or federal labor law. This case was decided in favor of the Secretary's petition, thus affirming that labor unions that deal with non-profit hospitals, as well as the non-profit hospitals themselves, are susceptible to the provisions of the Landrum-Griffin Act.[10,11]

CONCLUSION

Anne R. Somers, in her recent book, *Hospital Regulation: The Dilemma of Public Policy,* notes that "except for a small proportion of proprietary institutions (and to some extent in their case), hospitals have historically been exempt from most taxes, labor legislation, and other burdens imposed on other enterprises of their size and wealth."[12]

Reflecting on the development of the federal labor law status of non-profit hospitals, several opinions can be advanced.

It appears that judges and legislatures have expected employes of non-profit hospitals to share in those institutions' charity. Sen. Tydings, in introducing the amendment to exclude non-profit hospitals from the provisions of the Taft-Hartley Act, noted that the exemption would be financially beneficial to a "large number of hospitals which are having difficult times." Presumably this financial benefit would be gained by a depressed wage level possible because of the lack of collective organization. Additionally, it has been assumed that, since these institutions are by definition charitable and "charity begins at home," employes of these establishments would be treated equitably as a matter of course.[13] Traditionally, this has not been the case.

Employes of non-profit hospitals have been considered along with government employes with respect to their exclusion from protection of the labor laws. Yet, they possess none of the benefits of public employment (e.g., guaranteed tenure, promotion review boards, job security review boards, and adequate pension plans). This logic does not parallel the rationale that hospitals perform a quasi-governmental function, which is one of the factors advanced in arguments for exemption from labor law coverage.

10 "Secretary of Labor Sues Minnesota Hospital Union," *Hospitals,* April 16, 1962, p. 181.

11 "Building Service Local Ordered To File Reports," *Modern Hospital,* June, 1962, p. 166.

12 Anne R. Somers, *Hospital Regulation: The Dilemma of Public Policy,* Princeton, N.J., Industrial Relations Section, Princeton University, 1969, p. xi.

13 *Trustees of Columbia University v. Herzog,* 269 App. Div. 24 aff'd., 295 N.Y.S. 605 (1945). Subquoted from: Judith Vladeck, "Collective Bargaining in Voluntary Hospitals and Other Non-Profit Institutions," *Proceedings of New York 19th Annual Conference on Labor,* ed. Thomas G. S. Christensen, Washington, D.C., Bureau of National Affairs, Inc., 1965, p. 279.

The critical issue regarding public policy toward hospital unionism appears to be whether labor law coverage of health care facilities whose functions are critical will invite labor strife or prevent it. This consideration has been treated in diverse ways by several legislatures and courts. Those courts and legislatures deciding that hospitals should be included under the jurisdiction of labor laws reason that exclusion will invite labor strife because collective negotiation of differences between employes and employers will not be protected or encouraged and disputant parties will resort to other mechanisms of conflict resolution (e.g., strikes and lockouts). Those courts and legislatures deciding against coverage reason that inclusion will invite labor strife because the protection of union activity may encourage strikes. The resolution of this issue will provide the foundation of an effective and efficient public policy regarding the recognition of, and collective bargaining by, unions in the health care arena.

Part 3: Proprietary Hospitals, Nursing Homes, and State and Federal Government Hospitals

In the early years following the passage of the Taft-Hartley Act, the federal labor law status of for-profit health care facilities was uncertain. A literal reading of the legislation tended to indicate that, since proprietary hospitals and nursing homes were not specifically excluded from the provisions of the Act (as were non-profit hospitals) jurisdiction would be granted if impact on interstate commerce could be demonstrated.

In a 1959 ruling, the National Labor Relations Board asserted jurisdiction over a hospital operated by Kennecott Copper Corporation. The company operated a hospital and branch dispensary in connection with a copper mining operation in Santa Ria, N.M. The NLRB determined that the company was engaged in interstate commerce and that the hospital and dispensary were operated primarily to provide security to the employer against on-the-job injuries. During the four years preceding the hearing, 86 per cent of the patients of the facility were employed by the company. In addition, it was noted that the health care facilities had no separate legal identity apart from the company.

Kennecott Copper Corporation had moved that a petition for union recognition election in the hospital be dismissed on the grounds that: 1. The hospital's operation was exempted from Section 2(2) of the Taft-Hartley Act (i.e., it was a voluntary non-profit hospital); and 2. the operation of the hospital was not involved *in* interstate commerce and did not *affect* interstate commerce. In deciding that the hospital and dispensary should be included in the coverage of the Taft-Hartley Act, the NLRB noted:

> "We find no merit to the employer's first contention because the Board has held that a hospital is exempted by Section 2(2) of the Act only if the corporation operating the hospital is, itself, operated on a non-profit basis. . . .We reject the employer's second contention, and in accord with the petitioners [the union seeking recognition], find. . .that the hospital is clearly an integral part of the employer's operations and thus in and affecting interstate commerce. . . ."[1]

A 1955 NLRB hearing asserted that a proprietary hospital operated at Hato Tejas, Puerto Rico, was subject to the jurisdiction of the Wagner Act. The hospital had a gross business of $431,000 per year, 98 per cent of which was realized from the treatment of veterans pursuant to a contract with the United States Veterans Administration. In asserting jurisdiction, the NLRB noted that the operation of the proprietary hospital, by reason of its contract with the Veterans Administration, was directly related to the national defense and thus should be covered by the provisions of the Taft-Hartley Act.[2]

PROPRIETARY HOSPITALS

On Jan. 13, 1960, the NLRB received a petition for an election and bargaining unit determination at Flatbush General Hospital, located in Brooklyn, N.Y. This case raised for the first time the question of whether or not the NLRB had legal jurisdiction over proprietary hospitals other than those in which: 1. The facility was located in the District of Columbia; 2. the proprietary hospital was directly related to national defense; or 3. the hospital was integrated with an organizational unit over which the NLRB had jurisdiction.

The NLRB recorded the following as statements of fact: Flatbush General Hospital was a 111-bed proprietary facility which employed 140 employes. The facility had an estimated yearly gross income of $1 million, and approximately two-thirds of its purchase of supplies came directly or indirectly from outside the state. Most of the hospital's patients were residents of New York State. The union had reportedly been engaged in recognitional picketing at the hospital for a period of four days. This action would have been an unfair labor practice under Section 8(b) (7) (c) of the Taft-Hartley Act if indeed the hospital could be considered under the coverage of the Act.

The union moved to dismiss the hospital's petition for an election (thus allowing it to maintain the recognitional picket) on the grounds that the employer was a proprietary hospital not engaged in interstate commerce, and that even if statutory jurisdiction were found to exist, the impact of the operation of a proprietary hospital such as the employer's was insufficient in dollar volume to warrant NLRB jurisdiction. The employer, on the other hand, opposed the motion for dismissal (thus allowing jurisdiction to be granted, whereby the picket would be declared unfair) on the grounds that the New York State Labor Relations Board had decided in three earlier cases that the operation of proprietary hospitals affected interstate commerce to such an extent that they should fall under federal control.

The NLRB, in declining to assert jurisdiction, stated:

> "We are satisfied that the employer has sufficient inflow of goods from out-of-state to meet the requirements for a finding of legal jurisdiction [e.g., the employer was *in* interstate commerce]. However, we are of the opinion that the operation of this class of proprietary hospitals, although not wholly unrelated to commerce, are (sic) essentially local in nature and, therefore, the effect on commerce of labor disputes involving such hospitals is not substantial enough to warrant the exercise of the Board's jurisdiction. Our conclusion that such hospitals are local in character rests primarily on the facts that they service local residents and that their operations are subject to close regulation by the states for the protection of the health and safety of their residents."[3]

Thus it appeared that, as of 1960, the NLRB would decline jurisdiction over proprietary hospitals unless they were in the District of Columbia, had an impact on national defense, or were integrated with an organization over which it had jurisdiction.

However, several cases decided by the NLRB in 1967 reversed the ruling handed down in the Flatbush General Hospital decision. The NLRB announced that it would assert jurisdiction over proprietary hospitals having at least $250,000 gross annual revenue and over nursing homes having at least $100,000 gross annual revenue.[4] In ordinary circumstances, activities of an employer whose business meets the appropriate annual dollar volume standard will be deemed to "affect commerce." However, the NLRB requires evidence to support its legal jurisdiction, in addition to proof that the gross-dollar-volume test is met. If an employer refuses to supply the NLRB with appropriate financial data, the Board will assert jurisdiction without a finding that the dollar guidelines have been met.

FEDERAL GOVERNMENT HOSPITALS

In defense of the traditional policies of unilateral management-employe relations, the Federal Government is usually identified as a "sovereign employer." Essentially, the sovereignty doctrine is founded on the notion that public employe pressure on the government (either in the form of collective negotiation or work stoppages) would represent a dilution of the integrity of public authority. In affirming this policy during his administration, Franklin D. Roosevelt stated:

> "The process of collective bargaining, as usually understood, cannot be transplanted into the public sector . . . militant tactics have no place in the functions of any organization of government employees."[5]

Congress specifically excluded federal employes from the coverage of the Wagner Act of 1935 and the Taft-Hartley Act of 1947 by noting in Section 2(2) of each statute that the Federal Government, any wholly owned government corporation, or any political subdivision thereof was not considered to be an "employer" under the Act. Furthermore, Public Law 330, passed by Congress in 1955, makes it a felony for any federal employe to participate in any strike or assert the right to strike against the government.[6]

Although given no legal protection regarding collective activities, the organization of federal employes is not a recent development. The degree of penetration of labor unions into government-owned hospitals is impossible to determine, although successes in other areas of government employment have been noted. Skilled craftsmen in naval installations have been organized since the early part of the twentieth century. In 1904, the International Association of Machinists established its District 44 to work exclusively with federal employes. The first union composed entirely of government workers was the National Association of Letter Carriers, organized in the late 1890's.[7]

THREE TYPES OF UNIONS

In each session of Congress between 1949 and 1961, legislation was introduced requiring agencies and departments of the Federal Government to recognize and negotiate collectively with their employes. However, the realization of federal employes' demands had to await the election of John F. Kennedy to the Presidency in 1961. Kennedy, while campaigning during 1960, stated in a letter to a postal union official: "I have always believed the right of federal employees to deal collectively with the federal departments and agencies in which they are employed should be protected."[8] On June 22, 1961, Kennedy issued a memorandum creating a task force to study the issues of union recognition and collective negotiation in the federal civil service. The task force made its recommendations to the President on Nov. 30, 1961.[9]

As an outgrowth of the task force report, President Kennedy, on Jan. 17, 1962, issued Executive Order 10,988, which clearly outlined for the first time the government's policy on union recognition and collective bargaining and established mandatory regulation regarding these matters. Essentially E.O. 10,988 gave all federal employes the right to join or not to join organizations of their own choosing that would represent them regarding terms of employment. Three types of union or association recognition were established, depending upon the proportion of organization membership in the appropriate unit: Exclusive, formal, and informal.

Exclusive recognition is granted when a particular organization can demonstrate that it represents a majority of the employes in the unit. In this situation, the union is granted the right to bargain and negotiate agreements with the particular agency or department on behalf of all the employes in the unit.

Formal recognition is granted when the employe organization can demonstrate that it has a stable membership of at least 10 per cent of the employes in the unit and when no other organization has obtained recognition. A formally recognized organization is entitled to confer with management "from time to time" on personnel policies and matters affecting working conditions; the particular agency or department is required only to discuss and not to negotiate with such units.

An employe organization that does not qualify for exclusive or formal recognition is entitled to informal recognition regardless of its membership strength or the status of other organizations in the unit. Informally recognized organizations are entitled to present their views to management (the right of any individual employe), but management is in no way required to seek their view or engage in negotiation.[10]

A supplementary order, issued by the President in May. 1963, was roughly equivalent to the unfair labor practices contained in Sections 8(a) and 8(b) of the Taft-Hartley Act, with two major exceptions: 1. Strikes and picketing by government employes were prohibited; and 2. employe organizations were forbidden to discriminate against any employe with regard to terms or conditions of membership because of race, creed, color, or national origin.

On Oct. 29, 1969, President Nixon issued Executive Order 11,491 which replaced E.O. 10,988. The White House stated that this order "will substantially strengthen the federal labor relations system by bringing it more into line with practices in the private sector."[11] The order created a central authority, the Federal Labor Relations Council (FLRC), to administer the government's labor program and to serve as the final arbitrator of policy questions and disputed matters. Also the Federal Service Impasse Panel was also created; it has the authority to settle deadlocks in contract negotiation if voluntary negotiations fail. E.O. 11,491 also abolished the formal and informal recognition categories. In addition, exclusive recognition can no longer be obtained by a card count in the bargaining unit; a recognitional election conducted by the FLRC is now required.[12]

STATE AND LOCAL GOVERNMENT HOSPITALS

State and local government hospitals are exempt from the provisions of the federal labor relations law by Section 2(2) of the Taft-Hartley Act, which states that a state or any political subdivision thereof is not considered an employer under the Act. Hence, the control of labor relations in such facilities generally has been undertaken by the individual states.

A serious question regarding the federal labor law status of state and municipal government health care facilities was raised in *Maryland v. Wirtz*.[13] In this case, the U.S. Supreme Court affirmed the authority of the Federal Government to require state-controlled hospitals and educational institutions to follow the minimum wage and hour guidelines of the 1966 amendments to the Federal Fair Labor Standards Act. The extension of jurisdiction was justified by the following facts: 1. Even when the state is the employer, goods for these government-operated facilities travel across state lines; and 2. the federal regulation and subsequent prevention of substandard working conditions may forestall labor disputes which could burden or obstruct the free flow of commerce between states.

The ruling observed that the court was required to differentiate between the state as a government, not subject to federal regulation, and the state as a trader, in no better position than any other commercial enterprise. The court noted that when a state government employs workers to perform the usual function of an educational institution or hospital, it is subject to the same regulation and control as any other employer whose activities similarly affect interstate commerce.

Since the U.S. Supreme Court has now affirmed the expanded jurisdiction of the Federal Government in regulating certain specific aspects of labor relations in state and municipal governmental hospitals and educational institutions, one may speculate on whether the rationale used for this expanded jurisdiction could be equally well applied to broadening the coverage of the Taft-Hartley Act. Arthur H. Bernstein, in a recent article, has noted:

> "Congress now has the recognized authority to impose collective bargaining upon state-owned institutions if it chooses, applying the same theory of impact upon commerce as it has already done in the case of commercial employers."[14]

SUMMARY

Proprietary hospitals and nursing homes, although not specifically exempt from the Taft-Hartley Act, have been subject to federal labor laws to varying degrees. The NLRB will now assert jurisdiction over proprietary hospitals and nursing homes with at least a gross annual revenue of $250,000 and $100,000 respectively. In addition, proprietary facilities that are located in the District of Columbia, are related to national defense, or are integrated with organizations over which the board has jurisdiction are covered by the Act, regardless of annual dollar volume.

Federal, state, and municipal government health care facilities are specifically excluded from the provisions of the Taft-Hartley Act by Section 2(2). The labor-management relations of federal hospitals are regulated by a series of executive orders that are similar in thrust to the Taft-Hartley Act, although they limit the right of employes to picket or strike. It is felt that Congress now has the legal foundation to extend federal regulation of labor relations to state and municipal institutions based on the reasoning provided in *Maryland v. Wirtz.*

FOOTNOTES

[1]*Kennecott Copper Corporation,* cited in 99 NLRB at 110 (1952).

[2]*Hospital Hato Tejas, Inc.,* cited in 111 NLRB at 155 (1955).

[3]*Flatbush General Hospital,* cited in 126 NLRB at 145 (1960).

[4]See: *Medical Center Hospital,* Case No. 20-RC-6698; and *University Nursing Homes, Inc.,* cited in 1968 NLRB at 52 (1967).

[5]Letter by Franklin D. Roosevelt to Luther C. Steward, president of the National Federation of Federal Employes, dated Aug. 16, 1937. Quoted here from William B. Vosloo, *Collective Bargaining in the United States Federal Civil Service,* Chicago, Public Personnel Association, 1966, p. 17.

[6]69 Stat. 642 (1955).

[7]Jack Stieber, "Collective Bargaining in the Public Sector," in *Challenges to Collective Bargaining,* ed. Lloyd Ulman, Englewood Cliffs, N.J., Prentice-Hall, Inc., 1967, p. 67.

[8]Subquoted from: Vosloo, *op. cit.,* p. 59.

[9]*Ibid.,* p. 59.

[10]*Ibid.,* pp. 68-71.

[11]"Labor Management Relations in the Federal Services," *Government Employe Relations Report,* No. 320, Washington, D.C., The Bureau of National Affairs, Inc., Oct. 27, 1969, p. 1.

[12]*Ibid.,* pp. 1-2.

[13]*Maryland v. Wirtz,* 392 U.S. 183 (1968).

[14]Arthur H. Bernstein, "Federal Impact on Hospital Labor Relations," *Hospitals,* June 1, 1969, pp. 93-96.

Labor Relations

NORMAN METZGER

Norman Metzger is Vice President for Personnel at the Mount Sinai Medical Center in New York City.

The strong position that hospital boards and hospital trustees have taken over the years to point out the unique nature of hospital operations has paid off rather poorly in the field of labor relations. The Labor-Management Relations Act of 1947 (Taft-Hartley), which amended the National Labor Relations Act of 1935, exempted from its coverage any corporation or association operating a hospital if no part of the net earnings inures to the benefit of any private shareholder or individual. This decision—hailed as a major victory by hospitals throughout the country—has put hospitals at a disadvantage when compared to the corporations that fall under the jurisdiction of the National Labor Relations Board.

The effect of the Taft-Hartley Act's exemption of hospitals was to leave such institutions under the regulation of the states in which they operated. Most state legislatures have chosen to remain silent on this issue. New York State, on the other hand, passed legislation in 1963, extending to employees of not-for-profit hospitals first in New York City and later throughout the state, the legal right to bargain collectively through a union.

The growth of unions in the hospital field probably is paralleled only by the growth of unions in the education field. Hospital unions, finally making a breakthrough, have recruited members at a rate equal to and surpassing the growth of many industrial unions after the enactment of the Wagner Act in 1935.

As a result of the ill-conceived fight for exemption from the national law, hospitals covered by state labor relations acts were faced with inconsistent and sometimes disadvantageous decisions by state labor relations boards or judicial decisions in states without labor laws. In New York State, certain administrative decisions made by the state labor relations board have had potentially explosive and disastrous consequences.

This situation can be illustrated by consideration of two related concerns that have developed from the New York State Labor Relations Act: What is an appropriate bargaining unit and, a tangential concern, where do security guards fit with respect to the larger bargaining unit?

UNDER NLRB JURISDICTION

In the early days of the National Labor Relations Act, the National Labor Relations Board (NLRB) directed its attention to the growth of industrial unions, and specifically to the question of appropriate bargaining units. The board could establish an *employer-wide unit* that would incorporate all employees within specific classifications located at all plants of an employer; or a more restricted *plan unit* that would incorporate only employees of specific classifications in a specific plant; or a *craft unit* or a *department unit.* There was little restraint imposed upon the board during the early days of the act until the advent of the Taft-Hartley Act in 1947. This amendment limited the board's authority in deeming the appropriateness of a bargaining unit in the following ways:

1. Notwithstanding the fact that particular employees organize into a union within a specific department, this no longer was controlling upon the board.

2. The role of self-determination for professional employees was recognized so that such employees could not be included in a unit encompassing nonprofessional employees unless a majority of the professional employees voted in a separate self-determination election for such inclusion.

3. Security guards could not now be included in a unit encompassing other classifications of employees. In fact, security guards could only be organized by unions that limited their membership to guards.

The Labor-Management Relations Act (Taft-Hartley) is quite specific on exclusions regardless of the type of unit constituted as appropriate. In general, employees clearly associated with management's interests are excluded—supervisory employees, confidential employees defined as those who "assist and act in a confidential capacity to persons who formulate, determine and effectuate management policies in the field of labor relations," and temporary employees, including students hired during school vacation. The national board has developed basic criteria that they consider in making their more important decisions as to the appropriateness of a unit. This is vital, since both management and unions have keen interest in the makeup of the employees who will be entitled to vote. The factors considered by the national board in determining the appropriate unit are:

1. Bargaining history in the company or in the industry.

2. Similarity of wage scale, duties, hours, and working conditions among employees involved.

3. Membership eligibility requirement of the union involved.

4. The extent and the type of union organization of the employees who will vote, although the board is forbidden by the act to make this the controlling factor.

5. The employees' own wishes in the matter. This is of specific relevance in the case of professional employees and certain craft employees.

6. The organizational structure of the company and its relationship to the proposed bargaining unit.

The stickiest question that the national board has had to consider over the years evolved from the appropriateness of any single craft unit. The *American Potash,* 107 NLRB 1418, decision in 1954 served as the guideline for the craft severance problem until 1966. In the past the national board ruled that a unit of craft workers might sever itself from a broader unit if it were indeed a true craft and if the union representing this craft was the "historical and traditional representative of employees it seeks." These rules were revised by the *Mallinckrodt Chemical,* 162 NLRB 387, decision in 1966. The board consequently broadened areas that it would consider in craft severance cases, to include those inumerated above—such as whether the unit proposed was a distinct group of skilled craftsmen, the extent to which the members have maintained their separate identity during their inclusion in the broader unit, and the qualifications of the union seeking to represent a severed unit. Of course, this later decision encouraged the balkanization of units in a single plant. Employers long have faced the problem of deciding whether to deal with a large unit encompassing most of its employees or with several narrow units. The temptation to gerrymander employees into units that may affect who will win or lose in an election often overrides the most logical approach to this decision.

The exclusion of supervisors from the coverage of the national act was effected in 1947. Supervisors now are expressly excluded from the act's definition of the term "employee," and no employer can be compelled to recognize a union of supervisors. The act is quite explicit in defining the term "supervisor" as "any individual having authority in the interest of the employer to hire, transfer, suspend, lay off, recall, promote, discharge, assign, reward, or discipline other employees or responsibility to direct them, or to adjust their grievances or effectively to recommend such action if in connection with the foregoing the exercising of such authority is not of a merely routine or clerical nature, but recognizes the use of independent judgment."

As to plant guards, the act prevents the certification of a union as the bargaining agent of guards if it includes in its membership, or is affiliated with any organization that includes in its membership, employees other than guards. Quite explicitly, guards may not be grouped in bargaining units with other employees, nor may they be affiliated with unions that include in their membership employees other than guards. It is clear that the national board has recognized the conflict of interest inherent in grouping supervisors and guards into unions with employees that they must supervise and guard. It is further noteworthy that the national act recognizes the untenable position of a supervisor whose "allegiance" is diluted by union membership. The New York State labor relations law is oblivious to these two inherent dangers.

UNDER STATE BOARD JURISDICTION

Section 705(2) of the New York State Labor Relations Act states:

"The Board shall decide in each case whether, in order to insure to employees the full benefit of their right to self-organization, to collective bargaining and otherwise to effectuate the policies of this article, but the unit appropriate for purposes of collective bargaining shall be the employer unit, multiple employer unit, craft unit, plant unit, or any other unit; provided, however, *that in any case where the majority of employees of a particular craft shall so decide the board shall designate such craft as a unit appropriate for the purpose of collective bargaining.*"

This provision clearly directs the board to designate separate craft units when a majority of craft employees so decide. The effect of this statutory obligation is the proliferation of bargaining units within the hospitals. In *Sloan House,* a New York State Labor Relations Board case, the board declared that "the board is not limited to finding only the theoretically perfect unit. Bargaining units are not immutable but may alter from time to time with changing circumstances. The quest is to find 'in each case' that unit which will best effectuate the policies of the act by encouraging the practice and procedure of collective bargaining. Many factors enter into each particular finding of unit and no single factor is controlling."

The board's insensitivity to the needs of the hospital and the peculiar operations of a medical care facility are obvious in the unlimited approach to this problem of designating appropriate bargaining units. As it is now operating, it is conceivable that the board could designate from a dozen to two dozen separate bargaining units within a hospital. Units found appropriate include: (1) service and maintenance, (2) clerical, (3) technical, (4) guards, (5) house staff, (6) staff R.N.s, (7) supervising R.N.s, (8) L.P.N.s, (9) physical therapists, (10) pharmacists, (11) dietitians, (12) social workers, and almost any professional group, without limitation. Under the original rules, the board could establish a bargaining unit embracing only two employees. Even this limitation was modified in a decision the board handed down in 1939 that entitled a single employee to designate a representative to act for him. The board believed that in light of practical experience it could find no reason to think that the New York State Labor Relations Act denies the board the power to establish a unit composed of a single employee.

CONFLICT OF INTEREST

Although the national act excludes supervisors from its provisions, the State Labor Relations Act provides that only hospital supervisors be excluded from units of nonsupervisory employees. The state board goes a step further by permitting the same union to represent both supervisory and nonsupervisory employees. It is obvious that the national act fully recognizes the conflict of interest in a situation in which a supervisor is represented by a union that also represents the employees supervised by such personnel. This conflict of interest again was recognized in the exclusion of guards from representation by unions that represented nonguard personnel.

The protection afforded General Motors, General Electric, and other industrial firms by the Labor-Management Relations Act (insofar as the act excludes supervisors from coverage by its provisions and excludes guards from being organized into unions representing nonguard personnel) is not enjoyed by hospitals in New York State. The state labor relations board considers units of supervising R.N.'s to be appropriate. These units are represented by the state nurses association, which also represents units of staff nurses supervised by these same supervisory R.N.s.

How does the board expect the hospital to maintain discipline, to improve performance, and to maintain control of the work force when its supervisors are included in such units? One need only consider the possibility of a supervisor, who is a member of the state nurses association bargaining unit at a specific hospital, bringing charges against an R.N. who is a member of the state nurses association bargaining unit for R.N.s for the same hospital. It is not unlikely that the association would bring pressure to bear and would find itself in a most peculiar position when it represented the staff nurse in her grievance against the action of the supervisory R.N. To take this a step further, one easily can imagine the chaotic nature of an arbitration ensuing from a situation in which an R.N. was dismissed by her supervisor, who was a member of a bargaining unit represented by the same association. The state nurses' association would represent the staff R.N., who was terminated, and question the action of the supervisory nurse, who also was a member of the association's bargaining unit.

The impossible nature of this dilemma is extended further by consideration of the board's action on guards. Can a guard who is a member of a bargaining unit represented by a union that also represents other employees in the hospital be expected to file charges against a fellow union member who is found pilfering supplies from the hospital? What happens when the service and maintenance unit of the hospital decides, in obvious violation of the provisions of the state labor relations act, to strike at contract termination time? Will the guards who are members of the same union, albeit a different bargaining unit, cross the picket line of their own union? Can they be expected to maintain order on the picket line? Can they be expected to prevent illegal activities of a fellow union member during such a confrontation? The state board appears oblivious to this inherent conflict of interest. The national law provides protection against the aforementioned conflict for industrial firms, while hospitals receive no such protection.

CONTINUING FRAGMENTATION

The board's liberal interpretation of the appropriateness of a given bargaining unit can be expected to result in an unparalleled proliferation of bargaining units. One need only look to the railroad industry and the newspaper industry to see the disastrous effects of multiunit bargaining. The whipsawing inherent in such a situation adds little to the effective operation of any institution. Within the next decade, many hospitals in the United States may well be bargaining with a half dozen separate units that may be represented by a half dozen separate unions, each competing for status, wages, and conditions of employment that will exceed the other units.

The restrictions imposed upon the New York State Labor Relations Board by Section 705(2) of the New York State Labor Relations Act, which provides that the majority of employees of a particular craft can determine whether that craft should be represented as a separate unit for the purpose of collective bargaining, must indeed be amended if the disastrous effects of the proliferation of units as experienced in the railroad and newspaper industries are to be avoided.

The present policy under the New York State Labor Relations Act tends to encourage the continiung fragmentation of bargaining units. In designating the appropriate bargaining units, two leading authorities in the field, Douglas Brown and George P. Schultz, Secretary of Labor, have suggested that more weight should be given to:

"1. The needs of industrial organization as a whole, which would lead to a shift in emphasis to include, not only the consideration of the desires of smaller groups of employees, but the views of employers and desires of larger groups of employees as well, thereby broadening our bargaining units and discouraging fragmentation.

"2. The probable effect of public policy on the effectiveness of bargaining so that obstacles to the efforts of the parties to improve their bargaining effectiveness are eliminated—that is, through the broadening of units which are of sufficient economic strength to represent the parties effectively at the bargaining table."[1]

[1] Brown, D. V. and Schultz, G. P. Public policy and the structure of collective bargaining in *The Structure of Collective Bargaining,* ed. A. R. Weber (New York: The Free Press of Glen Cove, Inc., 1961) pp. 318-319.

OTHER STATES

That hospitals in general are excluded from the coverage of the Taft-Hartley Act is indeed no small concern to administrators around the country. Section 2(2) of the Labor-Management Relations Act specifically excludes not-for-profit hospitals from its jurisdiction. It is interesting to note that government-owned hospitals also are excluded and, as to for-profit hospitals, the National Labor Relations Board has taken jurisdiction only if they are vital to national defense or are located in the District of Columbia, where the NLRB acts as a local agency, or are operated in connection with an interstate business.[2]

The problem of unequal coverage as to labor relations law is not one peculiar to New York State. In Minnesota nearly all hospitals are covered by the Charitable Hospital Act. In Wisconsin, the Employee Relations Act covers not-for-profit hospitals. In California the State Conciliation Service may involve itself at the request of the parties. Such states as Oregon, North Dakota, Michigan, Massachusetts, Hawaii, and Kansas have, in one manner or another, prescribed regulations that bring some or all of their employees under state laws regarding representation and collective bargaining.

Fourteen states have labor relations laws similar to the National Labor Relations Act and for-profit hospitals are covered by all of these: in the case of not-for-profit hospitals, eight states provide for coverage of such employees while the remaining six specifically exclude such employees. In the case of New Jersey, which has no labor relations statute, the State Supreme Court upheld a lower court decision in 1965 that guaranteed to employees of not-for-profit hospitals the right to organize and bargain collectively.[3]

The fear of unionization that the large majority of unorganized, not-for-profit hospitals throughout the United States have maintained has driven hospitals into a position of extreme vulnerability. By running for the cover of exclusions from the Labor-Management Relations Act (Taft-Hartley)—forever pointing out the uniqueness of hospitals and maintaining an uncompromising antiunion posture—hospitals have brought themselves to a position of inequality vis-a-vis the industrial world. A careful reevaluation of our position obviously is needed at this time.

The lorica-like exclusion under the national law and lack of inclusion under state laws no longer can be considered sufficient protection against the newly revitalized organizing efforts of hospital unions.

It is interesting—and foreboding—that Local 1199 Drug and Hospital Employees Union, based in New York City, has opened satellite offices in Philadelphia and Baltimore and has embarked on a strike at two institutions in Charleston, S.C. What is most interesting is that Pennsylvania, Maryland, and South Carolina are not among the states that provide for collective bargaining for not-for-profit hospitals employees. The

---

[2]Northrup, H. R. and Bloom, G. F. *Government and Labor* (Homewood, Ill.: Richard D. Irwin, Inc., 1963).

[3]Gamm, S. *Towards Collective Bargaining in Non-Profit Hospitals: Impact of the New York Law* (New York State School of Industrial and Labor Relations. Cornell University, Ithaca, N.Y., Bull 60. Oct. 1968).

*See: Plan proposed to prevent strikes of hospitals. *Hospitals,* J.A.H.A. **44**:119 Feb. 16, 1970.

state laws now operative in the area of labor relations do not provide sufficient protection in dealing with union organizing efforts and collective bargaining in the hospital industry. The court rulings in some states that seem to regulate such activities are poor substitutes for a labor relations act. The sad lesson to be learned by the unorganized hospitals, both in those few states that provide for coverage of their employees and in the majority of states that exclude such employees, is that by maintaining our fractionated posture and by championing individual sovereignty of hospitals and states, hospitals have backed themselves into a cul-de-sac that has effected inequities and inadequate protection.

Hospital administrators and individuals in the labor relations field should seriously undertake to lobby for labor legislation that would apply to not-for-profit hospitals.* Such legislation could be similar to the Railway Adjustment Act, which is based upon the Labor-Management Relations Act but is specifically directed to the railroad and airline industries. When hospital spokesmen maintained that their particular industry was unique and had special problems, were they asking for less than equal treatment? It is time that the hospital industry and the American Hospital Association review their policies regarding hospitals and the Taft-Hartley Act. Hospitals should have, at the very least, protection under the law similar to that afforded the industrial community.

CONCLUSION

The much-lobbyed position of exclusion from the Labor-Management Relations Act, which removed not-for-profit hospitals from the jurisdiction of the National Labor Relations Board, has brought with it many disadvantages unrecognized in the heat of the battle over maintenance of such exclusion. The balkanization of bargaining units and the proliferation of unions in hospitals may well continue even under the coverage of the national act. The basic equality with industry discussed is in the area of exclusions from bargaining units of supervisors and guards, and a much broader definition for the exclusion of confidential employees. In addition to these exclusions, the availability of redress for the hospitals in the face of unfair union labor practices is certainly no less a need than that available to General Motors and General Electric under the national law. If this position is correct and hospitals are indeed a unique industry (which is quite clear from their function—patient care), then hospitals need at least as much protection as that afforded to industrial firms in interstate commerce. It is ironic that the small proprietary hospitals, uninvolved in research and teaching programs and providing a minimal range of health services, have been able to find more protection under the law in some instances than have the large majority of voluntary hospitals in the United States.

Some hospital administrators feel that their exemption from the Taft-Hartley Act has proved to be of little disadvantage in their own states. It has, they claim, saved hospitals from many a strike and costly bargaining sessions because the unions had no rights (or assistance from a labor relations agency). This protective advantage is short-lived, as the situations in South Carolina, in Baltimore, and possibly in Philadelphia and Pittsburgh, indicate. This advantage may have been present while the unions fractionated their approach. With the growth of Local 1199 Drug and Hospital Employee's Union, AFL-CIO, both in numbers and in financial support, it appears that all hospitals are fair game, whether protected by law or not.

The advantages of a national labor relations act for hospitals are clear. Organizational strikes would be outlawed. Unfair labor practices would be clearly defined for unions as well as management. The question of establishing bargaining units would be proscribed as it is under the national act and the Railway Adjustment Act. An orderly procedure for adjusting negotiating impasses could be established with specific relevance to the unique nature of our field. Amending present statutes in those states that provide for collective bargaining for not-for-profit hospitals is a most difficult job. The whole hospital field should direct its efforts toward obtaining maximum legal protection in its dealings with labor unions. A national labor law for not-for-profit hospitals would concern itself with the interest of the employees while providing due consideration to the interest of the hospitals and their patients.

Taft-Hartley Exemption

WILLIAM J. EMANUEL

William J. Emanuel is an attorney and partner in the firm of Musick, Peeler and Garrett in Los Angeles, California.

The exemption of not-for-profit hospitals from the coverage of the Taft-Hartley Act[1] recently has been the subject of controversy and criticism within the not-for-profit hospital community. A number of hospital executives, apparently situated primarily in New York State, are convinced that obtaining this exemption was a serious mistake. A leading exponent of this viewpoint is Norman Metzger, a prominent hospital executive and labor relations expert, whose views are set forth in the March 16, 1970, issue of *Hospitals, J.A.H.A.* It is the purpose of this article to present the other side of this controversial question in rebuttal to Mr. Metzger's article.

Mr. Metzger does not assert that the exemption is unjustified from the viewpoint of public policy but rather that it is ill-advised from management's viewpoint, because it deprives not-for-profit hospitals of the "protections" of the Taft-Hartley Act. He claims that the exemption has driven not-for-profit hospitals into a position of extreme vulnerability and has put them at a disadvantage when compared to corporations that fall under the jurisdiction of the National Labor Relations Board. He asserts that, by obtaining this exemption, not-for-profit hospitals have "brought themselves to a position of inequality vis-a-vis the industrial world" and have "backed themselves into a cul-de-sac that has effected inequities and inadequate protection."

Mr. Metzger urges the not-for-profit hospital community to lobby for labor legislation that would apply to not-for-profit hospitals so that they would be provided legal protection similar to that of the industrial community. He advocates labor legislation specifically designed for hospitals, as in the case of the railroad and airline industries under the Railway Labor Act.

ASSISTANCE FOR UNIONS

The main fault in these arguments is their characterization of the Taft-Hartley Act as a law designed *to protect management.* Although Taft-Hartley attempted to correct some of the imbalances in the Wagner Act, the avowed and primary purpose of the national labor law remains *to assist unions in the organization of employees.*[2] Any proposal to alter the exempt status of not-for-profit hospitals under this law should be evaluated critically in light of this central purpose.

The same would be true of any effort to obtain labor legislation designed specifically for hospitals. The recent experience of the agricultural industry in attempting to obtain enactment of such a law and the general reluctance of labor and management to confront the question of new labor legislation at this time[3] indicate little chance of success for such efforts. However, even if special legislation were adopted, its central purpose would be to assist unions in organizing hospital employees.

Although Taft-Hartley does provide some protection for employers, Mr. Metzger overrates the significance of such protection. For example, while many labor relations experts share his concern over bargaining unit fragmentation, Taft-Hartley is anything but a panacea for this problem. Although the extent to which employees organize themselves into a fragmented unit is not supposed to be a controlling factor in an NLRB unit determination,[4] it all too frequently is. While an organized work force sometimes is insulated from fragmentation, depending on the nature of the work force and the type of operation involved, an unorganized work force remains vulnerable. A union usually can obtain a fragmented unit in such circumstances merely by showing that the unit consists of an identifiable group of employees with a separate community of interests.[5] Fragmentation is encouraged further under Taft-Hartley by special unit rules for professional[6] and technical[7] employees and by other rules that permit the severance of craft and departmental groups from an existing unit if a separate community of interests is shown and certain other requirements are met.[8]

It should be clear, therefore, that employers subject to Taft-Hartley are by no means impervious to bargaining unit fragmentation. To the contrary, although it is hoped that the NLRB would not do so, there is no guarantee that under some circumstances it would not permit a hospital to be divided into separate units covering dietary, laundry, housekeeping, office personnel, technicians, registered nurses, pharmacists, lab technologists, and a number of others. Thus, the disquieting prospect of not-for-profit hospitals being split into multiple bargaining units would exist regardless of whether they are covered by Taft-Hartley.

SUPERVISORY CONFLICTS OF INTEREST

Another Taft-Hartley "protection" that Mr. Metzger overemphasizes is the exclusion of supervisors from the definition of "employee"[9] and, therefore, from voting eligibility in board-conducted elections. In particular, much emphasis is placed on supervisory conflicts of interest that often arise when registered nurses or other professional groups are represented by professional associations for bargaining purposes. From a hospital's viewpoint, there can be no quarrel with the proposition that supervisors should be excluded from bargaining units and that supervisory conflicts of interest should be avoided. Mr. Metzger errs, however, in suggesting that Taft-Hartley would afford hospitals total protection in this regard.

The best case in point is the RN bargaining unit, which typically is represented by a professional nurses' association. Because the great majority of RNs supervise other nursing personnel, it can be cogently argued that almost every RN should be considered a supervisor within the Taft-Hartley definition.[10] However, the NLRB has rejected this interpretation. Even under a fairly liberal interpretation, every RN at or above the charge nurse level should qualify as a Taft-Hartley supervisor. Although the NLRB adopted the latter interpretation in excluding LVN (LPN) charge nurses from broad service and maintenance units in nonexempt institutions,[11] it has refused to exclude RN charge nurses from RN units.[12] Apparently the NLRB has done this because it realizes that the exclusion of RN charge nurses would impede the effective organization of an RN unit, as a large part of the unit could be excluded. As a result of this approach, which the board justifies by a dubious distinction between professional supervision and Taft-Hartley supervision, relatively few RNs now are excluded as supervisors from RN units.

Even to the extent that RNs are excluded as supervisors, conflicts of interest nevertheless will continue to exist whenever such a supervisor is a member of a professional organization representing RNs for bargaining purposes, because she must deal on a management-labor basis with her own professional organization. In this situation, the hospital is confronted with the choice of allowing her to handle grievances filed by her own professional association on behalf of other RNs or forcing her to resign from that organization. This problem is intensified if, as often happens, the supervisor holds a position of responsibility in the professional organization. In short, Taft-Hartley does not cure the conflict of interest problems inherent when a professional organization operates as a labor organization.

OTHER PROTECTION

Although Mr. Metzger's proposed hospital labor law would prohibit organizational (recognition) strikes, he fails to explain that unions are, within certain limitations, free to engage in such strikes under Taft-Hartley.[13] Moreover, while the proposed law would establish an "orderly procedure" for adjusting bargaining impasses, Mr. Metzger fails to elaborate on how this would be accomplished and neglects to mention that both Taft-Hartley and the Railway Labor Act have been notably ineffective in this regard. He emphasizes the Taft-Hartley exclusion of guards from nonguard units,[14] but this protection, although important, is hardly worth the disadvantages of coverage under the Act.

Furthermore, it is significant to note that one of the most important protections afforded employers under Taft-Hartley, the secondary boycott law,[15] is available to not-for-profit hospitals notwithstanding their otherwise exempt status. Although a not-for-profit hospital is not considered an employer under the Act, the secondary boycott law protects "persons," not merely employers. Therefore, a not-for-profit hospital is entitled to this protection, whether it is the primary object of the labor dispute and some other person is a secondary object, or whether it is a secondary object embroiled in someone else's labor dispute.[16]

Many hospital executives are understandably perplexed at being urged to lobby for a law that would greatly facilitate union organization in return for a few legal protections, some of which are rather dubious and almost all of which are unnecessary unless union organization actually is achieved. They reason that this can be likened to jumping overboard in order to take advantage of the "protection" of the nearest life raft. The explanation is found in the fact that not-for-profit hospitals in New York are subject to a state "little Wagner Act," an anachronistic law that is slanted completely in favor of unions, and that they would prefer to be covered by Taft-Hartley. It is easy to appreciate their concern over this situation and to understand why they would want corrective legislation. However, they make the mistake of arguing that the entire not-for-profit hospital community would benefit from such legislation, which simply is not true.

CONCLUSION

Not-for-profit hospitals that do not share the plight of the New York hospitals stand to lose, not gain, by being subjected to the Taft-Hartley Act or similar legislation. The New York hospitals are indeed unfortunate in being subject to an unbalanced and archaic state labor law. However, the remedy for problems with state legislation should be found in the state legislature, not in Congress, where they would drag all other not-for-profit hospitals under the "protective" umbrella of the NLRB, or some other agency, to escape from a local problem.

REFERENCES

[1] National Labor Relations Act (as amended) S 2(2), 29 U.S.C. S 152(2).

[2] NLRA S 1, 29 U.S.C. S 151.

[3] Address by Secretary of Labor James D. Hodgson, *Labor Relations Reporter*, p. 355 (Bureau of National Affairs, Inc., Aug. 17, 1970).

[4] NLRA S 9(c) (5), 29 U.S.C. S 159(c) (5).

[5] For example, *Bagdad Copper Co.*, 144 NLRB 1496 (1963).

[6] NLRA S 9(b) (1), 29 U.S.C. S 159(b) (1).

[7] *Sheffield Corp.*, 134 NLRB 1101 (1961).

[8] *Mallinckrodt Chemical Works*, 162 NLRB 387 (1966). NLRA S 9(b) (2), 29 U.S.C. S 159(b) (2).

[9] NLRA S 2(3), 29 U.S.C. S 152(3). The definition of "supervisor" is set forth in NLRA S 2(11), 29 U.S.C. S 152(11).

[10] *Sherewood Enterprises, Inc.*, 175 NLRB No. 59 (1969); *Diversified Health Services, Inc.*, 180 NLRB No. 26 (1969).

[11] *University Nursing Home, Inc.*, 168 NLRB No. 53 (1967); *Rosewood, Inc.*, 185 NLRB No. 87 (1970). The Board refused to exclude LVNs who apparently functioned as charge nurses in *New Fern Restorium Co.*, 175 NLRB No. 142 (1969).

[12] *Sherewood Enterprises, Inc.*, 175 NLRB No. 59 (1969), as modified by *Doctors' Hospital of Modesto, Inc.*, 183 NLRB No. 94 (1970); *Diversified Health Services, Inc.*, 180 NLRB No. 26 (1969).

[13] For restrictions on the right to engage in strikes and picketing for recognition, see NLRA S S 8(b) (4) (B), 8(b) (4) (C), and 8(b) (7), 29 U.S.C. S S 158(b) (4) (B), 158 (b) (4) (C), and 158(b) (7).

[14] NLRA S 9(b) (3), 29 U.S.C. S 159(b) (3).

[15] NLRA S 8(b) (4) (B), 29 U.S.C. S 158(b) (4) (B).

[16] *International Brotherhood of Teamsters, etc.*, **153 NLRB 993 (1965)**; *Suffolk County District Council of Carpenters, etc.*, **173 NLRB No. 188 (1968)**; *International Longshoremen and Warehousemen's Union*, **176 NLRB No. 121 (1969)**; Etelson, *NLRB Jurisdiction over Secondary Boycotts in the Public and Other "Exempt" Sectors*, **20 Labor Law Journal 771 (1969)**.

Hospital Unionization

This section treats the subject of hospital unionization, its causes and effects. Historically the hospital has been isolated from organized labor. However, the last decade has witnessed substantial unionization activity among hospital employees. Today's administrator must not only ascertain the effect of a union on his organization, but also have a basic understanding of why employees desire to bargain collectively.

In *THE EFFECT OF UNIONS ON HOSPITAL MANAGEMENT,* it is pointed out that hospitals have lagged behind industry in recognizing the need for the industrial relations staff function. In addition, it is mentioned that hospital unions have traditionally been resisted by administrators because of four basic fears. They are the fears of strikes, costs, loss of control, and the resulting complication of the personnel administration functions. Arguments against hospital unionization are presented along with a more liberal philosophy toward unions by administrators. Moreover, the stimulating and inhibiting factors of unionism are discussed. The article cites that a new liberal view is emerging due to the fact that the hospital must compete in the labor market, must present attractive careers, and must also recognize its responsibility to employees.

In *GRIEVANCE PROCEDURES: OUTLET FOR EMPLOYEE, INSIGHT FOR MANAGEMENT,* the grievance procedure is presented as a safety valve which functions as an upward communication channel. Whether or not the hospital is unionized, a systematic method of solving employee grievances assists in improving employee relations. Should the hospital not be unionized, the institution of a grievance procedure will greatly assist in reducing employee dissatisfaction.

The Effect of Unions on Hospital Management

LEO B. OSTERHAUS, PH.D.

Leo B. Osterhaus, Ph.D., is the Director of the Center of Business Administration at St. Edwards University in Austin, Texas.

As organized labor has increased in numbers and scope, not only has it affected every individual in the United States, but the ramifications of its influence are evident in organizations and institutions that have traditionally been isolated or specialized in their functions, if not in their activities. Such an institution is the hospital.

In spite of deeply rooted traditions which surround hospitals with an almost religious-like aura, significant trends in public opinion and acceptance of unions as democratic institutions lend validity to the doubts of some and wishes of others that hospitals are prime targets for accelerated union activities.

Attracting organized labor to the hospital field are 7,123 hospitals employing almost two million people.[1] Related activities such as nursing homes, clinics and other medical treatment facilities swell this total.

It is generally conceded that working conditions and wages in the hospital have not kept pace with industry, even for the same skills; rather a reliance has been placed on appeals to the "will to serve humanity." Although this has been successful to a limited degree, these conditions beckon the unions. Sloan, in describing hospital labor problems, stated that although hospitals have paid low in the past, they must pay more and must eliminate possible causes for demands or unions will make them do it.[2]

Much of the organization of labor in the hospitals has occurred since World War II. A few hospital employes like engineers were organized loosely in the thirties, but the major drives have been in the past 10 years. One of the reasons for the delay in unionization in the hospital is probably the fact that the Labor Management Relations Act of 1947, usually referred to as the Taft-Hartley Act, specifically excludes nonprofit hospitals from its provisions which protect or encourage collective bargaining. Voluntary hospitals are also generally excluded from the provisions of state laws.

[1] Statistics were obtained from *Hospitals,* Part II, Guide Issue, Aug. 1, 1966, p. 428.

[2] Raymond Sloan, *This Hospital Business of Ours,* New York, G. P. Putnam's Sons, 1952, p. 216.

It would be a mistake to attribute the existence of unions today to any single cause; they resulted from a combination of many historical circumstances which existed in the hospital environment. In general, hospitals have lagged far behind industry in recognizing the need and providing for the industrial relations staff function. Hospital administrators have handled grievances poorly. They have failed to provide comparable wages and salaries, and the training in communication and supervision has failed to be effective in many cases.

SCOPE OF THE STUDY

It is generally stated that hospital costs are closely related to many of the labor-management problems. Costs in nonfederal short-term general and special hospitals have been increasing faster than the costs of any other segment of the medical care area. The proportion of the total cost represented by payroll expenses has increased from 50 per cent in 1946, to 70 per cent in 1964. Two-thirds of the increase in total expense per patient day between 1946 and 1964 can be accounted for by the increase in payroll expenses.[3]

With the increasing influence of labor unions on hospitals, and the pressures being placed upon hospitals to improve their manpower practices, the hospital is being forced to meet industrial employment conditions by increasing hospital wages and fringe benefits and shortening the workweek. Industrial employers have been able to meet some of their increasing labor costs through increased productivity; therefore, the author studied the potential of productivity increases in hospitals to see if they can compensate for higher labor costs.

The type of labor hospitals employ is a function of their employment conditions and creates certain manpower problems such as high turnover, absenteeism and high supervisor-employe ratios. Although the type of labor employed may result in low labor costs, it is necessary to include the effects of these problems in an evaluation of total actual cost and to estimate whether changed employment practices allowing for improved labor standards might not lead to an actual reduction in labor costs.

CONSISTENT DATA LACKING

Because of the critical relationship of manpower problems, labor unions and hospital costs, and the growing impact of these problems on hospital operation, research leading toward possible solutions and the development of effective policies is urgently needed. Data on which the research would be based, however, is not available. Studies have been made of specific manpower problems in individual institutions or small groups of institutions. But no comprehensive, consistent data has been collected from enough institutions over a wide area to provide the researcher with a base of correlated and verified information on patterns and trends of hospital personnel practices, policies and problems. After the author collected and organized these descriptive data, he then evaluated the effects of current practices on hospital efficiency and costs.

[3] *Hospitals,* Part II, Guide Issue, Aug. 1, 1965, p. 438.

While manpower and industrial relations problems in hospitals fall directly within the purview of the applied disciplines of personnel administration and labor relations, the techniques of labor economics, cost accounting, and industrial management have also been used to analyze the significance of hospital operations on specific policies and practices. The most productive approach to hospital manpower and industrial relations problems seemed to be an interdisciplinary approach capable of using the relevant information and techniques of both basic and applied disciplines and of the medical care field.

PHILOSPHY OF LABOR RELATIONS

Although most industries have probably thought at one time or another that "they were different," and organized labor "did not have a place" in their establishments, hospitals do seem to present other than routine labor-management problems.

The basic labor relations philosophy of the hospital field is shaped by hospital management, hospital associations, and other professional groups closely allied to the hospital and medical care field.

Hospital management is a diffused and varied group without a unified, concise stance on common problems. It is difficult to determine anything specific concerning hospital management. Not only is the ownership of hospitals diverse, but hospitals themselves are identified so closely with the general public that it is difficult to isolate public opinion from hospital management opinion. The direct public influence is immediately experienced.

The American Hospital Association, the unofficial voice of most hospitals, states as a policy: "It is for the hospital governing board to decide the hospital policy toward union recognition and collective bargaining."[4] The same organization states further: "It is hoped that such a hospital will approach the problem with due regard for: 1. the law, 2. sound personnel policies, 3. proper management principles, and 4. accepted community practices."[5]

As indicated from a review of recorded statements from leaders and other individuals in the field, attitudes toward unions vary from: 1. Violent opposition,[6] 2. toleration as long as individual union members do not interfere in any way with hospital operations and management,[7] 3. acceptance as bargaining equals to management,[8] and 4. acceptance because the ownership of the hospital or union represents a sizable portion of the clientele.[9] The majority opinion seems to cluster around the second attitude which may possibly be explained by the size and location of hospitals in this country. Undoubtedly, this attitude toward unions has been

[4] American Hospital Association, *Hospitals and Employe Groups,* Personnel Relations Series No. 2, Chicago, American Hospital Association, p. 5.

[5] *Ibid.,* p. iv.

[6] Grandville L. Jones, "Unions in Hospitals Are Wrong and Unnecessary," *Mental Hospitals,* September, 1957, p. 27.

[7] E. D. Barnett, "Satisfied Employes Promote Good Hospital Care," *Hospital Council Bulletin,* June, 1949, p. 19.

[8] San Francisco Bay Area.

[9] Hospitals owned by unions and hospitals furnishing hospital services to union groups.

influenced by the fact that most hospitals have less than 100 beds and are located in small communities where organized labor is weak.

The management philosophy of these rather conservative administrators is based on the following factors:

1.   The granting of control of employes and/or activities in a hospital to a union which knows little about the problems of the care of the sick is incompatible with safe patient care.

2.   Hospital operation is a continuous one, and to interpose any force that would tend to destroy its continuity would be harmful.

3.   Hospital activity, unlike industry, must strive for 100 per cent efficiency in its professional elements and cannot accept any interference that might appear if seniority, tenure, etc., were used primarily as a basis for selection of employes in the nursing units and treatment and diagnostic areas.

4.   Because hospitals are nonprofit organizations, no profits are available to share, or with which to bargain.

5.   Unions divide the loyalty of employes between management and unions.

6.   Hospital employes enjoy a high status in the community without union aid.

7.   Unions are powerless if the weapons of strikes, work stoppages and slowdowns are removed. As these weapons cannot be tolerated in hospitals without endangering life, unions would be unnecessary appendages.

8.   The right of employes to organize is secondary to the right of human beings to receive adequate attention when ill or injured.

9.   The Taft-Hartley Act is the law of the land—a public mandate, and since hospitals were specifically exempted from this law, unions should not attempt to organize in hospitals.

10.   Unionization in hospitals is not in the public interest.

11.   As it is assumed that with unionization comes additional labor costs, some leaders point out that this additional cost would have to be borne directly by the patients. The vital difference in the purchasing of hospital services is that the patient does not have a real choice of whether to purchase or not to purchase—he must buy hospitalization.

FOUR FEARS

The above theories (or expositions) are based on four fears:

1.   Strikes. Management realizes that hospitals are helpless against strikes if desired health care standards are to be maintained. Endangering lives and/or delaying the relief of suffering is unthinkable. Past records of strikes, in spite of their paucity, have magnified this fear.

2.   Unionization will cost money. A study of the wage rates confirms this fear. As hospital costs are reaching alarming proportions, administrators appear to be condoning, currently at least, a lower hospital charge at the expense of hospital employes' wages.

3.   Control will be lost. Management has a fear that unions will assume an unnecessary number of management's prerogatives. A divided control would be disastrous in a hospital if exhibited to any degree.

4. Organized labor will complicate administration and require that a central control be established to insure that personnel administration is consistent. Detail procedures will have to be given the supervisors on how to handle simple disciplinary problems and complaints. All actions will have to be documented completely so that the case can be supported if it goes to arbitration.

A MORE LIBERAL VIEW IS EMERGING

Enlightened writers have been warning for years that hospital management should re-evaluate the philosophy of purchasing labor, and vitalize hospital personnel policies. These warnings, stripped of their more highly theoretical (but probably more important) discussions, are based on hard reality that can be ascertained by even the most recalcitrant. These are:

1. Unionization is now generally accepted as a way of life, and this trend may affect the favorable public reaction enjoyed by the hospital in the past in hospital-labor disputes.

2. Noneconomic incentives accruing to hospital employes are currently over-rated. Gordon in commenting on this states:

> There appeared to be a general acceptance of the proposition that nonmonetary incentives have sometimes been over exploited and are not a substitute for a fair wage scale that is equitable within the hospital and that provides a necessary standard of living for the worker and his dependents. [10]

3. A social revolution has taken place that should be considered in the over-all operation and relationships of hospitals. This change is best illustrated by the following comment:

> In the fields of wages and salary administration, many new concepts have been introduced. In this field, as in the field of relations with organized labor, we are dealing with group pressures, and we have as yet not resolved the dilemma of conflicts between individual and group aspirations.[11]

4. Sound personnel policies and a modern personnel department are needed with or without a union; they are not a luxury or a frill but a necessity in these enlightened times. Hospitals must quit vacillating and establish these departments or this will be just another defenseless weakness. Everett W. Jones states:

> The constant upgrading of administrative abilities and leadership and the development of sound personnel and public relation practices may well determine the ultimate fate of our voluntary hospital system.[12]

Many people connected with the hospital field complain that the worker today is more interested in the monetary return than in service to the sick. These and similar

---

[10]Paul J. Gordon, "Why Anyone Works in a Hospital," *The Modern Hospital,* June, 1954, pp. 76-78.

[11]B. A. Lindberg, "Looking in on Hospital Personnel Administration," *Hospitals,* May, 1953, p. 65.

[12]Everett W. Jones, Hospital Consultant at the National Board of Methodist Hospitals and Homes Convention, Indianapolis, Ind., 1945.

statements are emanating from both the conservative and the liberal side of the question as evidenced by the following:

1.   Hospitals are competing with industry for personnel in the face of a diminishing labor pool, particularly since the change in status of women workers after World War II. To meet competition, wages and other benefits must approach parity with industry.

2.   Hospitals must present an attractive career program for the three-quarter million new workers entering the labor market every year, or fall heir to the castoffs from industry.

3.   Hospitals should recognize that they have a basic obligation to both their employes and the public in their employe relations.

The above facts, reinforced with a new philosophy, have resulted in enlightened efforts to accept unions,[13] and writings such as those of the AHA, Stevens,[14] Freeman,[15] and Metzger[16] have furthered the cause.

A very limited number of administrators have advanced the theory that unions actually benefit hospital operations. This attitude, as limited in converts as it may be, is found in the mental hospital field,[17] but it is not entirely limited to this area.[18] The limitation of the scope of this attitude is emphasized since one of the two major problems that contribute to limited unionization in mental hospitals is the fact that hospital administrators are slow to recognize unions. Today, for an administrator to advocate that unions do benefit hospital operations is an undertaking of some trepidity.

In summary, the majority of hospitals are conservative in their thought and action toward unions, but a trend to a more liberal view is indicated.

FACTORS STIMULATING UNIONIZATION

The magnitude of the nonunion labor force in the hospital industry apparently has been one of the factors attracting the eyes of union organizers during recent years. In 1964, there were 7,127 hospitals in the United States employing a total of 1,886,839 fulltime personnel with an annual payroll of $7,974,623,000.00.[19] Of all the hospitals this vast industry, only 435 hospitals in 1965 had contracts with labor organizations.[20] This fact certainly provides an incentive to the labor organizer, especially in light of recent declines in over-all labor union membership.

[13]Ray Bruner, "Toledo Plan' Supported by Hospitals and Labor," *The Modern Hospital,* July, 1959, pp. 76-77.

[14]R. D. Stevens, "How Administrators Can Negotiate with a Union," *Southern Hospitals,* December, 1956, p. 26.

[15]John R. Freeman, "You Can Too Learn to Live with Unions." *The Modern Hospital,* November, 1964, pp. 95-98.

[16]Norman Metzger, "Living with a Collective Bargaining Agreement for the First 100 Days," *Hospital Management,* October, 1964, pp. 49-52.

[17]Pamphlet entitled *Mental Health Story,* published by the American Federation of State, County and Municipal Employes, AFL-CIO; Jack R. Ewolt, "Employes Union: Pro and Con; Unions Can Benefit Hospital Administration," *Mental Hospitals,* September, 1957, pp. 26-27.

[18]Arthur Hare, "Hospitals and Union in Harmony." *The Modern Hospital,* February, 1948, p. 74.

[19]*Hospitals,* Guide Issue, Aug. 1, 1965, Part II, pp. 431-451.

[20]Interview with Edward W. Weimer, director, Administrative Services, AHA, Aug. 2, 1965.

Poor labor relations practices are thought to be one of the major factors contributing to the general labor movement. This condition has apparently provided a major boost in the unionization of employes in the hospital industry.

> In general, hospitals have lagged far behind industry in recognizing the need for, and providing, the industrial relations staff function. In many hospitals of several hundred employes, the personnel function is performed as "the other hat" of an already harried administrator, or his assistant.[21]

Inadequacies in personnel or industrial relations have been especially noticeable in the area of grievance procedures in hospitals. "In some hospitals, there is little provision made for the settlement of grievances, an oversight that stimulates interest in unions."[22] In recognition of this shortcoming, concerted efforts of the American Hospital Assn. have been directed toward personnel relations during the past several years. These efforts have taken the form of numerous workshops and institutes conducted for hospital administrators and their assistants on the subjects of labor relations, as well as publications aimed at improving personnel policies of member hospitals, especially in the areas of employe handbooks and grievance procedures.[23]

Another factor which would seem to contribute to the encouragement of labor unions in hospitals is the matter of wages.

> A disproportionate chunk of the charity of too many hospitals has been involuntarily carried by underpaid employes who supply the hospital with essential services.[24]

The Bureau of Labor Statistics' survey of hospital wages conducted during 1963 showed a number of hospital employes receiving less than what is usually considered to be the minimum wage. Almost 130,000 of the one million workers covered by the survey were receiving less than $1.25 per hour.[25] Another factor to keep in mind is that this survey was limited to hospitals in metropolitan areas with populations in excess of 250,000. A much larger percentage of low-paid employes can normally be expected in hospitals in smaller cities and in rural areas.

Even though the wage issue is usually not the greatest motivating factor for union membership, it would seem to rank high in importance for workers in the hospital industry. The difference between the wages of hospital workers and those employed in work outside the hospital industry is such that hospitals sometimes have been accused of "exploitation."[26] The mere mention of this word, of course, strikes at the very heart of the labor union movement, and it provides additional impetus for the drive to unionize hospital employes.

[21]James L. Centner, "Hospitals and Collective Bargaining," *Personnel Journal,* November, 1959, p. 203.

[22]Walter L. Daykin, "The Hospital and Employe Organizations," *Hospital Administration,* Fall, 1958, p. 7.

[23]For example, see the following pamphlets published and distributed by the AHA. *Suggested Employe Dissatisfaction Procedure, Preparing an Employe Handbook, and Hospitals and Employe Groups.*

[24]Carl I. Flath, "Hospitals and the Labor Movement," *Southern Hospitals,* July, 1960, p. 26.

[25]U.S. Department of Labor, Bureau of Labor Statistics, *Industry Wage Survey: Hospitals,* June, 1964, p. 12.

[26]George Kirstein, "Why Hospitals Exploit Labor," *The Nation,* July 4, 1959, pp. 3-6.

FACTORS INHIBITING UNIONIZATION

Although many hospitals have long had a small number of employes who belonged to unions, the unions have been slow to develop in hospitals for a variety of reasons. Foremost among them is that unions were preoccupied with more lucrative fields and thus delayed their action in this particular field. Some of the other more important reasons which prevented unionization of hospital employes are discussed below.

Dispersion and size of hospitals are factors which inhibit unionization. Of the 7,127 hospitals registered by the AHA in 1964, 4,009 had less than 100 beds. The average institution had approximately 260 fulltime employes.[27] These hospitals were dispersed throughout the United States, and the majority of the small hospitals were located in small communities. This fact made unionization difficult except where employes could be included with other organized groups from other industries in the community.

The nature of the hospital force itself has been a major inhibiting factor.

> Many hospital employes are women whose work is a temporary interlude between school, marriage and the rearing of a family. In other words, these female employes lack permanency, and it is a well-established principle that it takes permanent employes to form a strong labor movement. Employes of this type customarily lack labor-consciousness and are inclined to view problems that arise as temporary. In addition, a sizable proportion of the employes in hospital work are older workers who are unfamiliar with union operations; many are pleased merely to have employment. Consequently, they often are reluctant to engage in any activity which might jeopardize their job status.[28]

The hospital also has a multiplicity of professional and semiprofessional employes. Tead, in addressing the American College of Hospital Administrators, stated that among the factors that highlight and complicate the jobs of administrators is the critical function of utilizing a wide variety of specialized vocational groups within the organization as well as by the organization itself, and the difficulty of keeping the primary social objective of the institution foremost in mind.[29] This problem would apply with equal force to the union officials as well as the hospital executive.

Hospitals, proportionally, have a greater number of varieties of professional, semiprofessional, skilled, and semiskilled personnel than any other organization. This factor, combined with the reluctance of many of these personnel to be identified with unions, has impeded progress of unions.

Both national and state labor legislation has been a major deterrent for hospital unionism. Although these laws generally do not prohibit hospital employes, neither do they encourage and protect either of these actions.

THE STRIKE HAS NOT BEEN EFFECTIVE

Another major inhibiting factor is the nature of hospital business, i.e., the voluntary, nonprofit status of the typical hospital. This unique position has molded the opinions of legislators, the courts, and the public to the extent that attempts at

[27]Figures computed from Tables 1 and 2c, Guide Issue, *Hospitals,* Part II, Aug. 1, 1965, pp. 431-452.

[28]Daykin, *op cit.,* p. 8.

[29]From an address by Ordway Tead to the ACHA, Aug. 17, 1958, Chicago.

unionization of hospital employes are met with hostile attitudes in many areas. The emotions connected with the service of the business of the hospital—caring for the sick—has been a factor. Any actions which might temporarily interfere with the operation of a hospital are thought of as being directed toward those persons lying ill in the hospital. An important deterring force is public sentiment which was illustrated in an organizational drive that was thwarted through an information campaign, including appeals in local newspapers.[30] In a leaflet prepared by the AHA for hospital administrators, one of the actions suggested to combat unionism was "Tell your story to the press."[31]

Finally, the strike—labor's ultimate weapon—has not been very effective in hospitals. In several instances, workers striking for union recognition have been victims of unfavorable public reactions, and they have failed to receive support from other labor unions or from the clergy. The available supply of volunteer workers to fill the vacated jobs, the refusal on the part of most other laborers to honor the picket line, and the hesitancy of strikers to insist that their picket line be honored have often made the hospital strike ineffective. These factors were instrumental in the defeat of the union in Chicago.[32]

SUMMARY

Many feel that hospitals are unique and, therefore, should be treated differently from other service and manufacturing industries when considering labor-management relations and other subjects. No unanimity of opinion exists, but in general the hospital administrators and hospital trustees are rather conservative and try to avoid any radical change from the past. Administrators and trustees receive support from professional groups (except for the nurses) which seem to be anti-union or anti-collective-bargaining-minded. However, as these groups mature and gain status, they will probably seek economic security as well as professional and educational benefits for their members.

A more liberal view of labor-management relations has recently emerged in the hospital administration field. The success of this group is rather limited at the present, but the group is increasing in number as the new and younger administrators assume leadership in the hospital field.

[30]John T. Foster, "Good Story Well Told Defeats Two Union Efforts at Wisconsin Hospital," *The Modern Hospital,* July, 1964, p. 36.

[31]"What to Do! A Checklist for the Individual Hospital," AHA, Chicago, Aug. 15, 1959.

[32]Robert B. McKersie and Montague Brown, "Nonprofessional Hospital Workers and a Union Organizing Drive," *The Quarterly Journal of Economics,* August, 1963, pp. 372-404.

Grievance Procedures: Outlet for Employee, Insight for Management

ROD CLELLAND

Rod Clelland M.B.A., is Administrative Superintendent of Central State Hospital in Milledgeville, Georgia.

In April 1966, 3500 registered nurses in New York City hospitals delivered an ultimatum threatening resignation if better working conditions and improved pay were not provided. Shortly thereafter, similar events occurred in Los Angeles, San Francisco, and Phoenix, Ariz. These events brought into sharper focus several questions about grievance procedures in hospitals and underscored the urgency of finding answers. Among these questions were: Are nurses and ancillary hospital personnel ready for union organization? How are hospitals preparing to deal with the new forces and new relationships that unionization suggests?

Heretofore, hospitals have been exempt from labor legislation requiring overtime pay and minimum wages. However, bills recently passed by Congress have put an end to these exemptions and suggest a need for reappraisal of all hospital personnel practices.

It is important to learn what is currently known, what is being done, and what is being planned in all areas of employee relations, but this is especially true in the area of grievance procedures, because such procedures are not only essential to a good personnel program, but also the best defense against unionization.

The need for a grievance procedure resides in the emotional makeup of human beings, particularly in their need for relief from frustrations. Unfair treatment of an employee, imagined or actual, can create an emotional block to his future usefulness. To relieve such situations, the best mechanism is a rare one, a supervisor gifted in human relations. Since more than half of hospital personnel are generally in nursing service, nurse training programs in hospitals and in colleges have a responsibility to emphasize supervisory techniques, but have not generally done so to any great extent to date. A newly appointed nursing supervisor usually has no training to help her deal with the complexities involved in the management of human resources.

Even if management subjects were taught in advanced nursing courses and hospitals did train nursing supervisors and prospective supervisors in the requirements of supervision, some means would still be needed to guarantee free expression of employee unhappiness.

THE PROCEDURE DEFINED

A grievance procedure usually consists of a series of steps through which succeedingly higher levels of authority are called upon to resolve an employee's expressions of discontent over his relationship with any element of his employment.[1] The following is an example of a simple grievance procedure now in use in several medium-sized western hospitals:

A personnel relations committee is created to give employees an opportunity to take their problems to an important committee.

When a problem arises, the employee first takes that problem to his supervisor. If it is not resolved satisfactorily, he next makes an out and presents it to the personnel director, who attempts to resolve it.

If the problem still remains unresolved, the employee writes it out and presents it to the personnel relations committee, which investigates it thoroughly and reports its findings and recommendations to the administrator. The decision of the administrator is final.

In company-union contracts the grievance clause is usually more complex, carefully defining the participants on each side and the level of authority at which the problem is to be settled. In addition, time limitations are specified for considering a problem at a given level. Finally, various means of impartial outside arbitration, binding on both union and management, are provided in the event of an impasse throughout all of the internal steps. Adopting these steps can be beneficial to hospitals also, for they assure ultimate and bilateral fairness and they will compete well with the grievance program of any union.

Too frequently supervisors fear that their abilities will be judged on the very existence of employee expressions of unhappiness. Such fearful attitudes, which may be founded on past criticisms by the administrator or board, lead to a suppression of personal communication of dissatisfaction. It should be made clear that a supervisor will not be judged merely on the existence of grievances but rather on the volume of grievances and more particularly on their nature and on a determination as to whether or not they have been handled consistently in a fair and judicious manner.

Wendell French, in his analysis of the personnel management process, recommends such procedures for their value in fulfilling certain basic human needs:

"(The) procedure may give expression to a variety of human wants and needs. The self-esteem needs (independence, dominance, and achievement in particular) and the need for the esteem of others (recognition and attention) find expression in filing a grievance against management and pushing the complaint to a satisfactory conclusion."[2]

The best known text on hospital personnel administration lists the functions of grievance procedures among those essential to an adequate personnel department.[3] In

[1] Evans, J. J. *A Program for Personnel Administration* (New York: McGraw-Hill Book Co., 1945), p. 57.

[2] French, W. *The Personnel Management Process* (Boston: Houghton-Mifflin Co., 1964), p. 388.

[3] Bailey, N. D. *Hospital Personnel Administration* (Berwyn, Ill.: Physician's Record Co., 1959), p. 8.

[4] Ibid, p. 200.

pointing out that employees need more than wages, it looks upon good grievance procedures as essential to upward communication.[4]

In rationalizing the need for hospitals to set up grievance procedures, the following description of the initial effects of union organization may serve as an added incentive to establish them:

"When a firm is first unionized, what are the effects? A basic social change occurs in the structure of employer-employee relationships. A wedge seems to have been driven between the company and its employees. Many of these employees now profess an allegiance to an outside organization that, if it is affiliated with a national union, has broader interests and problems than those confronting an individual employer. In the initial stages of union relations, therefore, conflict is more probable than cooperation, especially if recognition of the union has followed a bitter period of name calling, electioneering, or possibly, a strike."[5]

THE SAFETY VALVE FUNCTION

A grievance procedure is also valuable as a safety valve, being a continuous means of avoiding arbitrary decisions and of providing justice. It can be an instrument for interpreting policy and perhaps discovering needs for policy changes. It is actually a formal expression of that much praised and desired thing—upward communication to management.

Edward W. Weimer has pointed out that some hospitals believe what is most unlikely—that their employees have no dissatisfactions.[6] A grievance procedure can enable first-line supervision to recognize anomalies in employee morale with the same kind of awareness that physicians possess in detecting symptoms and syndromes in patients. It permits them to find means to minimize the ill effects of grievances once they are discovered, for hospitals and industry both know that unrest is an overwhelming factor in the loss of productive effort. With Medicare, increased bed demand, chronic nurse shortages, and public reaction to increased hospitalization cost, administration must travel every path that can lead to a higher ratio of production per employee.

Robert E. Finley says we *need* some grievances. Forecasting what the enlightened personnel men of the future may bring about, he says:

"Labor relations men will not nearly as often be faced with grievances and troubles caused by managers who have no policies or objectives, who are not organized properly, who are arbitrary and insensitive leaders, or who perceive so poorly what is going on in their departments that they unjustly evaluate the work of certain people. There will, of course, always be grievances and to have a few is healthy. Some kinds of grievances, however, that now occupy so much . . . time, will dwindle as managers become more knowledgeable."[7]

Not only does Finley believe that some grievances are needed, if for no other reason than to allow all personnel a channel of individual communication, but he also believes

[5] Pigors, P. and Myers, C. A. *Personnel Administration* (New York: McGraw-Hill Co., 1965), p. 188.

[6] Weimer, E. W. Grievance procedure. *Hospitals, J.A.H.A.* 38:36 Aug. 16, 1964.

[7] Finley, R. E. *The Personnel Man and His Job* (New York: American Management Association, 1962), p. 404.

that trained, knowledgeable, nonarbitrary, sensitive, organized managers and supervisors whose objectives are supported by policies are essential to grievance handling. It is now important that hospitals hold similar beliefs.

A limited survey among medium-sized hospitals in the western part of the United States on grievance procedures in use produced a number of informal procedures. Some institutions had no procedure; some are planning to develop one. At least two who had abandoned grievance procedures are preparing to reinstitute them. Of the procedures studied, none showed an awareness of the time urgency involved. The importance of this can be seen in formalized grievance procedures that provide for outside arbitration, where due to a delayed decision the employer can be required to reinstate a previously discharged employee, even after having filled the position during the discharged employee's absence.

There is need to learn the techniques for handling grievances that are most helpful. Some dangers in the application of such procedures should be noted and avoided. The trick of avoidance may lie in the drafting of the procedure, but more likely it lies in enlightened, alert administration.

BEGIN WITH SUPERVISOR

The supervisor or department head must not be bypassed in handling grievances unless one wishes to cut the ground from under him, with a resultant increase in the number of grievances. Employees must know the channels available to them in presenting a grievance and it has to begin with the supervisor.

The open-door policy sounds good to some, but it can rip the bottom out of the grievance procedure. For one thing, it can waste a remarkable amount of the administrator's time and it can embarrass and weaken the position of the supervisor.

In preparing to deal with unions, particularly with regard to handling the grievance clause, there are a great many tactics to anticipate: Unions may make use of the procedure as a "slowdown" weapon by encouraging the filing of multiple grievances; an employee may fail to state the real grievance, causing a second or third handling; grievances related to an outdated event of the past may be brought up; and grievances may be put forward that are really only efforts to bargain for a more advantageous condition of work than the contract provides.

SUMMARY AND RECOMMENDATIONS

The current situation makes it urgent that attention be given to the following:

1. Adequate training in supervisory skills should be given to all supervisory personnel, both in academic curriculums and on the job.

2. Workable procedures should be devised to allow employee expression of dissatisfactions.

3. Administration should study many related labor-management areas in preparation for the potential need to deal with employees through a union representative.

It is recommended that hospital associations and the larger hospital councils learn and teach the formulation of objectives, policies, procedures, methods, and the training needed to develop these skills in hospitals.

Part IV

QUANTITATIVE METHODS IN DECISION MAKING

This part of the book presents the subject of decision making from a quantitative point of view. The concept of Operations Research is presented along with specific examples of some of the OR techniques and their application to problem areas within the hospital organization. The hospital administrator is a decision maker. When basic alternatives can be quantitatively and systematically evaluated better decisions result. The administrator need not be familiar with the detailed mechanics of each evaluation technique, however, an understanding of their use is becoming more crucial in today's complex environment. As a result, the two following sections present a conceptual and general approach to quantitative decision making.

The first section, OPERATIONS RESEARCH, presents various OR techniques such as queuing theory, simulation, and resource allocation models as they apply to the hospital organization. The computer is also presented as a tool which is available to the administrator for assistance in decision making. Finally, an indication of the future role of OR in the hospital organization is presented.

The second section, DECISION MAKING, presents the vital elements that should be recognized in the process of making decisions. A methodology for quantifying alternatives is presented. In addition, a means of assigning values to health care benefits is discussed in relation to capital budgeting.

Operations Research

This section presents the subject of Operations Research and its use in the hospital organization. OR is basically the application of scientific methods and techniques to problems with the purpose of providing a quantitative basis for making decisions. The development of OR techniques has been fostered by the computer age and they have been successfully applied to military and industrial problems. In a similar manner, they are currently being applied to problem areas within the hospital organization. While the administrator need not be an expert in the statistical, programming, and simulation techniques, an awareness of their application to his organization enables him to recognize the value of and benefits that can be derived from their application.

In *OPERATIONS RESEARCH IN HEALTH AND HOSPITAL ADMINISTRATION,* the are of Operations Research is described. OR is viewed not only as a way of thinking but is also viewed as the application of specific techniques to hospital areas such as inventory levels, resource allocation, waiting time, and scheduling problems. A key characteristic of any OR technique is the evaluation of alternatives relative to specific criteria. Those criteria may consist of minimizing patient waiting time, maximizing facility usage, or the allocation of scarce resources to achieve some objective such as patient care. An indication of the future role of OR in the areas of facility design and communication systems is also presented.

In *COMPUTER TECHNOLOGY: A CHALLENGE FOR HOSPITAL ADMINIS-TRATORS,* the point is raised that administrators need to be more systematic in their decision making. The computer is presented as a tool which facilitates the use of OR techniques. In addition to preforming routine tasks such as payroll, census, and accounts payable, the computer simulation of areas of the hospital organization enable the administrator to predict future resource needs and/or more effectively utilize current resources. A brief model of a simulated emergency room is presented as an example of the use of an OR technique and the progressive use of computer facilities.

Operations Research in Health and Hospital Administration

RONALD L. GUE, PH.D.

Ronald L. Gue, Ph.D., is a Professor of Hospital Administration at the University of Florida in Gainesville.

What can operations research (O.R.) mean to hospitals? Some hospital administrators may be well familiar with the field; others may view it as some foggy area of endeavor that is cited once in a while in the literature and mentioned in a convention every now and then; a few may have been involved, in one way or another, with an operations research study. In any case, because O.R. can have an indelible impact on hospitals, it is important for the hospital administrator of the present—and of the future—to become as familiar with it as possible. To this end, we present a brief sketch of operations research as a discipline, illustrate its use in several problem areas in the health field and discuss its potential in the future growth of health and hospital administration.

Hospitals have felt the impact of scientific and technical developments in industry, the military and related areas throughout hospital history. The industrial revolution, based on the development of power-generating equipment and machine tools, has benefited hospitals in many ways. Large scale production and the development of national transportation have allowed new economies. The concept of division of manual labor felt so strongly in industry has prompted redefinition of the duties of nursing and ancillary activities.

The division of manual labor in industry was followed by a division of managerial labor. A parallel development has been seen in hospital administration. In industry the continued development of technology and managerial segmentation caused new problems concerning control and decision-making, the complexity of which continues to grow. This complexity has caused a keen awareness that the changes in management and developments in technology in the past have not been followed by parallel advancements in administration and in the executive function.

Throughout these developments, parallel progress in the health field has lagged behind similar progress in industry and the military. In this paper we will attempt no rationalization of this, but will only point out that in the late forties and early fifties

---

operations research was born in response to the need to handle some of these new and complex problems in industry and the military, and that the health field is just beginning its parallel development of O.R. and its application to complex problems of coordination and control. As an example of the time lag involved, one needs only note that papers similar to this one were appearing in various industrial and trade journals about ten years ago (12, 13).[1] It's interesting to note that one of the earliest references to the use of "scientific management" in hospitals comes from the military (21).

During and since World War II hospitals have suffered from severe public pressures from without, as well as troubles from within. Flagle (10) has cited rising costs, shortage of key professional personnel, internecine strife between physicians and administration, inadequacy and decay of physical plant as being among the more acute problems facing hospitals since World War II. The development of operations research in the health services has been in response to the growing complexity of the administrative function in the face of these problems.

OPERATIONS RESEARCH AND DECISION PROCESSES

Operations research has several characteristics that serve to differentiate it from other disciplines. Its most distinguishing feature is its concern with whole problems or its system orientation. The idea here is that activity by any part of an organization has some effect on other activities within the organization. We all are aware of the occasional conflict of opinion among the medical staff, nursing service and administration in a hospital system. For example, some hospitals in the country have recently been examining the feasibility of using disposable bedpans. From the standpoint of nursing, their use seems to be highly desirable since it replaces the undesirable task of emptying and handling soiled bedpans. Administration, on the other hand, while aware of the implications to improved nursing satisfaction and improved nursing care must consider the cost of the disposables. If the unit cost of the disposable bedpan proves to be more than that of the reuseable bedpan there may be some question in the administrator's mind about the value of adopting the disposables. There could be a basic conflict between nursing and administration in deciding whether or not to use disposable bedpans. In making a decision that is oriented toward the hospital as a system, rather than nursing satisfaction or dollar cost, both factors must be considered.

The basic concept of the systems orientation, while accepted in theory, is seldom used in practice. This is generally due to practical limitations on time and resources, or due to the fact that the theoretical techniques available for use are not sufficiently developed to be applied under a systems orientation.

MIXED RESEARCH TEAMS

A second characteristic of operations research frequently cited is that the research is conducted by a mixed team of scientists from many disciplines. This mixed character of the research teams was necessitated during the early years of O.R. because there was no one formally trained to do operations research. The value of this mixed approach

---

[1] Numbers in parentheses refer to references in the Bibliography at the end of the paper.

to problem-solving that was born of necessity has come to be recognized as the heart of any operations research effort. In O.R. studies in the health field we may find physicians, administrators, engineers, statisticians, economists and many other disciplines. For example, a recent article on the evaluation of recurrent medical examinations (28) was authored by a mathematician and a physician. There are many such examples in the literature of the wedding of health service personnel and other diverse disciplines.

A third distinguishing characteristic of O.R. is its method and approach to problem solving. Operations research is generally concerned with complex decision problems—problems related to determining how people should act in order to reach a satisfactory or best decision. Decisions are usually made because the decision-maker wants to attain some goal or objective. Generally he will choose an action that will help him attain his objective. The word "decision" implies a choice, and there must be more than one course of action available to the decision-maker; otherwise, there is no choice.

Consider, for example, the hospital administrator who must decide what quantities of linen inventory he should keep on the hospital floor. His objective might be to minimize the total cost to the hospital. How should the administrator choose one course of action (a single supply level) from all the courses of action (all possible supply levels) available to him? How does operations research help him make his decision?

In order to make his decision the administrator must have some measure of the effect of choosing each course of action—a measure of effectiveness. In our example, this would probably be an expression of the dollar cost to the hospital for each course of action. However there are certain uncontrollable factors which may affect the total cost to the institution. For example, the demand for linen is uncontrollable since it is governed by such things as census on the floor and the nature of the patients' ailments. Thus, the measure of effectiveness will depend on the administrator's choice of a course of action and the state of various uncontrollable factors in the system.

The operations researcher usually resorts to the use of a model of the system that expresses the measure of effectiveness as a function of the alternative courses of action and the uncontrollable variables in the problem. This might be a mathematical model of the form:

$$E = f(C_i, U_j)$$

This equation says symbolically that the measure of effectiveness (E) depends upon the controllable variables, or courses of action (C_i), and the uncontrollable variables (U_j). Operations research, as a discipline, helps the decision-maker to decide which course of action (C_i) will yield the "best" measure of effectiveness. In our example, it would help the administrator to determine which linen supply level would minimize the total linen supply cost to the hospital.

The decision-making framework and the example discussed above are admittedly oversimplified, but they do serve to illustrate the framework used in O.R. Operations research is not only concerned with how to make best decisions, but is concerned with every facet of the decision-making process from actually defining the problem to determining what the best decision really is. The reader who would like to do more study of the framework for decision-making is referred to Miller and Starr (8) or Ackoff and Rivett (2).

Although operations research is a distinct discipline in its own right, its presence in a research activity is usually in combination with certain associated areas of science and engineering. For example, the quantitative measurement techniques of industrial engineering are frequently used in the data collection phase of the O.R. study. The theory of mathematical statistics is frequently used in designing the data collection system and in the analysis of the data. Digital computers are often used in facilitating computations in the data analysis, as well as playing a significant role in storing, retrieving and processing information in the management system that evolves as a consequence of the operations research study. Because of its close association with these and other disciplines, any discussion of the applications of O.R. will necessarily include studies in some of these related areas. In the problem areas discussed below, these related studies as well as research that is clearly O.R. will all be classified as operations research. Certainly each piece of work cited has played, or will play, an integral part in an O.R. study.

DECISION PROBLEMS

There is no single classification of problems that falls in the realm of operations research, but there are certain problems that have repeated themselves in the past few years. Ackoff and Rivett (2) have suggested that many of these problems seem to fall in a classification similar to the eight areas listed below:

1.	Inventory	5.	Competition
2.	Allocation	6.	Replacement
3.	Waiting Lines	7.	Search
4.	Scheduling	8.	Sequencing

We will use these areas to discuss the types of problems of concern to O.R. and then discuss selected applications in the health field. The applications mentioned do not constitute an exhaustive list of health research, but only serve to indicate the character of past and current activity.

INVENTORY PROBLEMS

Inventory has been defined as idle resources, and resources "are anything that can be used to obtain something else of value" (2). Men, drugs, supplies and equipment are resources that hospital administrators are involved with. Decisions in inventory problems are made in terms of time and quantity, and in response to the following questions:

1. When should the inventory be replenished?
2. How much should be added to inventory?

Time and quantity are usually controllable variables, while such factors as demand and time between order and delivery are uncontrollable.

The administrator will see certain obvious inventory problems in a hospital system related to drug inventory, supplies, stores and linen. In the most thorough study of these problems to date, Smalley *et al.* (25, 34 and 35) have been studying the inventory problems that exist in hospital supply decisions. They have studied cost factors, design of cost prediction instruments, hospital inventory policies and the various costs associated with these policies. Differential costs associated with a shift in usage from one supply item form to another (e.g., reusable to disposable) have been identified and measured. Methods of establishing reorder points, economic lot sizes and other inventory policies in a multi-item hospital inventory system have been studied and compared. Various methods for measuring order costs and carrying costs have also been examined.

In a less traditional application, Rockwell *et al.* (33) have formulated the demand and supply of whole blood in a hospital as an inventory problem. They have analyzed the effect of various ordering policies on the blood inventory level. Attempts have been made to minimize the risk of storage and to maximize the effective utilization of available blood within a community.

ALLOCATION PROBLEMS

An important class of decision problems is concerned with the allocation of limited resources so that some measure of effectiveness is maximized or minimized. If there are enough resources to go around, the problem is greatly simplified. Usually the resources are limited in such a way that they cannot be used in the most effective manner.

Studies at The Johns Hopkins Hospital (23) have been concerned with the allocation of nursing resources to meet the variable demands of patient care. Their initial concern was with the amount of bedside care a patient actually received from nursing personnel of all types. After concluding that the demands of an individual patient vary with his degree of illness, a classification scheme was developed that categorized patients into three homogeneous classes. The average amount of bedside care required by patients in these classes was found to vary widely from one category to another. Using this classification scheme, a bedside care index was developed to indicate the total amount of time required for bedside care in an eight-hour day. Once nursing requirements are thus established, nursing personnel are allocated among the hospital floors.

A group at Tulane University (18) has studied the allocation of basic food ingredients in hospital menu planning. Their efforts have been toward the planning of menus that satisfy basic dietary and taste requirements, while minimizing the total cost of the meal to the hospital. It is hoped that research in this area will lead to a system for planning menus through the use of digital computers, that will be practical for use by many hospitals in the country.

WAITING LINE PROBLEMS

Queuing, or waiting line problems, are concerned with the design and planning of facilities to meet a randomly fluctuating demand for services. If service facilities are not adequate to meet demand, this causes congestion to occur at the service facility and incurs certain associated costs. However, increased service capacity to reduce congestion usually causes increased idleness in the service system, thus incurring a cost of idle service facilities. Waiting line problems usually strive to design systems that balance the aggregate costs of idleness and congestion and minimize the total cost of the service system.

Analysis in this problem area of health research has been more extensive and probably more sophisticated than any other. Outpatient departments, as service facilities, have been analyzed in this country (43) and abroad (14). Several appointment systems have been considered in an attempt to reduce the time patients spend waiting for service while maintaining a low level of physician idle time.

The hospital system itself may be viewed as a large and complex service facility. Congestion occurs in the form of waiting lists or patients who go to another hospital when they cannot be immediately admitted. Increasing the capacity of the hospital may cause an excess of idle service facilities in the form of idle beds, excess staff and other services. Balintfy (17) and Young (44) have developed explicit descriptions of the hospital as a service facility and have examined the effect of various admission and service policies on reduction of waiting lists as well as a reduction in idle facilities.

SCHEDULING PROBLEMS

Scheduling problems are concerned with the timing of arrivals (or departures) of units at a service facility in such a way that costs associated with total time taken to complete a project, idle service facilities and waiting time for service are minimized. There is a good deal of similarity between waiting line and scheduling problems. In fact some authors (1, 2) have classified both as waiting line problems. We personally feel that separating the two will make our arguments a little easier.

Studies at the University of Florida Hospital (24) have been concerned with the scheduling of operating room staff and facilities in the face of highly variable demand. Statistical methods have been devised so that the variation between predicted and actual operating room utilization is reduced along with subsequent costs.

Two relatively new techniques are currently being considered for scheduling and isolating key activities in planning construction and in research and development. The techniques are called PERT (Program Evaluation and Review Technique) and the Critical Path Method. They may be used by architects, engineers and administrators to plan construction and finance large scale hospital projects in such a way that costs are minimized, time schedules are maintained and potential bottlenecks are located. A recent article by Nalon and Ballinger (30) discusses the use of these techniques by hospitals.

COMPETITION PROBLEMS

Competition problems involve two or more individuals or organizations with conflicting objectives trying to optimize (maximize or minimize) some measure of effectiveness. These are problems where a decision made by one decision-maker can affect a decision made by one or more of the remaining decision-makers. Examples of competitive problems range from two players struggling to win at chess to two large companies striving for a greater share of their market.

An important extension of the competition problem is the consideration of Nature and its effect on decision-making. These are viewed as competition problems with one or more decision-makers in competition with Nature. This formulation has evolved to handle the random and uncontrollable character of certain variables in decision problems. Ledley and Lusted (28) have suggested the formulation of the diagnostic process as a competition problem against Nature. Warner (39) has reported the application of these concepts in the diagnosis of congenital heart disease. Flagle and Lechat (27) have reported on the use of the concept of competition against Nature in the selection of diagnostic and therapeutic strategies in public health. All of these studies have taken a step forward in increasing the accuracy and developing a better understanding of diagnoses.

OTHER DECISION PROBLEMS

The remaining decision problems in our classification of problem areas in operations research have seen limited application in the health services. In order to complete our discussion of the nature of O.R., we will just briefly summarize the character of the remaining areas.

Replacement problems are of two general classes, depending on whether the equipment involved deteriorates gradually or does not deteriorate but is subject to failure. In the case of deteriorating items, the problem is concerned with balancing the cost of new equipment against the cost of maintaining the efficiency of the old equipment. For items that fail, the problem is one of determining which items to replace and how often to replace them.

Search problems are concerned with looking for "things" where the search is subject to two kinds of errors: (a) failure to find the "things" and (b) failure to find the "things" although one has looked in the right place. These "things" can be symptoms of a disease, information in a medical record and others.

Sequencing refers to the order in which units requiring service at some service facility are serviced. In terms of queuing problems, the order in which members of the waiting line are served is called the queue discipline. The sequence of units to be served is chosen in such a way that the sum of the pertinent costs is minimized.

Very few problems found in operations research fall uniquely into one of the categories above. O.R. problems may include many of the decision models discussed. For example, the work of Connor *et al.* (23) at The Johns Hopkins Hospital on the allocation of nursing resources included problems in scheduling, replacement and waiting lines, among others. In their work on the reasoning foundations of medical diagnosis, Ledley and Lusted first define a diagnostic problem as a competitive problem and then formulate certain search problems in order to efficiently apply the analysis through the use of data processing.

The sketch of decision problems in O.R. that has been presented above can offer, at best, only a gross indication of the nature of the field. A recent book by Ackoff and Rivett (2) is recommended to the administrator who wishes to learn more about operations research.

CONTENT OF FUTURE RESEARCH

The decision problem framework in the discussion above was used primarily as a method of presenting the nature of operations research. In summarizing the accomplishments of operations research and associated areas, and in projecting the content of future research, we will use a classification that is probably a little more familiar to the hospital administrator.

NURSING

Previous work in this area has firmly established the character of nursing activity or time allocation (e.g., 23, 39). Measures sensitive to variations in the amount of self sufficiency of the patient population have been developed and subsequently used to allocate nursing time to various patient areas (23). Current research at The Johns Hopkins Hospital is concerned with developing a method of distributing nursing tasks among nurses, students and aides in such a way that the effectiveness of nursing care is maximized. The random and variable nature of nursing care has been studied and the effect of this variation on patient waiting time and the allocation of nursing resources has been predicted (42). Studies related to the measurement of patient care are underway at Ohio State University (27).

A research project at the University of Florida Hospital is concerned with a quantitative analysis of a unit manager system: a system that assigns many administrative and non-professional tasks formerly performed by nurses to a non-nurse. Exploratory studies are underway to examine the effect of the unit manager system on the allocation of nursing time, supply consumption and personnel costs associated with patient care. The long-run goal of the project is to establish a quantitative basis for the evaluation of the unit manager and similar systems throughout the country.

Most O.R. studies in nursing eventually point out the need for a measure of the effectiveness of nursing care. This measure has been called a measure of the quality of nursing care with increasing frequency. In order that more advanced decision problems related to nursing can be solved, this measurement problem must be tackled. Studies of the quality of nursing care and related areas are underway at a few hospitals in the country (e.g., 31, 32). The future should see an expansion of research in this area. Once adequate measures of effectiveness of nursing care have been formed, research activity in nurse scheduling and allocation, assignment of tasks and other related activities can proceed at full speed.

HOSPITAL PLANNING AND DESIGN

With increased federal support of hospital expansion and growing community health needs, the need for advanced concepts in the planning and design of health facilities becomes more apparent. The utilization of existing hospital facilities has received extensive study (14, 38, 45). These studies have concerned themselves with more efficient use of the hospital system. For example, Young (45) has predicted the effect of various admissions policies on the hospital census. In a related piece of work, Balintfy (17) has predicted daily discharges and admissions and has examined the effect of seasonal and chance fluctuations in occupancy levels.

LACK OF COMMUNICATION

Although there have been several articles in the literature concerning the use of operations research in planning new facilities (e.g., 20, 38), there is little evidence that O.R. has had a profound effect on hospital planning and design. There is a distinct need for improved communication between the researchers in this area and those doing the hospital planning. On the other hand, operations research in this area is still in a virgin stage. Still to be answered are questions such as: What criteria should be used in deciding where to locate a hospital? When is a hospital too large? Where should ancillary services be located within the hospital?

LOGISTICS

Problems in this area are concerned with the demand for and supply of quantities of people, equipment and auxiliary supplies. The relationships between highly variable demand, limited supply and its movement, and consumption have not been fully explored. Problems related to optimum inventory levels of supply, distribution systems and purchase quantities have been studied and in a few cases implemented (33).

Unlike most of the problem areas discussed in this paper, there is not an overwhelming need for new theoretical developments in the study of logistics; there is simply a need to apply the existing knowledge of operations research in the area. Smalley, *et al.* (34, 35) have led the way with their work on supply decisions mentioned earlier. The future should bring an increased concern for supply and logistics and the implementation of research results to analysis of optimum inventory levels and purchase quantities.

COMMUNICATIONS

Flagle (10) cites three major areas of concern for communication in hospital systems: management information, electronic monitoring of patient conditions and computer-aided diagnosis.

Hospitals, like other organizations, require adequate and rapid communication to facilitate the management function. Although some claim that hospital systems are unnecessarily bogged down with paperwork (the physical form of communication), they are probably no more bogged down than similar organizations found in industry or the military. Regardless, there is currently deep concern in the health field for management information systems. Automation of these systems has been a frequent subject of discussion. The so-called "total system" concept has evolved through a concern to automate the entire hospital communication system. One of the more noteworthy studies in this area is taking place at Bolt, Beranek and Newman, Inc. (19). Their effort is to "design, construct, apply and evaluate" a computer system specifically for use in a general hospital. They are in the process of developing computer programs that will allow efficient communication between the various parts of the hospital system and the computer.

ELECTRONIC MONITORING OPERATION

The advent of space medicine technology has fostered a growing interest in the electronic monitoring of patient conditions. The monitoring operation has been limited to certain vital signs, including temperature, pulse rate, and respiration rate. The efforts in this area are aimed at precision in patient care, more precise ways to diagnose illness and more precise ways to anticipate treatment needs (36).

Medical data processing presents a problem of increasing magnitude to hospitals throughout the country. New data is formed continuously by the physicians' daily examinations and interviews. These visits to the physician generate other data including doctors' orders, medication records, X-rays and laboratory reports. This flood of information filtering into the medical records system causes enormous problems in both storage and retrieval of medical information. Current research is concerned with utilization (in terms of quantity of records and what information in the record is used), prediction of space requirements, and the design of automatic data processing systems (33).

The computer obviously plays an important role in future plans for research in hospital system communication. A recent article by Spencer, *et al.* (36) summarizes past work in the automation of hospital functions and projects the need for future research. They point out that operations research is needed to study the decision processes in hospital operation and the implications of these decision processes on the requirements for communication systems.

SCREENING AND DIAGNOSIS

A recent and most intriguing application of operations research has been in the logic of screening and diagnosis. Mathematical models of diagnosis have been formulated by Ledley and Lusted (30). Their original concern was caused by an increasing interest in the use of computers in medical diagnosis. Before computers could be used there was a need to know more about how a physician makes a diagnosis. As an example of the use of these mathematical models, together with the digital computer, Warner (39) has reported their application to the diagnosis of congenital heart disease.

The screening of patients in hospitals with large out-patient facilities presents a major problem. Walton (33) has developed models of the decision processes involved in ascertaining the need for medical attention and has used these models to direct patients to proper specialty clinics.

Of all the problem areas discussed, modeling the diagnostic process stimulates the imagination more than any other. A concentrated effort is certain in this area in order to increase the accuracy of diagnosis, to develop an understanding of diagnosis and to facilitate the use of computers in the diagnostic process.

RESEARCH LEADERSHIP

Without question, national leadership in the application of operations research in the health field has come primarily from the federal government. Specifically, the Hill-Burton Act of 1954 provides that:

... the Surgeon General shall encourage, cooperate with, and render assistance to appropriate authorities, scientific institutions, and scientists, in the conduct and coordination of research, investigations, experiments, demonstrations, and studies relating to cause, diagnosis, treatment, control, and prevention of the physical and mental diseases and in impairments of man.

A good part of the operations research activity, partly in response to this government support, has developed in various academic institutions in the country. Operations research projects in universities such as The Johns Hopkins University, Case

Institute of Technology and Yale University are supported, in part, by grant funds from the Public Health Service. Other universities, such as the University of Florida, have fostered a spontaneous interest in the use of O.R. in health problems without grant support.

UNIVERSITY LEADERSHIP

We must look to the universities of the country for future leadership for at least two reasons: first, the existence of the required physical facilities such as hospitals and clinics, libraries, computing facilities and competent researchers, together with the atmosphere and traditions of research excellence, all in one geographical location, make the university the ideal setting for health research activity. Secondly, the dearth of competent health researchers is concomitant with each day's growing needs; the university, while participating in a health research program, will take a step in the direction of fulfilling the research needs of the country and in the direction of training researchers in the proper laboratory setting.

On the other hand, the wedding of the federal government and the university in a health research partnership breeds problems. For example, at least one experienced consultant in the field has said that he could count on one hand the number of hospital research studies conducted at various universities in the country that have actually been implemented. This is a danger signal. The root of the problem is found in the basic properties of this government-university partnership. First, the fact that the research activity in the university hospital is usually not dependent on the hospital for financial support may cause a lack of incentive to achieve practical results through implementation. Secondly, hospital administration, while realizing that there is a lack of implementation of the research activity in the hospital, may feel that the prestige that accompanies having an O.R. group outweighs this lack of implementation. Thus, the O.R. group may be tolerated without solid accomplishments.

Another point to be considered is that operations research groups in the university setting are staffed primarily by academic personnel. These researchers tend to seek problems of intellectual interest as well as problems that merit publishable research. However, many problems of practical significance to the hospital will satisfy neither of these requirements. A related problem is that many of the university O.R. groups employ graduate students. As a consequence of the limited resident time of these students, many research activities lack continuity and follow-through, thus compounding the problem of lack of implementation. We don't claim to know the answer to these problems, but we do feel that the implementation of certain O.R. studies may be sufficiently rewarding to hospitals in the country to justify the expenditure of hospital funds for operation research and related research activity. A second method of stimulating implementation may be for the operations research group to have certain non-academic staff members—who are primarily concerned with implementation of research projects and with certain pragmatic problems that are of little interest to faculty and graduate student—participating in the project.

These problems of implementation and continuity are indicative of the rapid expansion of operations research in the health field, and of the awareness of hospital administration to the need for new techniques to aid decision-making in the increasingly complex executive function. This is reason enough for optimism; these problems will ultimately be resolved.

CONCLUSION

Although operations research is intimately associated with decisions and decision problems, its major contribution to the health services has not been the identification of optimal or best decisions. Flagle (5) points out that where operations research has made a contribution

... has often been in revealing to administrators the true nature of the system with which they are dealing. Most often than not, the "true nature" has been the (chance) aspects, which have been misunderstood or not formally recognized in the existing management systems. The criteria for decision and change have not been in mathematical optimization, but simply a motivation for compatibility between the management procedures and the organizational phenomena they seek to control.

Advances that have been made are advances in understanding rather than in the identification of best decisions. A benefit of improved understanding is an ability to better formulate and define the real decision problems facing the health administrator. Hopefully, the future will bring a more explicit definition of decision problems in health administration together with subsequent solutions.

BIBLIOGRAPHY

This bibliography is intended to suggest further reading in operations research to the health or hospital administrator. Most publications cited have been chosen for their clarity, brevity and lack of technical detail. In the case of certain articles concerning applications, technical detail is unavoidable. These cases will be noted.

Introductory Reading in Operations Research:

1. ACKOFF, RUSSELL L. "The Development of Operations Research as a Science,"*Journal of Operations Research Society of America,* Vol. 4, No. 3, June 1956.
2. ――― and PATRICK RIVETT. *A Manager's Guide to Operations Research.* New York: John Wiley and Sons, Inc., 1963.
3. BOEHM, GEORGE. "Helping the Executive Make Up His Mind," *Fortune,* April 1962.
4. CAYWOOD, THOMAS E. "Operations Research as a Management Resource," *Hospital Administration,* Vol. 3, No. 2, Spring 1958.
5. FLAGLE, CHARLES D. "Operations Research in Community Services," Chapter 13 in Hertz, David B. and Roger T. Eddison. *Progress in Operations Research.* Vol. II, New York: John Wiley and Sons, Inc., 1964.
6. ―――, WILLIAM H. HUGGINS and ROBERT H. ROY. *Operations Research and Systems Engineering.* Baltimore: Johns Hopkins Press, 1956 (See Chapters 1, 2 and 6).
7. MCCLOSKEY, JOSEPH F. and FLORENCE TREFETHEN. *Operations Research for Management.* Vol. 1, Baltimore: Johns Hopkins Press, 1954 (See Part I).
8. MILLER, DAVID W. and MARTIN K. STARR. *Executive Decisions and Operations Research.* Englewood Cliffs, N.J.: 1960 (See Chapters 1-4).
9. WAGNER, HARVEY M. "Practical Slants on Operations Research," *Harvard Business Review,* Vol. 41, No. 3, May-June 1963.

General Reading with a Little Mathematic Sophistication:

10. FLAGLE, CHARLES D. "Operations Research in the Health Services," *Journal of Operations Research Society of America,* Vol. 10, No. 5, 1962.
11. ―――."Operations Research in a Hospital," Chapter 25 in reference 6.

Applications of O.R. in Industry:

12. ACKOFF, RUSSELL L. "Operations Research—New Tool of Industrial Science," *Industrail Laboratories,* November 1953.

13. HICKS, DONALD. "Operational Research in the Coal Industry," *Operational Research Quarterly,* December 1951.

Case Studies in Health and Hospital Administration: (Starred numbers indicate those articles with technical detail.)

14. BAILEY, N. T. J. and J. D. WELCH. "Appointment Systems in Hospital Outpatient Departments," *Lancet,* May 31, 1952.

15. ———. "Operational Research in Hospital Planning and Design," *Operational Research Quarterlv,* Vol. 8, No. 3, September 1957.

16.* ———. "Queueing for Medical Care," *Applied Statistics,* Vol. 3, No. 3, November 1954.

17.* BALINTFY, JOSEPH L. "A Stochastic Model for the Analysis and Prediction of Discharges and Admissions in Hospitals," *Management Sciences,* Vol. 2, New York: Pergamon Press, 1960.

18. ——— and C..RALPH BLACKBURN. "A Significant Advance in Hospital Menu Planning bv Computer," *Institutions,* July 1964.

19. BARUCH, J. J. "Hospital Research and Administration with a Digital Computer," *Circulation Research,* VoL 11, No. 3, September 1962.

20. BLUMBERG, MARK S. "D P F Concept' Helps Predict Bed Needs," *The Modern Hospital,* Vol. 97, No. 6, December 1961.

21. BLUMBERG, MARK S. "Hospital Automation: The Needs and the Prospects," *Hospitals,* Vol. 35, No. 15. August 1961.

22. BECKMAN, MAJOR FRANKLIN P. and CAPTAIN ROLAND C. KENNEDY, "Pioneering 'Scientific Management' in U.S. Army Hospitals," *Hospital Management,* Vol. 70, No. 5, 1950.

23. CONNOR, ROBERT J., *et al.* "Effective Use of Nursing Resources: A Research Report," *Hospitals,* Vol. 35, May 1, 1961.

24. DAVIS, GORDON J. and RUDDELL REED, JR. "Variability Control is the Key to Maximum Operating Room Utilization," *The Modern Hospital,* Vol. 102, No. 4, April 1964.

25. FREEMAN, JOHN R., *et al.* "Carrying Costs," *Hospital Management,* Vol. 97, No. 5, May 1964.

26. FLAGLE, CHARLES D. "Criteria of Effectiveness for Selection, Training, Motivation of Hospital Personnel," *Journal of Operations Research Society of America,* Vol. 5, No. 4, August 1957 (Abstract).

27. ——— and M. F. LECHAT. "Statistical Decision Theory and the Selection of Diagnostic and Therapeutic Strategies in Public Health," presented at the meeting of the International Federation of Operations Research Societies, Oslo, July 1963.

28. HOWLAND, DANIEL. *The Development of a Methodology for the Evuluation of Patient Care,* Progress Report, Systems Research Gioup, Ohio State University, 1961.

29.* LINCOLN, THOMAS L. and GEORGE H. WEISS. "A Statistical Evaluation of Recurrent Medical Examinations," *Journal of Operations Research Society of America,* Vol. 12, No. 2, March-April 1964.

30.* LEDLEY, ROBERT S. and LEE B. LUSTED. "Reasoning Foundations of Medical Diagnosis," *Science,* Vol. 130, No. 3366, July 3, 1959.

31. NALON, PAUL F. and ROBERT I. BALLINGER, JR. "Critical Path Method of Scheduling and Financing for Hospitals," *Hospital Management,* Vol. 97, No. 5, May 1964.

32. Nurse Utilization Project Staff, State University of Iowa, *An Investigation of the Relation Between Nursing Activity and Patient Welfare,* 1960.

33.* Operations Research Division, The Johns Hopkins Hospital, *Progress Report,* 1962.

34.* ROCKWELL, THOMAS H., *et al.* "Inventory Analysis as Applied to Hospital Whole Blood Supply and Demand," *Journal of Industrial Engineering,* March-April 1962.
35. SMALLEY, HAROLD E., *et al.* "Cost Factors in Purchasing," *Hospital Management,* Vol. 97, No. 2, February 1964.
36. ———, *et al.* "Inventory Policies," *Hospital Management,* Vol. 97, No. 3, March 1964.
37. SPENCER, W. A., *et al.* "Requirements and Applications of Automation in Hospital Functions," *Journal of Chronic Disease,* Vol. 17, 1964.
38. THOMPSON, JOHN D., *et al.* "How Queueing Theory Works for the Hospital," *The Modern Hospital,* Vol. 94, No. 3, March 1960.
39.* TORGERSEN, PAUL E. "An Example of Work Sampling in the Hospital," *Journal of Industrial Engineering,* May-June 1959.
40.* WARNER, HOMER R., *et al.* "A Mathematical Approach to Medical Diagnosis," *Journal of the American Medical Association,* Vol. 177, No. 3, July 1961.

Dissertations and Theses:

41. DAVIS, J. GORDON. "A Model for Improvement of Operating Room Utilization," Master's Thesis, University of Florida, 1961.
42. GUE, RONALD L. "A Stochastic Description of Direct Patient Care and Its Relation to Communication in a Hospital," Doctoral Dissertation, Johns Hopkins University, 1964.
43. SONNENDECKER, J. R. "A Model for Forecasting Whole Blood Requirements of a Hospital Blood Laboratory," Master's Thesis, Ohio State University.
44. SORIANO, A. "A Comparative Study of Block and Individual Appointment Systems in the Outpatient Department, Wilmer Opthalmological Clinic," Master's Thesis, Johns Hopkins University, 1960.
45. YOUNG, JOHN P. "A Queueing Theory Approach to the Control of Hospital Inpatient Census," Doctoral Dissertation, Johns Hopkins University, 1962.

Computer Technology: A Challenge for Hospital Administrators

FRANK GREENWOOD, PH.D. AND CHARLES R. KENDRICK

Frank Greenwood, Ph.D., is Director of the Computer Center at the University of Detroit. Charles R. Kendrick is Manager of the Hospital Consulting Services, McDonnell-Douglas Automation Company, St. Louis, Mo.

Hospitals are very complex organizations of specialized resources, problems, and motivation. Hospital administration, consequently, is one of the most difficult areas in the practice of management. Technological—and other—changes of the last two decades have compounded the problems.

Computers often are associated with the most critical changes affecting hospitals. For example, with the coming of Medicare many administrators have found their cost data inadequate to support reimbursement claims. Their studies to improve cost accounting frequently lead to investigating whether or not to computerize in-patient billing, and this inquiry logically is extended to census, payroll, accounts payable, and the like.

As computers become more widespread, computers will themselves cause changes. (Improved techniques of equipment sharing, where several hospitals use the same hardware, almost guarantee their increased use in the health care field.) One such change is that surviving hospital administrators soon will be required to be more precise and less intuitive in their decision-making. Decision-making can be more exact because computers can be used to evaluate the effects of a wide range of alternative actions before a decision is made. This article, as an example, discusses how to use computers to help produce recommendations for improving emergency room performance in a municipal hospital system. It illustrates the change whereby administrators will be forced to abandon decision-making by instinct, and will, instead, have to quantify the relationships between the hospital and its environment in arriving at decisions. Reports by McDonnell Automation Company, St. Louis, provided much valuable information for this paper: Kirkpatrick and Whitehair, *Computer Simulation of an Emergency Room Facility* (April, 1967), and *Emergency Room Report for Department of Health and Hospitals, City of St. Louis* (July, 1967).

STOCHASTIC SIMULATION MODELING

Operations research (OR), or management sciences, is the application of mathematical models to management problems. World War II gave it a big push as management science techniques were applied to such problems as the best size for convoys crossing the submarine-infested Atlantic and the most efficient schedules for aircraft maintenance.

In the absence of a compelling national emergency, however, operations research languished after the war—until the spread of computers. A computer's capacity to handle huge volumes of routine, repetitive computations makes it an ideal tool for many management science problems, and, therefore, computers now make OR techniques broadly feasible.

One frequently used OR technique is stochastic simulation modeling. A "model" is a mathematical likeness of an existing physical system, such as an emergency room. It is a set of mathematical instructions addressed to a digital computer. When executed, these instructions produce sets of numbers which are the solutions. Properly constructed mathematical models react exactly as would the system being imitated, and they are, therefore, called "simulation models." An emergency room model simulates patient arrivals, waiting times, and treatments. The type of patient arriving or being treated at a particular time depends on chance. Careful study of the actual emergency room reveals the overall pattern of the hour of the day patients arrive and the types of emergency treatment rendered. If the simulation model is designed to randomly choose patient arrival times and treatments from this overall pattern, it is called a "stochastic simulation model." The word "stochastic" recognizes the randomness factor ("stochastic" is derived from *stochos,* the Greek word for "guess").

Small changes can be made in the model to correspond with minor procedural changes in the emergency room, or major changes can be made in the model that are analogous to drastic changes in the facilities. Therefore, with the stochastic simulation model plus the computer, the merits of small or large changes can be studied without interfering with health care in the actual emergency room. To generalize: sophisticated hospital administration will soon be characterized by computerized information systems using such (steadily improving) models to help make management decisions. The hospital's objectives won't change, but day-to-day operational decision-making will change, requiring administrators to use a quantitative approach, as opposed to an intuitive method, for decision-making.

THE EMERGENCY ROOM SIMULATION

Let us now consider the application of stochastic simulation modeling in the hospital situation.

There are four basic components to an emergency room simulation model that must be identified accurately before a set of mathematical instructions can be created: facilities, load, logic, and queue. These are the building blocks of a satisfactory model and should be clearly understood before data gathering from the real system is begun.

Facilities in the emergency room that will be represented in the model (physician/nurse team, registration desk, X-ray facilities, etc.) must be inventoried. All facilities have performance characteristics which must be observed in the real system and incorporated in the model as service time distributions.

Load on the real system comprises arrival time of patients and their treatment needs following examination. These arrivals and treatment types must be observed and categorized. Later they are used in the model as distributions for the stochastical generation of patient probabilities.

Logic, the procedure of assigning patient priorities and routing of patients to facilities, must be defined in a flow chart for each type of patient. The simulation logic ties together the *load* and *facilities.*

Queues (patient waiting lines) that can possibly develop in the real system must be provided for in the model. It is the status of these queues that is important to report during computer simulation runs. A typical queue report contains:

> Number of patients entering the queue;
> Number of patients leaving the queue;
> Average stay time of patients in the queue;
> Maximum time a patient waited in the queue;
> Clock time that this patient left the queue;
> Maximum length of the queue;
> Clock time when the queue length became maximum;
> Present queue length.

To accurately reflect the random properties of the emergency room, three types of data are observed in the real system for formulation into patterns, or frequency distributions:

> 1. Patient arrival rates by time of day;
> 2. Patient treatment type by time of day;
> 3. Facilities service times.

These are obtained with specially installed time clocks while observing the operation of the emergency facility.

These data show that this emergency room typically receives about 260 patients per day and has a capacity of 12.4 patients per hour. Most patients arrive in the late afternoon or early evening; during these periods, the number of patients waiting and the time to get treatment increase greatly. Of all the patients visiting the emergency room, only 29.3 per cent are acute or urgent (i.e., true emergencies) and 70.7 per cent are non-urgent. About four per cent of the latter are alcoholics.

After collecting the above information, the model is built in three steps;

1. Identifying the events that affect the model (e.g., a physician coming on duty, patient arrivals or departures, or the temporary absence of a doctor to examine a patient in the ambulance);

2. Analyzing how each event alters the model status;

3. Programming this analysis (i.e., instructing the computer to operate the model).[1]

The changes in the emergency room that this model can test include:

1. Increasing and decreasing patient loads (both overall and for particular types);
2. Referring non-urgent patients to a clinic for treatment;
3. Adding physicians;
4. Adding a physician in a particular specialty such as pediatrics, etc.;

---

[1] Patient arrivals are described by a Poisson distribution, treatment type patterns by a probability matrix (treatment types vs hour of the day), and treatment services times by flat distributions.

5. Adding facilities such as additional treatment room, etc.;
6. Revising physician's schedules;
7. Adding nurses;
8. Revising procedures.

Therefore, the model can help administrators evaluate various solutions to emergency room problems and can reveal unanticipated future problems rapidly, economically, and without disrupting patient care in the actual emergency facility.

WHAT CAN COMPUTERS CONTRIBUTE?

Among the conclusions the model alone helped to develop for this particular emergency room are:

1. The need for an X-ray facility immediately adjacent to the emergency room.
2. The need for the addition of a pediatrician.
3. The need for additional treatment rooms.

Based upon information provided by the model and upon systems analysis, from an industry knowledge standpoint, the consultant made many recommendations including:

1. Provide a triage officer to separate the urgent from the non-urgent patients upon arrival at the emergency room;
2. Provide a separate general or screening clinic to be operated 24 hours a day, as an interface between the overloaded emergency room and the overcrowded daytime, weekday, out-patient clinic, to manage the non-urgent patients;
3. Develop an admitting department separate from the emergency room;
4. Establish a single administrative responsibility for coordination of all ambulatory services in the Department of Health and Hospitals;
5. Consider the ultimate total replacement of all outmoded emergency room and out-patient clinic facilities with a modern, more efficient physical plant.

Here, then, are the kinds of results that can be achieved through the use of computer applications to hospital problems.

The U.S. computer population has exploded from near zero to about 38,000 in a decade. The health care field is experiencing its part of this growth in computers, particularly since hardware-sharing techniques are improving so that smaller hospitals can enjoy the economics of electronic data processing. Most current computer applications are for hospital accounting. The hardware has the capacity to contribute much more to hospital management. That we are beginning to realize this potential is evidenced by the preceding discussion. Administrators who survive the management changes computers are triggering will minimize decision-making by the "seat of the pants" and will learn how to quantify the relationships between their institutions and their environments so their judgments will be more precise and less intuitive.

Decision Making

This section presents the area of decision making. For the most part, the decision making process involves the identification of feasible alternatives which can be applied to the solution of a given problem. Once the alternatives are identified they must be evaluated according to specific criteria. Although the decision making process is used by all managers in all organizations, the hospital administrator has unique constraints typically not imposed on his industrial counterpart; specifically, the necessity of frequently establishing subjective criteria to be used in the evaluation of alternatives.

In *THE ANATOMY OF A DECISION,* the administrator is presented primarily as a decision maker. His responsibility is to allocate the hospital's limited resources in such a way so as to achieve maximum goal attainment at minimum cost. The vital factors of a decision are presented as maximum-minimum criteria, resources, risk, and payoff. More than just a decision making process, the quantitative approach of evaluating alternatives provides a systematic way of thinking.

In *CAPITAL BUDGETING DECISION-MAKING FOR HOSPITALS,* a hybrid methodology for evaluating capital decisions is presented. Mixing the industrial capital budgeting technique and health care cost benefit technique, a model is presented for the systematic evaluation of individual hospital capital expansion programs. Various assumptions are made which attempt to quantify the realm of health care benefits. Regardless of one's interpretation of the validity of the assumptions, the capital budgeting technique presented provides a simple and useful tool for administrators to use in deciding among alternatives.

The Anatomy of a Decision

EDWARD J. SPILLANE

Edward J. Spillane is Assistant Director of The Catholic Hospital Association.

In the complex situation of today's hospital, there is a great need to identify the administrator's primary function in terms of his objectives or output. Too often, in practice, if not in theory, hospital management specialists consider the administrator's *work* more important than his *objectives*. His identity seems to "melt" into and become synonymous with certain activities–loosely labeled management functions–such as planning, coordinating, delegating authority and reviewing financial statements.

But the administrator is primarily a decision-maker. He is not adequately described in terms of specific tasks. Rather, he is concerned with achieving results, with accomplishing objectives. His principal goal is to allocate the hospital's limited resources in such a way as to achieve maximum payoff at minimal cost in terms of realizable hospital objectives. To accomplish this task he must continually make decisions. Decisions, then, comprise the major part of an administrator's output. Through them he either achieves or fails to achieve his and the institution's objectives.

Because decisions *per se* are so important, they must be carefully analyzed. An analysis of a past decision can furnish guidelines for the future; an analysis of a "constructed" or "in-the-making" decision can often mean the difference between success or failure of a yet-to-be-launched project.

ANALYSIS VITAL TO UNDERSTANDING DECISION-MAKING

This article attempts to identify and briefly describe the vital factors which comprise a managerial decision. Unless these parts are understood the administrator and his subordinates will be unable to:

1. Analyze a decision or learn from such an analysis.
2. Be certain that the decisions they "construct" meet the requirements of a complete decision.
3. Fully understand, let alone use, the new concepts, techniques and procedures of the management sciences as recommended by management specialists.[1]

Conversely, an understanding and appreciation of the essential elements of a decision will enable the administrator to more correctly identify and concentrate on his role (decision-maker), and thus better fulfill his responsibility (achieving results). Moreover, it will help him to better coordinate and evaluate his efforts of allocating available resources and thus achieve more efficiently his and the organization's goals.

Included with a brief description of the essential elements of a decision model will be a question outline that the administrator can use to judge the adequacy of each part of a decision. Elementary, but hopefully adequate, examples of each vital element will also be given.

THE ANATOMY OF A DECISION

The following paragraphs may appear to deal only with the decision itself to the exclusion of the administrator's real challenge of implementing the decision. However implementing the decision as well as abstracting relevant facts from the empirical situation are correlative activities and dependent upon effective decisions. Since the success of these activities depends directly on a decision(s), the decision is the key or initiative factor. Admittedly, it is often difficult to distinguish *the* decision from the many supporting decisions that precede and follow the major, output-oriented "go" or "no go" decision. Once again, it is not the activities *per se* that need analysis and emphasis. It is the decision(s), or more correctly the construction of the decision model, that in most instances really spells success or failure in the administrator's efforts to achieve his and his organization's many and varied objectives.

The anatomy of each management decision model is comprised of five vital elements. They are:

1. A clear idea of what is to be maximized or minimized based upon a problem or question.
2. An identification and appreciation of the resources to be allocated.
3. An identification and appreciation of non-resource constraints.
4. An identification of risk factor(s)—imperfect knowledge situation.
5. A comparison of payoff "value" with input "costs."

Although these elements are essential to every decision, they are not all-inclusive. In concentrating on the vital elements, one must not lose sight of the whole. No part is meaningful by itself and each is fully understood only in its relation to the other parts. Likewise, no decision should be made and/or acted upon apart from its relationship to other decisions made or contemplated.[2] A decision lacking one or more vital elements may result in an inefficient allocation of hospital resources in terms of potential payoffs.

---

[1] For a more detailed application of some of these tools and techniques to hospital administration, see the excellent article "Modern Management Concepts, Tools," by George R. Wren, Ph.D., *Hospital Topics,* January, 1968, p. 37.

[2] "Rational decision-making depends on having a full range of rational options from which to choose. Successful management organizes the enterprise so that this process can best take place." Robert S. McNamara.

MAXIMIZATION-MINIMIZATION

The focal point of every decision is the determination of that factor which is to be minimized or maximized. Describing and understanding this factor is the most difficult aspect of "constructing" a decision. This factor must be subject to some degree of quantitative or qualitative measurement and translated into terms of output or objectives. In making this determination, community analysis (market research), exit interviews, attitude surveys, sampling techniques and many other data-gathering tools are helpful. An understanding and utilization of such managerial concepts and techniques as value analysis, management by objectives, payoff tables, simulation and systems management is not possible unless the administrator can clearly define that which he is attempting to maximize or minimize in each decision situation. Vague platitudes (e.g. maximize the quality of patient care, minimize the costs of patient care, good personnel policies), stated in purely descriptive terms, are too general; only precise definition will meet the requirements of determining the maximization-minimization factor.

The Anatomy of a Decision

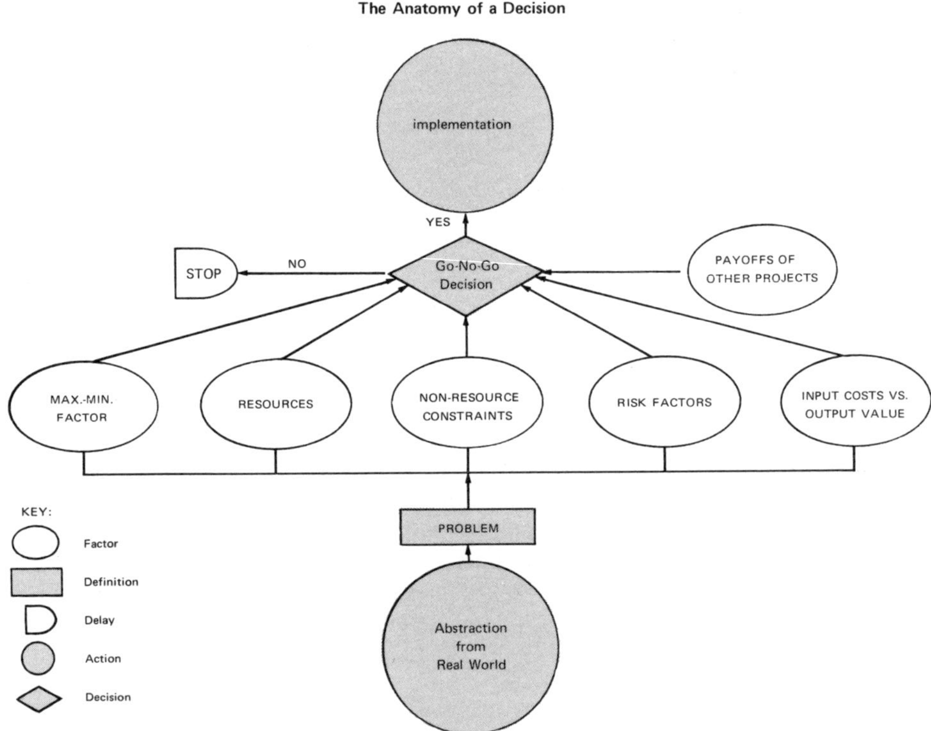

In identifying this factor, the administrator should attempt to answer the following questions: What is to be maximized or minimized, and to what degree? For example: 1. Labor turnover *(what)* is to be minimized to a target level of two per cent *(degree)* a month; 2. Medication errors *(what)* are to be minimized to a target level of 12 *(degree)*

per month; 3. The productive time of all physicians while in the hospital *(what)* will be maximized so that no physician will ever have to wait *(degree)* for an open line in order to dictate medical records information.

Although strict definition is necessary, the dynamics of the situation also require flexibility. The maximization-minimization factor can and will be changed as other parts of the decision take shape. Its significance lies in two areas: 1. Its relation to the other parts of the decision model and its ability to furnish the administrator with a clear objective or base upon which to proceed in the decision-making process, and 2. its use as a standard for future evaluation and control.

LIMITED RESOURCE ALLOCATION

This decision factor is used to identify the quantitative and qualitative characteristics of the resources available and required. In each decision, limited (scarce) resources will be programmed for allocation via some type of organizational structure to some project or activity. These limited resources must be calculated in terms of cost, quantity, quality, possibility for and degrees of substitutability. In addition, the relation of payoffs in terms of output resulting from various mixes of resources (together with associated input costs) to that which is to be maximized or minimized should be identified and analyzed. Understanding what is needed to accomplish this part of the decision will make industrial engineering science and such managerial concepts as linear programming, break-even, labor-capital substitution and discounted cash flow analysis more meaningful and useful to the administrator.

In analyzing this part of a decision, the administrator must answer the following question: What least expensive mix of scarce resources will achieve a payoff that is consistent with the maximization-minimization requirement?

LEAST EXPENSIVE MIX OF SCARCE RESOURCES

An example of a limited resource allocation could be algebraically expressed as follows: To achieve a given target of 1000P level of clean linen inventory (output) during an eight-hour period, two possible combinations of resources (inputs) and production functions can be proposed, which will achieve the same output.

$$A. \ 1000P = f(1800L + 300X + 8Y + Z)$$
$$B. \ 1000P = f(1200L + 800X + 4Y + Z)$$

Where

L = Linen at a unit cost of \$1.
X = Labor at a unit cost of \$2.
Y = Capital equipment (allocated expense) at a unit cost of \$50.
Z = Other indirect costs of \$5 per eight-hour period.

Assigning costs to the variables (inputs) in the above equations (production functions) and solving the equations will give the lowest cost needed to achieve the target output of 1000P per eight-hour period.

One can readily see from the payoff analysis that combination A is the preferred mix of resources. Substituting capital (L and Y) for labor resources (reduction in units of labor) makes the difference in costs possible. Without such a substitution analysis the administrator may overlook various options and a less than efficient allocation of the hospital's scarce resources could result. This assumes, of course, a "payoff at minimal cost" rationale.

NON-RESOURCE CONSTRAINTS

Each decision usually includes certain identifiable constraints on the allocation, organization and use of resources that are non-resource in nature. These non-resource constraints can be classified as legal, social, psychological, religious or political in nature, and, often, they do not lend themselves to quantification or certain prediction. The administrator must recognize these constraints, estimate their impact on other parts of the decision and the final output and then incorporate this knowledge into the decision model.

Various federal, state and local laws regulating the use of labor resources are tangible examples of non-resource constraints. The psychological impact of change on labor units is less known and more difficult to estimate. Another possible constraint would be the significance that findings and recommendations of local planning agencies, in terms of the need or lack of need for additional hospital beds, might have on the administrator's decision to expand or not expand the inventory of hospital beds. In terms of labor resource allocation and use, union contracts present a definite constraint on the administrator's decision-making.

RISK FACTOR

Every decision-maker attempts to achieve certainty in the decision-making process, but seldom in major decisions is this goal realized. Neither the constraints nor the chances of achieving the objective as reflected by the element to be maximized or minimized are known with certainty. The administrator must make estimates and base subsequent actions upon them. An understanding of the aspect of risk will make such things as the Bayesian probability theory, decision trees and joint probability tables more meaningful and useful to the administrator.

Being aware of the degree of risk is the first step toward reducing the risk factor. The administrator must determine the degree of risk by attempting to decide whether the activity or project will actually meet or surpass the desired payoff. One example of the element of risk or uncertainty facing the administrator can be seen in the following situation: A proposal to purchase a pulmonary function test machine costing $1,500 has been made. The risks involved in this project might include, but are not limited to, some of the following: Will the physicians use the machine enough to recover the cost before the machine becomes obsolete? Can necessary personnel be obtained to help the physician in the operation of the machine? Will other hospitals purchase these machines and reduce the volume of use? In deciding whether or not to purchase the PFT machine, the risks or uncertainties must be analyzed, evaluated, considered and incorporated into the total decision.

COMPARISON OF THE PAYOFF VALUE WITH THE INPUT COSTS

In constructing this part of the decision the administrator is actually asking: "Given the costs of inputs (resources) and the value of the output factor to be maximized or minimized is the allocation of resources to this project justified?" In other words, the payoff must be equal to or greater than the costs of the resources allocated to achieve this payoff. The probability of success factor will, of course, alter this balance. For instance, in the laundry production example given previously it was found economical to substitute capital for labor. However, the probability of success factor could change the picture drastically. If the probability of achieving 1000P by substituting capital for labor was only 50 per cent (A) because of machine downtime and lack of an adequate maintenance department, while the probability of achieving 1000P in the labor intensive situation (B) was 90 per cent, one would naturally reconsider the choice of resource mixes.

An administrator would not readily incur X costs for a payoff value of X-1, especially when the same combination of resources could be allocated to other projects and achieve an X + 1 value payoff.

An example of the cost input vs. value output analysis is as follows: labor turnover in a given situation is calculated to cost a hospital $500 per terminating employe. Thus the total value to the hospital for a reduction in turnover could be expressed $500X (X being the reduction in turnover units). An estimate is made that labor turnover can be reduced by 10 units or roughly 12 per cent for a 200-bed hospital during a 12-month period. If the cost to achieve this objective, in terms of a better employe selection program, increased salaries and fringe benefits and more inservice education, was equal to or greater than $5,000, one would question the wisdom of the allocation of resources. Although other factors might indicate that reduced turnover, inservice education, department head meetings, etc., would be desirable, they should not be initiated because such action cannot be justified, in this instance, by the cost of input-value or output-analysis.

"GO" OR "NO GO" OUTPUT

All of the decision factors coalesce in the action or no action judgment. In making this judgment, the decision-maker must compare the payoff resulting from the allocation of the resources to one project with the payoff that might result from allocating the resources to another project or activity. An example of this would be as follows: Assume that $3,000 worth of resources could result in a $5,000 payoff via reduced labor turnover. But assume also that the $3,000 worth of resources could be allocated to improve the doctor's parking lot with a payoff value of $8,000. Under a results-oriented management with limited resources, and assuming that computations of cost and payoff values are correct, the labor turnover project would in all probability be put aside in favor of the parking lot project.

SUMMARY

Better decisions through improved technology result in increased hospital efficiency. Improved technology can be explained as follows:

$$OP = f(A, B, C, D) \text{ when}$$
$$(A + B + C + D) = X \text{ costs (present situation)}$$
$$OP = f(A_1, B_1, C_1, D_1) \text{ when}$$
$$(A_1 + B_1 + C_1 + D_1) = X - Y \text{ costs}$$
$$\text{(improvement through technology)}$$

That is, the same payoff using less resource input costs or a required greater payoff using the same or less resource input costs is essential to improved technology.

This article has analyzed the decision-making process and has given the manager a brief conceptual framework within which the various concepts and tools of modern management can be fitted and understood in relation to the decision-making process. Without such an outline the newer "scientific" methods of managerial problem-solving will not be understood, let alone utilized. Although analyzing decisions and using modern management techniques cannot solve all of the administrator's "real world" problems, such activities can give him a new way of looking at his job—the job of making decisions capable of achieving objectives. A better understanding of the nature of a decision can help him achieve his primary goal—allocating the hospital's limited resources in the most effecient way possible. This is what technology and increased efficiency in hospital operations is all about.

Hospital decision-making must be considered within the context of reimbursement formulas. Unlike the competitive environment, the hospital environment does not demand adherence to maximization and minimization requirements. Reimbursement formulas tend to allow a decision-making process not subject to unlimited resources. Changes in the reimbursement formulas requiring more efficient uses of hospital resources via technology in the future will make this decision-making process more relevant to hospital decision-makers.

Capital Budgeting Decision-Making for Hospitals

RICHARD F. WACHT, PH.D.

Richard F. Wacht, Ph.D., is an Associate Professor of Finance at Georgia State University in Atlanta.

There has been a considerable amount of work accomplished in the area of cost-benefit analysis applied to health programs. Some of the more notable efforts have been by Weisbrod[1] and Mushkin,[2] and other authors who have made contributions in supporting areas, such as Reynolds in his study of the cost of road accidents in Great Britain.[3] Most of this work, however, has been directed toward the aggregate costs and the aggregate benefits to society of eradicating disease and saving lives, and the main interest has been concentrated on the problem of valuing the benefits per life saved or per illness avoided.[4]

EXPENDITURE BY SOCIETY AS A WHOLE

Implicit in these efforts to develop a theory of human capital formation and the attempts at statistical measurement of the benefits to be derived by allocating economic resources to health programs is the assumption that their primary concern should be with the analysis of an expenditure *by society as a whole* earmarked for the elimination or cure of a specific disease. This assumption, however, suggests that the application of cost-benefit analysis is performed by what may well prove to be the wrong unit; instead of analyzing an expenditure by *society*, the unit that should perform the analysis is the individual *hospital*—the ultimate investor of society's health program funds and the ultimate dispensor of health services to society. This follows from the fact that hospitals are financed at the margin by public-type funds (e.g.,

[1] B. A. Weisbrod, *Economics of Public Health: Measuring the Economic Impact of Diseases* (Philadelphia: University of Pennsylvania Press, 1960).

[2] Selma J. Mushkin, "Health as an Investment," *Journal of Political Economy*, Vol. LXX (Supplement), October 1962.

[3] D. J. Reynolds, "The Cost of Road Accidents," *Journal of the Royal Statistical Society*, Vol. 119, Part 4, 1956.

[4] A. R. Prest and R. Turvey, "Cost-Benefit Analysis: A Survey," *The Economic Journal*, Vol. LXXV, December 1965, p. 721.

Reprinted by permission from *Hospital Administration: Quarterly Journal of the American College of Hospital Administrators,* Chicago, Vol. 15 (Fall 1970), 14-27. Copyright 1970 by the American College of Hospital Administrators. All rights reserved.

public grants, gifts, donations, etc.) and they attempt to serve the health needs as demanded by the communities in which they are located. In addition, the hospitals generate income by billing patients for services rendered and, consequently, are sometimes in a position to supplement public funds with their own internally generated funds which may be made available for additional investment in health programs. Therefore, it would appear that the individual hospital, rather than society, ought to be charged with allocating those resources placed at its disposal among health programs not presently provided by it or else provided on only a minimal basis.

A SET OF DECISION RULES

Since a change in focus may in fact be required, and since the current state of the art of hospital capital budgeting can be described as primitive at best, the purpose of this paper is to develop a set of decision rules for applying existing cost-benefit theory and technique to the problem of maximizing the return on health program investment (made by hospitals). The applications in the field are legion, but the scope of the following discussion will be limited to investment in plant and equipment.[5]

THEORETICAL FRAMEWORK

Cost-benefit analysis, which is also known as investment planning and project appraisal, is a practical way of assessing the desirability of public projects in terms of short- and long-run benefits accruing from all affected economic entities.[6] It has as its counterpart in the private sector what is termed capital budgeting theory. With the aid of this similar approach, the profit-seeking corporation assesses its proposed capital investment expenditures in order to eliminate from consideration those projects which fail to meet some predetermined *profit* criterion.[7] The aim of both approaches is identical; i.e., to maximize the present value of all benefits less that of all costs, subject to specified constraints.

NEITHER APPROACH ADEQUATE IN ITSELF

In spite of the very great similarities between cost-benefit analysis and capital budgeting, neither approach is adequate in itself to provide the basic framework for capital budgeting decision-making in hospitals. This is because of the unique position hospitals occupy in our economy—halfway between the public sector and the private sector. Hospitals operate on the margin with public funds and mainly for the public good; therefore, cost-benefit analysis is especially applicable in the area of measuring non-monetary benefits derived from saving lives and from correcting mental and

[5] Included here under the term *plant* and *equipment* will be project planning, which encompasses necessary outlays for and benefits from capital and non-capital (e.g., personnel, medical and non-medical inventories, etc.) items for installing a new health service.

[6] Prest, *op. cit.,* p. 683.

[7] See Ezra Solomon, ed., *The Management of Corporate Capital* (Chicago: The Free Press of Glencoe, 1959), and Harold Bierman and Seymour Smidt, *The Capital Budgeting Decision,* 2nd ed. (New York: The Macmillan Co., 1966).

physical disabilities of people so that they may become more productive members of society.

It must also be recognized that, to a great extent, hospitals act like profit-seeking corporations. Hospitals must attempt to cover operating costs in order to survive and in order to continue to improve the health services that the public demands of them. Society may be willing to pay for the health care of people who are unable to pay for it themselves, but it should not be asked to bear the burden of waste or inefficiences in the management of hospitals. Thus, maximum benefit (in both the financial sense and social sense) should be sought for each dollar of expenditure by each hospital. Consequently, capital budgeting, designed as a microeconomic tool where money costs and money returns are involved, is just as applicable for hospital financial management as cost-benefit analysis.

Given that a combination of both approaches is needed, it is now necessary to spell out as precisely as possible the general principles of this hybrid approach, which shall be called *hospital capital budgeting.*

Very briefly, the object of analyzing an expenditure within the framework of hospital capital budgeting is to determine the numerical value of the ratio of the present value of benefits expressed in dollars to the present value of money costs. In order that society realize a net gain from the investment, this ratio should be greater than unity; that is, the present value of the benefits should exceed the costs.

As a practical matter, the major difficulties in applying this tool will be in defining and measuring the benefit; and costs associated with a hospital project. In most cases the scope and nature of the projects which are to be submitted for analysis are clear, but *for the sake of definition,* it might be well to enumerate the various elements that would go to make up these costs and benefits:

CAPITAL BUDGETING COSTS

(a) *Costs.* There are two types of costs with which hospital capital budgeting will be concerned: (1) the cost of acquiring, assembling, and making ready for operation all the necessary material required by the project, which cost shall be referred to as the *investment;* and (2) the costs associated with the normal functioning of the project once it has commenced operation. The latter costs will be called *operating costs.*

Investment is defined here to include the delivered cost of the plant and equipment, installation costs, any increase in inventories and accounts receivable attributed directly to the functioning of the project under consideration, and any other expense that would normally be capitalized and subsequently written off over the expected life of the equipment.[8]

Operating costs are those expenses which are directly associated with the project's operation, such as wages and salaries, electricity, and any increase in overhead expenses brought about by the adoption of the projects. Non-cash expenses, such as depreciation, are ignored however, since most hospitals are either state-supported institutions or non-profit corporations. Consequently, the effect of depreciation on tax liability need not be considered.

---

[8]The total of these items is the amount which is analogous to the principal or market value of a bond or certificate of indebtedness which should be returned to the investor (with interest) at maturity.

(b) *Benefits.* The benefits from new projects can be separated into two parts: (1) monetary benefits; and (2) non-monetary benefits. The *monetary benefits,* obviously, accrue from offering a service to the public at a price and collecting a sum of money once the service has been rendered. It is hoped that the money thus collected would be sufficient to cover the operating costs. If so, the *net cash benefits* arising from the investment in the project will be positive and can be expressed in terms of dollars received monthly, quarterly, or annually. If, however, operating costs exceed the collections, net cash benefits will be negative, but they will still be expressed in the same terms, but will be deducted from total benefits.

The *non-monetary benefits* arising from hospital investments are those with which cost-benefit analysis is mainly concerned; that is, the benefits to society arising out of saving lives or correcting some sort of malformation or malfunctioning of human bodies either totally or in part. One very definite result of this type of activity is that society retains (or gains) a productive member or realizes a gain from a productive member being made even more productive. Such benefits should be included in hospital capital budgeting, even though they are not directly expressed in money terms.

VALUATION OF COSTS AND BENEFITS

Hospital capital budgeting is concerned with costs and benefits which are either directly expressible in terms of money or, are capable of being expressed in terms of money. In applications such as these, all items should be valued at their *current* market value without adjustment for expected changes in the general price level. The reasoning here is that the valuation of all costs and benefits must be determined on the same basis, and for convenience the current price-level is generally employed.[9]

The more difficult problem, however, is to measure the value of those non--monetary benefits accruing to society from the investment in plant and equipment by hospitals. The basis for this type of measurement for health care benefits in general has been the subject of much of the literature of cost-benefit analysis, and the concensus is that economic resources devoted to health care represent in some part an investment in health; the resource gained as a result of dollars spent in order to prevent or cure sickness (including injury) is human labor. Thus, the attempt to value this resource gain in dollars must necessarily be directed toward estimating the output added by health care.[10]

Unlike much of the previous work in this area, the effort here must be directed toward labor product measurement not in the aggregate but as it applies to a given capital expenditure by an individual hospital.

RELATIVE WORTH ANALYZED

The effects of sickness or injury on human labor available for productive purposes can be classified under three headings: (1) death (permanent loss of labor); (2)

[9] Prest, *op. cit.,* p. 691.

[10] Mushkin, *op. cit.,* p. 138. For a more complete discussion of labor product measurement in the aggregate, see S. J. Mushkin and Francis d'A. Collins, "Economic Costs of Disease and Injury," *Public Health Reports,* LXXIV (September 1, 1959), pp. 795-809.

disability (temporary or permanent loss of labor); and (3) debility (temporary or permanent decrease in the productivity of labor).[11] In order to measure the value that hospital capital spending provides, an estimate of gain in productive work time brought about by the capital expenditure must be made, and a money value must be assigned to the output that this added work time represents. The resultant dollar figure will be an estimate of the non-monetary benefits arising out of the capital expenditure which, when added to the net cash benefits, will provide a figure that can be used to analyze the relative worth of the proposed capital acquisition.

MAN-YEARS AS A MEASUREMENT

The gain in resources derived from human labor made available for productive purposes through hospital capital expenditures must first be stated in terms of some basic unit which can then be assigned a value. Perhaps the most convenient unit of measurement would be man-years added to production since any smaller unit would tend to compound the arithmetic without making a corresponding contribution to the accuracy of the estimates. Reduction in deaths and long-term disabilities can be expressed directly in terms of additions of man-years on the job, and, in the case of debility, an improvement of efficiency on the job can readily be converted to full-time equivalents.[12]

EARNINGS AS A GUIDE

The estimate of the dollar value of the economic benefits from saving lives begins by determining earnings of the average person whose life is saved (productive capacity is enhanced) as a result of the capital expenditure being made by the hospital. The use of earnings, defined here to exclude any income resulting from a return on property or capital, can be justified on the grounds that the product of human labor benefits society and that this benefit should be measured by the market value placed on the units of labor.[13] The use of the earnings of the average person is also justified since the facilities acquired by hospitals will continue to yield benefits over a number of years by serving a cross-section of those people who are likely to succumb to the particular disease being treated.

The value of the total benefits, expressed as an annual figure, will therefore be

$$(1) \qquad B_t = B_m - C_o + \sum_n (e_t\, Y)\, (1 + r)^{-n}$$

where B_t represents total benefits at time t; B_m, monetary benefits received per year; C_o, annual operating costs; e_t, annual earnings at time of the average person benefiting from the capital expenditure; Y, estimated number of man-years added to production per year; and r, the rate of discount used to determine the present value of future

---

[11] *Ibid.*

[12] *Ibid.*, p. 140. Full employment can be assumed since there can be no loss of production in an unemployment situation and since unemployment should be considered as having its own costs.

[13] The value of the *product* is not used since this value is the result of the joint efforts of land, capital *and* labor. The benefits to society from saving lives is only that part of the product created by labor and should be valued by what labor receives in compensation.

earnings over the next n years, n being the number of years remaining of the life expectancy of the average person mentioned above.

PRESENT VALUE OF TOTAL BENEFITS

Equation (1) requires that the *present value* of future earnings of the average man be used as the non-monetary benefits. In addition, the estimated future benefits from the capital expenditure must be discounted at some rate of interest in order that all costs and benefits be reduced to comparable terms. In other words, what is required is the present value of total benefits, B_t. In equation form, this would be

$$(2) \qquad \text{Present value of total benefits} \; = \; \sum_t B_t (1 + r)^{-t}$$

where t would equal the expected economic life of the capital investment. Thus, there are two requirements for which an interest rate is needed to discount future benefits.

The literature on selecting the proper rate of interest for *public* investment projects is voluminous, and what is infinitely clear from a survey of this literature is that the proper method of determining this interest rate is at present unclear.[14] If such a method could indeed be developed, it would no doubt be of great value. But lacking such a ready-made tool, the best anyone can do is depend on a value judgment in selecting an interest rate.[15] It would appear satisfactory, however, to use the cost of acquiring borrowed funds for hospital capital budgeting purposes since this rate of interest is (1) meaningful to the individual hospital in terms of real costs, (2) easily determined or determinable, and (3) convenient. No defense of this rate on theoretical grounds will be offered here since, as Prest and Turvey so aptly put it, "whatever one does, one is trying to unscramble an omelette, and no one has yet invented a uniquely superior way of doing this."[16]

HOSPITAL CAPITAL BUDGETING TECHNIQUE

The technique of hospital capital budgeting can best be described with the aid of a hypothetical situation. The case problem that will be examined is one involving the establishment of a new hospital wing designed to cure hemophilia by means of organ transplant.[17]

---

[14]Otto Eckstein, "A Survey of the Theory of Public Expenditure Criteria," in James M. Buchanan (ed.) *Public Finances: Needs, Sources, and Utilization* (Princeton: Princeton University Press, 1961), pp. 458-460.

[15]For purposes of hospital capital budgeting, the problem of finding r becomes at once simpler and more complex than that for strictly public expenditures. On one hand, the monetary returns to the hospital take the form of corporate earnings which, in this sense, should be discounted at the hospital's cost of acquiring capital funds. This is simply the cost of borrowing for private institutions or, for state-supported institutions, the cost of funds borrowed by the state at the margin. On the other hand, the non-monetary benefits are actually returns to society expressed in money terms and should be discounted at a social rate of interest, which figure cannot be agreed upon. Thus, the choice of r must be a value judgment.

[16]Prest and Turvey, *op. cit.,* p. 700.

[17]No claim is made for the accuracy of any dollar figures presented here, nor should these figures be considered as even rough estimate of actual cost and income. The figures are for illustrative purposes only.

NET INVESTMENT REQUIRED

TABLE 1
CASH OUTFLOW FOR INVESTMENT IN PLANT AND
EQUIPMENT FOR ORGAN TRANSPLANT PROJECT

($000)

ITEM	YEAR 1	YEAR 2
Construction Costs	$1,052	$ 80
Equipment Costs	48	168
Installation Costs	0	42
Working Capital	0	10
TOTALS	$1,100	$300

The first step is to determine the net investment   required in order to build, equip, and otherwise ready the new wing for the acceptance of its first patient. It is important to determine both the total cash outlay for the project and the timing of such outlays. For example, it can be assumed that the new wing will take one year to build and another year to accumulate and install the necessary equipment once the decision has been made to undertake the project. The expenditures on the building and equipment contracts are to be paid continuously over the two-year period, except for the supplies inventories (which will be called working capital), so that the initial cash outflow can be shown in Table 1.

OPERATING COSTS

The next step is to estimate the operating costs which would likely be incurred at the projected level of activity for the new wing. These would consist of all utilities for the wing, personnel (both staff and administrative), housekeeping, supplies, etc. In other words, any actual increase in current operating costs associated with the new wing and its functioning should be considered. Allocated costs, however, such as administrative overhead, should be ignored unless these costs actually increase as a result of the project. For present purposes, let it be assumed that annual operating costs total $120,000 (and are incurred and paid continuously throughout each year, beginning in year three).

Another important consideration is to estimate the useful life of the combined investment. The building may last forever, but since it was designed for a special purpose (organ transplant) its maximum utility is realized only so long as it is used for the purpose for which it was designed. The equipment, on the other hand, will last for only a relatively short time before it will have to be replaced. But replacement of existing equipment is an investment decision in itself, so the useful life of a project extends from the time the first patient is accepted until the facility can no longer serve its primary purpose because of deterioration or obsolescence. In the present example, this period will be from year three through year ten or an expected useful life of eight years.

ESTIMATING THE RESULTING BENEFITS

The final bit of information needed is an estimate of the benefits—both monetary and non-monetary—that will result from the investment in the project. Measurement of the monetary benefits is relatively simple. It is merely the estimated annual number of non-indigent patients times the expected per patient charges. An estimate of the average length of postoperative care must naturally be made, along with the ancillary services that will be provided during the patient's stay. To these billings should be added any receipts from other sources on behalf of indigent patients. For the present case, it can be assumed that total monetary benefits are estimated to be $3,500 per average patient (including indigent for determining the average) and that it is expected that twenty patients per year will be treated successfully in the new wing.

MEASURING NON-MONETARY BENEFITS

Several steps are involved in measuring non-monetary benefits. The first is to determine the characteristics of the patients who will directly benefit from the investment expenditure made by the hospital. Hemophilia, for example, is almost exclusively a male disease. The disease can cripple as well as kill, and although its crippling effects can be treated on a temporary basis, no method has yet been devised to prevent their recurrence. As a consequence, a person with hemophilia, if he avoids the crippling effects of the disease and survives long enough to enter the labor market, is limited as to the type of employment he may engage in and probably will not reach the maximum productive capacity he would have achieved without the disease.

MAKING AN ESTIMATE

If it can therefore be assumed that the organ transplant will cure the hemophiliac, the investment in the project will result in preventing death, disability, and debility (in some ratio) in twenty people per year. It can also be assumed here that the time to perform the organ transplant for the patient would be at as early an age as practical, since the slightest bump may be fatal or permanently damaging to the hemophiliac. Finally, let us assume that a search of existing data shows that 5 per cent of all those suffering from the disease enter the labor market, 65 per cent die partially as a result of the disease prior to entering the labor market, and the remaining 30 per cent become permanently disabled.

Based on these assumptions, an estimate of the non-monetary benefits can now be made. The first step is to determine the average annual earnings at each age (for males only in this case) beginning from the age of the average patient, and discount these earnings to the present at the proper rate of interest.[18] The *present value* of the lifetime earnings of an average American male, age one year, discounted at 7 per cent

---

[18] The rate used here is 7 per cent.

is $19,266.[19] Without the organ transplant, 19 of 20 males would never enter the labor market, and the one who will, will earn, say, only two-thirds of his potential. Thus, the annual non-monetary benefits of investing in the new hospital wing will total about $378,000. Table 2 summarizes the timing and size of all the costs and benefits over the relevant period.

BENEFITS OVER COSTS

The final step in the process is to discount the net benefits (and costs) at the proper interest rate and compare the present value of the net investment with the present value of the net cash benefits plus the non-monetary benefits.[20] In this case, the present value of the net investment, discounted at 7 per cent is $1,362,000, and the present value of the net benefits from years three through ten total $1,498,000. The excess of benefits over costs is therefore $136,000 and the project should be undertaken, since the rate of return on investment by the hospital exceeds the cost of acquiring the funds. If the present value of the net investment had exceeded that of the benefits, however, the project should be rejected on the grounds that this particular allocation of resources would tend to make society less well off in the long run.

TABLE 2

COSTS AND BENEFITS ASSOCIATED WITH
ORGAN TRANSPLANT PROJECT

($000)

Year	Investment*	C_o Operating Costs	B_m Monetary Benefits	e_tY Non-monetary Benefits	B_t Net Benefits (Costs)
1	($1,100)†				($1,100)
2	(300)				(300)
3		($120)	$70	$378	$ 328
4		(120)	70	378	328
5		(120)	70	378	328
6		(120)	70	378	328
7		(120)	70	378	328
8		(120)	70	378	328
9		(120)	70	378	328
10	10‡	(120)	70	378	338

*From Table 1.

†Parenthesis denote costs or cash outflows.

‡Represents the retention of working capital after project life is ended (See Table 1).

[19]Based on 1960 census figures. U.S. Senate, 88th Congress, 1st Session, *Hearings Before the Committee on Labor and Public Welfare on Bills Relating to Equal Employment Opportunities,* July-August 1963, p. 334.

BEST APPLICATION

Again, it should be stated that perhaps the best application of this tool would be in deciding among alternative investments, given a budget constraint or otherwise mutually exclusive projects under consideration by a hospital. In this type of application, the hospital would select the project(s) which promised the greatest excess present value or the greatest ratio of the present value of net benefits to present value of investment.

SUMMARY

In summary, the steps that one should take in applying the technique of hospital capital budgeting developed in this paper are as follows:

1. Determine the size and timing of cash expenditures on the required investment in plant and equipment.
2. Estimate the operating costs involved in the project.
3. Estimate the life of the project.
4. Estimate the monetary and non-monetary benefits.
5. Discount the costs and benefits with the proper interest rate and compare.

This technique will provide the hospital with an objective criterion that can be used in capital budgeting decision-making processes. Existing criteria on which such decisions are now being based, such as need or urgency,[21] persuasiveness or bargaining skill of individuals, and other similar approaches, obviously are not totally responsive to the hospital's environment as expressed in terms of the economics of health and medical care of the community which it serves. This is not to suggest, however, that the technique of hospital capital budgeting presented here should be used as the sole criterion for such decisions. The hospital's policy statements and long-run objectives should provide the framework for all activities, regardless of their nature, but it must be recognized that objective criteria are also necessary for rational decision-making.

SUGGESTED FURTHER READING

Robert Dorfman, ed., *Measuring Benefits of Government Investments* (Washington, D.C.: The Brookings Institute, 1965). Outlines some of the current thinking about criteria useful in measuring returns in the Public Sector.

Samuel B. Chase, Jr., ed., *Problems in Public Expenditure Analysis* (Washington, D.C.: The Brookings Institute, 1968). A much broader approach to the problems discussed in the Dorfman book.

Burton A. Weisbord, *Economics of Public Health* (Philadelphia: University of Pennsylvania Press, 1961). The most often quoted book in the field—a real classic.

Herbert E. Klarman *Economics of Public Health* (New York: Columbia University Press, 1965). Another classic.

[20]The present value tables used here are found in Jerome Bracken and C. J. Christenson, *Tables for Use in Analyzing Business Decisions* (Homewood, Illinois; Richard D. Irwin, Inc., 1965).

[21]*American Hospital Association, Budgeting Procedures for Hospitals* (Chicago: AHA, 1961), p. 38.

Part V

HEALTH CARE POLICY AND TRENDS

This part of the book presents various health care issues and trends. Today the health care system and its hospitals are being criticized. Governmental participation is increasing along with a rise in expectations and demands from society. Various policy issues are currently being raised that have a spectrum range from health care as a right to public financing of benefits. The resolution of these issues and trends will have a significant impact on the future role of the hospital organization and its management.

The first section, RESPONSIBILITY, presents this issue from an internal and external point of view. The determination of the hospital's responsibility to itself can only be ascertained from critical self evaluation. By the same token, the hospital's responsibility to society must be established through the value judgments of administrators and the public. It is pointed out that the hospital's responsibility to the public should only be made after a comprehensive examination of the total delivery system has been conducted.

The second section, INSTITUTION AND AREA-WIDE PLANNING, presents the subject of planning within and among health care institutions. Being a prerequistie for efficient operation and allocation of resources, planning must be undertaken systematically, rationally, and in light of the hospital's responsibility to the public.

The third section, HEALTH CARE POLICY ISSUES, presents a critical examination of the delivery and financing systems. The trends of the hospital being the focal point in delivery and public financing of health care services are identified. The promotion or impeding of these trends requires that policy decisions be made. The task is not simple. However, since they affect the hospital organization and its management, administrators should actively participate in their resolution.

Responsibility

This section presents the subject of the hospital organization's responsibility both to itself and society. The demands on the health care delivery system have strained its institutions to the point where it is now necessary for the hospital to identify its future role. The role identification must not only be viewed in terms of society, but also with respect to itself, its management, and its efficiency.

In *A TRUSTEE VIEWS THE VOLUNTARY HOSPITAL SYSTEM,* the non-profit hospital system is presented as one of America's most precious assets. The point is made that inadequate attention has been given to promoting the efficiency of the hospital organization and that continued neglect could lead to its gradual liquidation. The time has come for the hospital to critically evaluate itself and its responsibilities. Viewing the hospital from a business man's point of view, answers must be sought to the problems of costs and efficiency, but not at the expense of services. Viewing the hospital from the trustee's point of view, answers must be sought to the problems of the proper mix of area facilities and the utilization of well informed trustee members.

In *THE SOCIAL RESPONSIBILITY OF GENERAL HOSPITALS,* the hospital is presented as an institution which is under pressure to expand its role and scope of services in order to respond to social needs. The social model requires the alteration of the current mission of the hospital and the focusing of efforts toward preventative care, concern for human values, and the provision of health care as a right. That is, social responsibility. It is stipulated that expanded missions may jeopardize the quality of medical care due to limited resources. However, it is constructively pointed out that the determination of the future mission of the hospital requires leadership and clear planning programs. The adoption of the social model by hospitals can only be permitted if a systematic evaluation indicates that the hospital organization is the proper vehicle.

A Trustee Views the Voluntary Hospital System

RAY R. EPPERT

Ray R. Eppert was formerly Chief Executive Officer and Board Chairman of Burroughs Corporation and is currently Vice-Chairman of Harper Hospital in Detroit, Michigan.

Last March, it was my privilege to be one of the American Hospital Association's witnesses on Public Law 89-97 (Medicare) at hearings in Washington, D.C., before the Ways and Means Committee of the House of Representatives. I was testifying as a hospital trustee in behalf of the voluntary hospital system.

What do we really mean when we speak of the voluntary hospital system? Several years ago, a committee of the American Hospital Association took a hard look at the nature of the system and defined it very well. In the light of current developments, it is important that we keep this definition fresh in our minds. The committee said that the distinguishing feature of our hospital system is "its dependence in large part upon the voluntary principle—that principle that emphasizes the individual rather than the crowd; that stresses freedom of choice rather than compulsion; flexibility rather than rigidity; quality rather than quantity; that provides a place for charity as well as duty; that is in essence freedom, and, in sum, the aggregate of free choices made by individuals through all other means than increasing the powers of government, which involves the use of involuntary taxing and police powers."[1] The statement went on to say that this voluntary principle code is most manifest and society is best served when the following criteria are most fully met:

1. The individual hospital has autonomy and local nongovernmental control.

2. The hospital is responsible for its own financing and receives its support from those who use it and from those who donate funds or services for its continuation and improvement.

3. The hospital is not operated primarily for profit.

I endorse this statement, including the last point: "The hospital is not operated primarily for profit." Not that I am opposed to for-profit enterprises. As I told the Congressional committee, "I am an advocate of the profit system. I have spent my life working within that system, and I believe I understand and appreciate the broad

[1] Voluntary hospital system: American Hospital Association Board of Trustees statement. *Hospitals, J.A.H.A.* 35:33 Aug. 1, 1961.

---

benefits that this country, and all of us as individuals, have derived from its motivation. Yet I seriously doubt that it is possible—or wise—for the health field to depend upon hospitals developed primarily as private for-profit organizations. These proprietary, for-profit institutions serve their communities well, and they provide an essential service; but it would be a mistake to leave the future of hospital care entirely in the hands of such organizations."

VALUE OF NONPROFIT HOSPITALS

I am proud to have been the chairman and chief executive officer of a very large *for-profit corporation.* I am equally proud to be the chairman of a *not-for-profit hospital.* These two statements are not in fundamental conflict.

Just what is it that businessmen dedicated to the profit motive see in nonprofit hospitals? They believe that the free enterprise system is something much broader than the producing of individual and corporate profits. They believe that it provides freedom to operate, freedom of incentives, freedom for change, and freedom to improve the quality of a product. In the operation of a nonprofit hospital, they recognize, as does the AHA statement, these same freedoms. These hospitals provide more than the basic, essential services. They offer their communities high quality care, and they do this not because they have to, but because they want to. Business leaders want the hospital to continue to have this freedom of action not for the sake of profits, but so hospitals can continue to innovate and improve and to keep their services at a high level of quality and efficiency.

But just because I and my fellows in the industrial and business community support and believe in our nonprofit hospital system doesn't mean that we believe in or support an unbusinesslike operation. There has never been a time when it was as necessary as it is now for these hospitals to be conducted in a businesslike fashion and to be able to demonstrate it. Today, hospitals are in the spotlight and that means they are on the spot.

At the present time, some 24 per cent of the patients in the non-profit hospitals are Medicare patients. And if the Medicare reimbursement is inadequate, and it is, it presents a serious threat to our voluntary short-term care institutions. You can't afford to be underpaid for 24 per cent of your business. No one has that kind of margin. Industry doesn't, and the hospital doesn't. Furthermore, any business enterprise that does not have sufficient income so that it can generate adequate retained earnings puts itself in a position of gradual liquidation.

A nonprofit hospital doesn't have retained earnings as such, but the problem is the same in the sense that we must be certain that we are not dissipating our capital. This business of earnings and capital is fundamental to the growth, even the survival, of our voluntary hospital system. I say in all earnestness that inadequate reimbursement, the ignoring of the need of the nonprofit hospital for earnings, could lead to the gradual liquidation of our system. We cannot lose capital faster than our ability to replace it and remain the viable, dynamic institutions that the public expects us to be.

COSTS A NATIONAL CONCERN

Perhaps we have all heard too much talk about costs. The unpleasant truth, however, is that we are going to hear more rather than less because we all know that costs are going to become higher, not lower. The hospital may or may not be the whipping boy, but it certainly is the principal object of the national concern with medical costs.

Whenever I speak of hospital costs, I try to stress the vital fundamental that any cost-cutting and efficiency drive must be performed within the context of maintaining and, if possible, improving patient care. We could cut costs tomorrow just by arbitrarily reducing the quality of the product—that which goes on with the patient while he is in the hospital. We could also reduce our teaching and research. Instead of moving forward in the health field, we could stagnate. It would be cheaper. But our goal, the goal of the board and the medical staff and administration, must be to improve and not to retrogress.

COST AND EFFICIENCY FACTORS

We must seek answers to the problems of cost and increased efficiency, but not at the expense of better service and greater progress in the health field. I doubt that, even in the face of outcries about costs, the public would let us do it. The citizens see the definite evidence of the results of our health care progress and they read about it every day and they like it.

I don't know of anyone who isn't in favor of better health, be he Republican or Democrat. We can be certain that the demand for high quality institutional care and for all the other components of comprehensive health care is going to increase. And so rising costs will keep us, we may be sure, in the spotlight and on the spot.

The not-for-profit health system is going to be called to account and it must be able to respond promptly and adequately. Therefore, it is urgent that we not stand idly by and wait for developments but rather take the initiative to determine what can be done better then we are now doing. How can we better discharge our responsibility and still, so to speak, be in the economic ball park? The time has come when the hospital must look at itself critically, analytically, and objectively.

For a moment, let's look at hospital administration. I think the time has come when the top administrator should be and must be recognized as the chief operating officer of the institution. At Harper Hospital in Detroit we deliberately adopted a corporate format. I am not the president of the board of trustees. I am chairman of the board. The executive who was director of the hospital is now its president and he is on the board of trustees. That doesn't mean that he is dictating policy unilaterally, but it recognizes his proper position, responsibility, and accountability.

The chief operating officer of a hospital requires great executive talent, sometimes more than in business because there is really more coordination of diverse elements and less direct control. For example, in dealing with the medical staff, the president or director or superintendent of a hospital cannot deal with the physicians as though they were subordinates in a manufacturing division or design division of an industrial company. He cannot just implement a procedure. He can't just demand. The top administrator must be more than a fine executive, he must also be a consummate diplomat.

Are there enough top hospital executives? A great deal is being done by the American Hospital Association, but is there a more direct method of upgrading top administrators, not just in title but in breadth of thinking, in knowledge, and in ability to make executive decisions?

ORGANIZATIONAL TECHNIQUES

How many hospitals do formal budgeting? It has been said that a budget is the point of departure, but the budgeting process does encourage operations planning.

Should the hospital have a profit improvement committee, looking at not the dollar profit—there isn't any as such—but at the profit in service to the community, and looking at it from all angles?

Should there be a program improvement committee, one in which the medical staff would play an important role? This would be apart from the joint conference committee, because at the moment I am looking at inside management, and the joint conference committee, quite properly, is made up of some trustees, medical staff, and hospital management.

Should there be an incentives study committee, and what phases of operations should be studied?

How closely are hospitals today measuring the balance between inpatient care and outpatient care?

How many hospitals have looked, from the management and medical standpoint, at the whole gamut of hospital-related medical services? Understandably enough, we tend to have an inhospital fixation. But there are health profits to be made in other ways and a soundly organized and efficiently operated hospital is our best method of realizing these advances.

Although it may not be too productive to seek pat comparisons between industry and the hospital, that is no excuse for ignoring some approximate resemblances. The balance sheet of a hospital is not like that of a for-profit corporation. Its principal asset, the bed count, is not shown. The bed count does not necessarily determine the quality of the institution. The point I strive to make is that good financial practice calls for recognizing the importance of "turnover" of our assets, whether they be food, drugs, accounts receivable, or beds.

A tissue committee tells us whether a particular operation was really necessary. Are we auditing our bed utilization factor similarly? I recognize that the primary purpose of a tissue committee and the primary purpose of the medical audit and of bed utilization review is to enhance quality of care. In this paper, I am looking at the hospital performance from the business standpoint and there is an undeniable and important fiscal factor in proper utilization. When a patient convalesces in an acute hospital bed rather than in an extended care facility bed or at home, it might be considered an improper use of the principal hospital asset. And the better the bed, and the better the hospital, the bigger the asset and, therefore, the greater the waste.

Proper bed patient turnover ensures that our invested capital serves the maximum number of people. Efficient utilization performance may permit the necessary price increases and at the same time effect a reduction in total cost to the patient. Proper bed utilization is not a program of downgrading the end health result produced. It is good for the patient, good for the doctor, and good for the hospital.

CONTROL BY THE MEDICAL STAFF

In the hospital, the conservation of this asset is not merely an executive decision. The true control in the hospital doesn't lie with the executive alone, it lies with the physician. It is the medical staff that is, in a very real sense, the marketing organization of the hospital. They don't say "come on in and try our beds," but the doctor is the input and he is also the output. He is the one who signs the patient out to home or to the extended care facility. No one is asking the physician to subordinate his professional judgment as to what is medically good for the patient to economic considerations. But it is the responsibility of the hospital, and, therefore, of administration, to make the physicians aware of their stake in this matter. The doctor must make the best possible use of this frightfully expensive instrument, the hospital, that we have put at his disposal. This calls for wholehearted cooperation with the hospital in attempts to do those things that will improve efficiency without impairing in any way the doctor's professional prerogative or the quality of the care rendered to his patient.

Nothing is more important to hospital management than people. But is hospital management managing people properly? Does the hospital have a clear, concise set of rules and procedures? Are they enforced? Are they in writing? Are they understood? Wages represent some two-thirds of the hospital costs. We must, therefore, ask ourselves: Are we doing everything we can from the standpoint of methods, procedures, and time studies to ensure maximum productivity without any loss of good patient care?

WAGE FACTOR IN POLICY

There was a time when wages were so low in hospitals that the employment scale had to be downgraded. You didn't have to tell those workers they were being underpaid. They knew it. And there was not the same feeling, probably, of performance, of giving a good day's work for a good day's pay. Now, things have changed. Hospital wages are rising. Have we really taken a good look at our personnel department, our personnel management and practices since this wage movement started coming closer to the community wage level? Or are we still receiving the same attitude that we used to get from employees and which we accepted because we were paying them less than that which would ensure maximum performance? Certainly, with rising wages, management has more latitude and more right and more obligation to insist upon high performance from personnel. This takes us right back to job descriptions and accountability. What do we expect? Do we really know? Let's not criticize our employees if they don't fully understand what they are expected to do, what constitutes a day's work, what is the most efficient way of performing their particular job, and their individual accountability.

COMPREHENSIVE PLANS NEEDED

It seems quite obvious even to one who is not involved in a direct way in the day-to-day operation of a hospital that the spotlight I mentioned earlier will focus its sharpest beams on how well the hospitals behave from the standpoint of sensible planning. This is as it should be, because when we talk about comprehensive health facilities, we cannot escape the necessity for good, efficient planning. I believe that the communities that purchase and use our services directly or indirectly through governments and third-party payers are going to insist on a form of policing. This may take the legislative route, as it did in New York, or it can take the voluntary route as it did in Detroit. But regardless of the device, it must have teeth. In Detroit, sanctions are applied through a united capital fund drive for hospitals. Every five years we have a capital fund drive for the social service agencies involved in our united fund and for the hospitals. The large prospective donors—corporations, for example—are exempt from further contributions during that five-year period. Thus, any hospital that attempts to raise capital funds without going through a regular procedure requiring documentation of need by the Greater Detroit Area Hospital Council doesn't have a mass market in which to raise capital funds.

We would still need areawide planning even if there were no insistence on it as a method of assuring hospital cost effectiveness because it is the only way we can achieve the proper type, the proper size, and the proper mixture of institutions. To use the language of business again, areawide planning is really sophisticated, community-wide market analysis and product planning for better health. It provides us with a means of product innovation, product improvement, a way of assimilating the research results that are pouring in on us from every side. I know of no more dynamic industry than the health industry. I know of none that requires more innovation, more product planning, more product change, more tooling for new production than the health complex. This is the aspect of areawide planning that is often overlooked. We are too inclined to look upon this technique simply as a way of preventing us from doing those things that we shouldn't do, rather than telling us the things we should do and ways of doing them better.

Forces are at work against areawide planning and I think we all know them: the administrator who believes there is a direct relationship between the size of his institution and the size of his paycheck and his prestige; the physician who discourages a patient transfer to an extended care facility because it is a few blocks or a few miles away and personal time is involved; the trustee who wants to create a veritable monopoly, who doesn't stop to determine this institution's proper role in the community, and then stick to it. Some trustees can become quite impatient, almost unbalanced, when they start thinking in terms of the great hospital they happen to be connected with. They lose perspective.

I have already said a few things about management and the medical staff from the viewpoint of a trustee wearing a businessman's hat. Now I would like to look at the hospital as a businessman wearing a trustee's hat and examine somewhat more searchingly the trustee in this complex enterprise of ours. I think the time is past when the hospital will take a trustee, or be willing to take a trustee, simply because he has a good name to put on a letterhead or because it's a chance to pick up some endowment money. If you are building a business, you would not elect a director to the board simply because he might make a voluntary contribution as a dividend payment to the stockholders. You want mature judgment on the board, not a promissory note for some future legacy.

DUTIES OF TRUSTEES

We have formal training programs for administrators and, everyone knows, it takes an increasingly long time to educate a doctor. But do we fall short when it comes to the education of the trustee? Can we honestly say that all trustees, even a majority of them, truly understand their job so that they can provide the proper—and I emphasize the word proper—backing for good administration, in such a way that their actions will also ensure the best possible institutional results?

You can have a fine administration, you can have a fine medical staff, but you can quickly get the hospital into serious trouble if the board is made up of well--intentioned but poorly informed trustees who treat the hospital as sort of a prestigious avocation and tend to make snap decisions without the kind of evaluative study they would bring to their own business board on important issues.

Actually, the hospital is just about the worst place in the world to make snap decisions because only too often that which has been done is irreversible. Are we being fair to the trustee when we put him in a position of assuming such great responsibility without proper preparation? Do we need something more direct than we have for the education and training of trustees? Most of them are sophisticated and successful men, and it may seem gratuitous to be talking about training and education for them, but trustees do need training and education. No man likes to expose his ignorance, especially when he has made his mark in his own world, and unless someone takes the initiative to inform and educate him to the full measure of his responsibility, he will never fully appreciate what a really splendid thing it is to be a working trustee of a hospital.

SYSTEM'S GREATEST STRENGTH

The more than, 30,000 trustees—the figure may be 50,000—in our voluntary hospital system are that system's greatest strength, but often they do not do the job they could do for their individual institution and they certainly are not doing the massive job they could do for the nonprofit hospitals of this country as a group. It isn't because they don't want to. I believe it is because too many do not have a true understanding and knowledge of how and why a hospital is a different kind of enterprise, of the problems of administration, of the problems of the medical staff, and the physician's separate and special personality. So we often deny the trustee a chance to adjust himself to the fullest to the hospital enterprise.

Often trustees serve on the boards of many companies and they know that they cannot serve as a director in the same way on any two boards because the purposes of one company differ from the purposes of another. In this corporate role, the trustee recognizes that he must understand the business before he can be a good director for the company. Now, I ask, is this recognition of the need for understanding less important when we're dealing with human life? A trustee has a responsibility to be more than just pleased with his membership on the board of an important hospital. He has a personal responsibility to understand enough about the operation so that he can be certain he is contributing to the best of his ability to the decisions that are made.

There is a radical difference between a corporate director and a hospital trustee. The board, in the case of a corporation, a business, or even a for-profit hospital, can measure the competence and performance of management on the basis of profit and loss results. If revenues and earnings are increasing, if dividends are increasing and retained earnings are satisfactory, the corporate director logically assumes that things are pretty much in gear. Those same yardsticks do not exist for a trustee of a voluntary nonprofit hospital to measure either the status of the institution or the performance of management. A greater depth of knowledge of operations is necessary. I'm certainly not suggesting that trustees get into operations or interfere in any way with management other than in a support and leadership role. But it should be an intelligent support and leadership role. There probably are some hospital administrators who do not want a too well-informed board or shirk their part in trustee training and education. Maybe the administrator believes it would downgrade his position or possibly he may even believe that he wouldn't be competent to deal with a better informed board. A really good executive believes just the opposite. He knows, and the good hospital trustee knows, that the only meaningful audit the board member can make of the hospital comes through knowing enough to be able to gauge the programs that come up for consideration, to evaluate the discussions and the pertinency of the points the administrator is making. The trustee cannot do it by snooping. Trustees should not bypass administration, especially in matters of medical staff relationships. The trustee who listens too much or talks too much with members of the medical staff other than through the formal joint conference arrangement is asking for trouble for himself, the administration, and the hospital.

JOINT CONFERENCE COMMITTEE

The joint conference committee is the proper method of communication among trustees, management, and the medical staff. There are physicians who believe that the doctor ought to be an actual member of the board. I, for one, believe that the physician who represents the medical staff at the board meetings—in the case of Harper Hospital it is the chief of the medical staff—is in a stronger position than one with a vote on the board. If I were a physician, I wouldn't want to be a voting trustee and certainly if I were the chief of staff, I would not want the medical staff represented by anyone but myself. The chief of staff is the link to the medical executive committee, and he is the proper spokesman for the staff at meetings of the board. That role should be given to no one else.

I want to emphasize that by and large, our hospitals and our people have been well served by governing boards across the breadth and length of this land and throughout the history of the whole voluntary movement. But the point I want to underscore is that, to a far greater degree than ever before, hospitals are going to be under the scrutiny of outside agencies, and what was sufficient in the past may not be good enough for the future.

At the local hospital level we can point to many great trustee accomplishments. I do not think we can do so on nearly the same scale at the national level. There are many trustees who are not yet aware of the impact that government now has and will have on the future of not-for-profit hospitals.

I do not believe that trustees and their hospitals fully realize the great power of trustee collective strength for good if this potential were fully mobilized. A list of all the trustees of nonprofit hospitals would be a veritable Who's Who in America. No single organization would even compare with it. Amplified properly and constructively through organization, that voice cannot be ignored.

The organization necessary to bring the amplification of our trustee voice for the preservation and enhancement of the values of our voluntary system is, I believe, the American Hospital Association, and to my mind this is one of its most important tasks. Almost all voluntary nonprofit hospitals are members of the Association. While it is the hospital's chief operating executive who participates most actively in Association affairs, we should remember that each trustee of a member institution can be considered an ex officio member of the American Hospital Association. I know the difficulties that face the Association in developing such an action program, but the importance of doing so cannot be ignored.

TRUSTEES' ACTIVITIES

In one of the Association's own reports.[2] it is stated that "the Association should encourage hospitals to involve trustees in activities beyond the traditional emphasis on finances and internal management, and to urge them to take a vigorous role in pressing external hospital problems such as areawide planning and relationships with government." The report goes on to say that "If the Association is to grow in usefulness, it must adapt to changes in hospitals and their environment. Such important changes are occurring so steadily that it is imperative that the Association's objectives and programs be broadened to meet the enlarged definition of the hospital's responsibility."

Never have changes so important to our hospitals been occurring more often than at present. Never has it been more important for the American Hospital Association to give urgent priority to the task of mobilizing the trustees of our nation, of marshaling the vast resources they represent in talent and accomplishment. Properly oriented and informed, the trustees will respond enthusiastically.

Our voluntary not-for-profit hospital system is one of America's most precious assets. That system must now welcome and meet the challenge of our national determination to achieve ever higher health standards for all our citizens. They must give leadership in these programs because we know, and I think Washington knows, that success at the national level can only be achieved through the continuing success of our voluntary nonprofit hospitals, which represent 75 per cent of the nation's short-term care hospital investments and facilities. Without them there could be no national program. It's just that simple.

The voluntary way is the American way, and I am very certain that the new health challenges will be accepted, not as insoluble problems, but rather as new opportunities to quicken our pace of forward progress. Our indicated action calendar is moving very fast. It is time to mobilize our boards. Suggesting this mobilization of trustees does not mean that I am advocating the formation of a pressure lobby. Rather, I am recommending the creation of a well-informed, influential, vigilant, voluntary army, dedicated to achieving the maximum advances in physical health and determined to maintain concurrently our vital institutional economic health, without which we will surely fail. This is a trustee responsibility that cannot be subcontracted or ignored.

[2] American Hospital Association, *Statement on the Changing Hospital* (Chicago: the Association, 1965).

The Social Responsibility of General Hospitals

BRIGHT M. DORNBLASER

Bright M. Dornblaser, is Director of the Graduate Program in Hospital Administration at the University of Minnesota.

The hospital field is under pressures from society to expand its missions, or to significantly alter how and where its missions are performed. What is the appropriate response?

OBJECTIVES

We recognize that the basic objective of the hospital as a social institution is to improve the quality of living—while working for life itself.

We further recognize that we can sharpen our ideas of ends of health care institutions from the honing action of experience in applying ideas within the context of the general hospital, its problems and realities. This is particularly so if cybernetics applies, if there is a feedback mechanism to the university or other sources of ideas which are being tested through application.

On the basis of experience, what should be the response to the question, "what is the mission of the hospital beyond beds and out-patient services?"

THESIS AND ANTITHESIS

One quick, if perhaps unpopular, answer to this question is "None!" The underlying rationale is that the hospital has more than enough to do to perform its medical care mission well, and "Whatever we undertake to do, we must do supremely well."

This position is, of course, the antithesis of a thesis with common currency today: That the quality of personal health care services for the middle class people now receiving such services is adequate; that the important unmet needs now are social; that hospitals have demonstrated a capacity to serve well; that they should expand their scope of service in response to social need; and that they are socially irresponsible if they do not. Is this thesis correct? Should the hospital become the hub rather than a medical care spoke of the health care wheel?

Reprinted by permission from *Hospital Administration: Quarterly Journal of the American College of Hospital Administrators,* Chicago, Vol. 14 (Spring, 1969), 6-17. Copyright 1969 by the American College of Hospital Administrators. All rights reserved.

MEDICAL CARE MISSION

Some traditionalists might respond by saying that to expand the general hospital's missions would jeopardize the quality of medical care. Our concentration, they believe, should continue on the quality of care provided to the individual patient who requests personal health services. The problems of continuing to provide care at the level of quality perceived possible by the producers of care are extensive, they are burdensome, and they are continuing. Subverting a specialized interest and skill to a more generalized concern, they feel, will exact too high a social price.

Proponents of this position suggest that the explosion of knowledge of the medical sciences and technology—with increased costs and shortages of dollars and competent manpower—can consume all the skilled health manpower and the fiscal, organizational, and managerial resources now available. These resources are subject to urgent demands today for improved efficiency, which suggests considerable change is manifest even within the medical model.

WRESTLING WITH SOCIAL ASSIGNMENTS

Those pressing for increased efficiency state that quality of care to the individual is not enough, that medical care excellence is insufficient—the least hospital people must admit is their obligation also to serve the community with efficiency, so that the highest benefits can be obtained for the medical care dollars expended.

It is hard to deny the reasonableness of this position.

This argument will be reinforced by management incentives—a summarizing test of management.

By one means or another, hospital management will be stimulated to "reduce" cost by increasing efficiency:

Through higher productivity, e.g., through establishing group practice and use of full-time physicians;
Through trade-offs of less skilled health manpower for the more skilled;
Through trade-offs of less costly programs for the more costly;
Through control of the construction of facilities, costly to construct and still more costly to operate.

The hospital will be a key social control point, even if choosing to remain in the medical care mode. As such, it will receive inexorable pressure in the name of efficiency to make significant and traumatic changes in the ways in which the accepted medical model missions are executed. Wrestling with these socially loaded "bear-by-the-tail" social assignments is a first full-time job. At this point we might identify with the farmer who protested to the Farm Bureau representative who wanted to instruct him on improved agriculture methods: "I ain't farming half as well as I know how yet!"

From these viewpoints we might well conclude that the hospital's first responsibility for service continues to be found in the medical model: Resources will be strained in order to continue executing these unique service responsibilities. Hospital representatives should be the leading advocates of continuing to perform them at a quality level. Furthermore, it is essential that hospital spokesmen not let others—who are clamoring for the general hospital to expand its mission—assume the continuance of past accomplishments, if added responsibilities are accepted.

SOCIAL MODEL VS. MEDICAL MODEL

It is the view of the general hospital mission from the perspective of a social model which contributes to the demands for increased service. These accelerated demands, of course, reflect rising public expectations. They reflect a concern for the well, as well as the ill. Furthermore, they reflect a belief that the poor should have the opportunity and be encouraged to use the health care system. Drawing from the models of the past, the hospital is today expected to be more than the haven or *hospitia* for the wayfarers climbing over the snow-covered passes of life. In addition, it is expected to send out the human equivalent of the St. Bernard dogs, to seek actively those who may be in need. The president of the University of Minnesota has coined the word "communiversity" to express this sense of social responsibility in terms of the university.

Assuming hospital efficiency will be increased, how will the "saving" from increased efficiency be used? To reduce taxes, unlikely. To increase medical care benefits, perhaps. To increase social model benefits, more likely.

What are these social model benefits?

FULFILLING SOCIAL DEMANDS

Basically, these benefits are intended to give substance to the accepted principle that health care is a right rather than a privilege.

We recognize this principle is more fiction than truth for perhaps 40 million Americans. We recognize, further, that those deprived of health services have advocates chanting, "we shall overcome."

The problems identified with our present health care non-system, which apply in varying degrees to all people presently served by our general hospitals, are familiar. They include:

1. Absence of program appropriateness, availability, accessibility, acceptability.
2. Absence of comprehensive care, of continuity of care.

From a social viewpoint, patient advocates state these deficits are intolerable, that they can be rectified if there is a will to do so, that they can be rectified without penalty if improvements in efficiency are made.

Patient advocates say, further, that the human costs gaps in health care services should be closed regardless of gains in efficiencies, despite the possible penalties of requiring a higher allocation of our gross national product, or of diminishing the quality of health care to our middle class society.

Patient advocates further assert that the general hospital has special capability to perform well the added health care missions of a social model, such as programs of "preventicare" and ghetto care. These characteristics and abilities include the needed philosophy of care, and the nucleus of the key health professionals needed to plan and execute such programs. It is natural that society, recognizing these strengths, and recognizing a heritage of a job well done, is asking hospitals to assume expanded missions of service to the community.

A second full-time job lies in fulfilling these social demands: To expand, relocate, and modify the manner of performance of general hospital missions.

OTHER SOCIAL MISSIONS

There are still other social missions which hospitals are asked to undertake in serving the community. They should be assumed, if the hospital as a social institution is going to advance the society of which it is a part as fully as possible. Lists of these needs are readily available from numerous sources. However, the Commission on Civil Disorders provides a convenient catalogue. Such pressing needs as eliminating unemployment and underemployment, improving inadequate education, and reducing disrespectful white attitudes are examples of monumental problems which general hospitals genuinely interested in serving their communities can help resolve. The difficult social demands in these areas require not so much in the way of finances, knowledge, or skills, as in attitudes.

CONCERN FOR HUMAN VALUES

Hospitals are being asked to provide their services in a human as well as humane fashion. While there are some penalties attendant in developing programs in response to social needs of this type—as against only those which reflect the health needs of our medical model, the cost/benefit ratio is probably highly favorable.

Society needs individuals with a concern for human values, and for social health, which lie beyond a concern for individual personal health. It is to be hoped, at least, that the humanitarian-oriented health field will prove a repository for human beings interested in the human being. This is particularly requisite when this end requires primarily a change of attitude. This can be considered a third major job of hospitals today.

It would seem that a possible responsibility of the hospital is to serve as a hub of the health care wheel, and in addition, to form part of the axle joining the health care wheel to the social welfare wheel. Indeed we have come a long way from our mission of service to the community solely as a medical care spoke of the health care wheel.

Some hospitals are accepting these responsibilities today; others very likely will tomorrow. Many, if not most, however, without questioning the statements of unmet need, may well challenge the assumption that hospitals should meet them.

This position questions the timing and asks for a social cost/benefit study of alternatives. It recognizes the spirit of compehensive health planning which pervades our land today asks, and even insists, that we examine alternatives in our planning process.

HEALTH CARE AS A RIGHT

Such study is needed. As one example, the costs of providing health care as a right to all, as some are privileged to know it today, is estimated as ranging on a gross basis as from \$125 to \$250 per person, for from 40 million to 200 million persons. Clearly, definitive study is needed of the economic consequences of implementing quickly and fully our stated natural health policy that health care is a right to all, rather than a privilege for the middle class of today. We should challenge the proclivity of some to promise benefits without resources to make them viable, except to ask those who have enjoyed benefits in the past to share them on the level of a greater common denominator. We should point out the problems of the "expectation gap" which are created by promises unfulfilled.

Clearly, the implications for health manpower requirements also need definition. The potential costs—or penalties, depending on our viewpoint—are also potentially large. Within this context, general hospitals can legitimately challenge the demands by public advocates by asking them to demonstrate the effective demand for health services from a large portion of the poor. For example, a stated need for improved health care service is conspicuously absent from the *Report of the National Commission on Civil Disorders,* which lists the twelve social problems identified as most important by the black community.

Further, it appears reasonable to challenge whether expenditure of funds to encourage effective demand for personal health services would provide the highest cost/benefit payoff. Environmental health expenditures, for example, might well have a higher payoff, socially and politically, as well as from a health viewpoint. So while allocation of savings from efficiencies to social model health programs is likely, the timing, appropriateness, and degree can be legitimately questioned.

We are entering an era when these now unanswered questions of cost/benefit relationships for personal health care services are of even greater importance. This is an era where personal health care services, or elements of such service, are increasingly going to be considered a responsibility rather than a right. A compelling case can be made for this principle. A proposal has been made that this principle be reflected in the health program in Minnesota's "Experimental City" by calling for compulsory annual multiphasic screening examinations. This requirement may well increase the consumers' effective demand upon providers of care to add or expand services, or both.

SYNTHESIS

The demand upon the providers of care from the social model for increased quantity of care could be the straw that bends the quality care back of the medical model camel. Public advocates of the social model may prove stronger than the champions of the medical model. Selected health care providers should provide leadership, in a response to conflicting demands, by demonstration and research.

The general hospital is the health care cutting edge on the interface between social science and evolving technology. Society can expect hospitals to be vitally concerned with the development and use of the knowledge, one of the most fundamental of social commodities. It is only through the heuristic application of new knowledge that it gains ultimate social significance.

Selected general hospital leadership needs to demonstrate the equality of right to health care by finding ways to make it viable, while recognizing the penalties of broadly promulgating one alternative before planning others and examining them comprehensively. We do need, and should encourage and support, social model demonstrations such as may be found in Roxbury and Columbia Point in Boston, in the Grovenure program in New York City, in the Watts area of Los Angeles, and others. This is not the same, however, as asking all hospitals, as they are presently constituted, to do likewise.

The current focus of attention on the appropriate future mission of the general hospital is basically a matter of social organization. Demonstration and research into different organization models for the delivery of health care therefore is particularly pertinent. This approach offers hope for the development of an organizational base to mount programs which synthesize the conflicting demands of our medical and social health care models.

It is not a question of the appropriateness of goals and objectives—what the consumers or their advocates want, they will, like Lola, get. Consumer power as expressed through the political system does and will prevail. The question is the degree to which existing social organizations such as the general hospital will provide the means to the ends—to the evolving social objectives. It is a social organization question which asks:

1. whether existing organizations, like the general hospital, will assume new program responsibilities, or whether new social organizations should be established which will be both more willing and able to do so.
2. whether new organizations should be established to manage the health care system—removing and centralizing some decision-making authority now held by the service organizations, i.e., hospitals.
3. whether new organizations should be established to perform existing programs to meet newly emphasized performance standards better than do existing organizations.

Hospitals, as we have seen, have a reasonable and perhaps even legitimate option of rejecting the social model to better serve the heavy demands of the medical model. Doing so efficiently releases resources to support other organizations endeavoring to meet the social model performance criteria for health care programs.

The general hospital has a further option within this context. It can choose to utilize programs developed by other community health care organizations, e.g., long term care, public health, Office of Economic Opportunity, model city organizations, rather than to plan and execute such programs within the general hospital organizational framework.

THE HOSPITAL'S OPTION

If general hospitals individually or collectively provide leadership in the planning and organizing of health services, if not in the actual performance of them, they can in this organizational sense become the community health center which is the self-established model widely held by hospitals today. Whether other health service organizations would grant such authority to hospitals is of course a question.

Should general hospitals select these options, they should recognize they are accepting a mission as a medical care spoke, rather than the hub of the health care wheel. Other organizations will be needed to serve as other spokes of our health care wheel, and may have hub organizational responsibilities as well. Government has filled service, coordinative and directive needs of society in the past, when not provided by the private sector, and is one viable alternative for doing so again.

Hospitals should have no complaints if society forms other organizations to perform additional missions which hospitals elect to forego. Conversely, society should not be critical of hospitals for electing to be the public advocates of quality performance of certain health functions that have and will need considerable support if they are to continue to be provided on a quality basis.

Hospitals have still another option: To form vertically integrated "health utilities" in which they could perform their specialized function. Other organizational sub-units of the health utility could plan and execute the health missions demanded and needed by our social model. These missions possibly could include responsibility for selected environmental health or welfare programs. The utilities could well be responsible for developing or assembling associated prepayment programs.

This organizational alternative to planning and executing expanding health missions is to be preferred, in the author's judgment. It provides the scale to accomplish both medical and social missions, permits the advantages of specialization while reducing the organizational fragmentation of our health care non-system, and lowers the need for centralization of program planning and execution under governmental auspices.

These organizations could form the needed bridge between programs for the middle class and the urban and rural poor; permit a "fresh start" towards the changes needed for efficiency; and ease the pressure on the hospital to reduce quality in order to reduce high unit cost.

The health utility would provide an organizational symbol for the change of role of the central personal health care delivery organization. It could assist the assembly of managerial talent and staff resources needed for improvement in both efficiency and effectiveness. It would permit the continuance of specialized functional interest and expertise in humanly compatible organizational sub-units.

"CORNER GROCERY STORE" ORIENTATION

The health utility with associated franchisement implies increased formal community responsibility and accountability, allocation of tax resources now reserved to governmental agencies, and centralization from a local perspective (but potential decentralization from regional and state governmental perspectives, and quasi-independence from their bureaucracies).

This organizational "tool up" may well be an essential foundation for the service and educational missions now being effectively demanded.

It is difficult to be sanguine that this organizational alternative will be adopted, except perhaps in such places as Minnesota's Experimental City, where it has been proposed. The existing hospital field still exhibits much of the "corner grocery store" orientation, in a chain store age. However, there are some hopeful signs. On this basis, as well as need, this alternative then is reasonable when endeavoring to define the general hospitals' future mission in service to the community.

FOCAL POINT FOR SOCIAL CONTROL

Regardless of the scope of the future mission, or the organizational context within which hospitals will operate, they will be a focal point for social control. The control will be concerned with both costs (efficiency) and benefits (effectiveness). The hospital's future missions will reflect judgments on costs and benefits, which in turn will reflect the criteria or standards used in making such judgments. The conclusions may well be expressed in franchisement of services. If hospital leadership wishes to have some control over the destiny of hospitals, for the quality and scope of hospital future missions, they need to be experts in the appropriateness of such standards.

This again will require a willingness to engage in collective effort. This could well be one of the most central and crucial missions of the general hospital in service to the community.

CONCLUSION

Society is demanding that further health missions be performed. Hospitals can legitimately consider their acceptance as alternatives, or their rejection so as to serve with excellence the continuing missions of the medical model. A preferred alternative is to develop health utilities. Such organizations could meet social needs for an expanded scope of service, while preserving the capability to perform on a quality, in-depth basis, the medical care functions which will need this concern in the future, as in the past.

Changes in the way existing health missions are performed, so as to increase efficiencies, can be anticipated. Allocation of the benefits of increased efficiency to expanded health/social missions can be expected. Both existing and expanded missions need to be performed with the social needs of minority groups in mind. Demonstration and research projects by selected general hospitals should show the way by synthesizing a response to the medical and social models. Translating the findings into standards of performance, for guidance of public expectations and decisions, is a basic mission.

Assiduous definition by public advocates of gaps in the meeting of health care needs should join with sedulous recognition of the "tooling up" effort needed to overcome these needs. The absence of qualified professional manpower is but one example of a long term obstacle even if organizational and financial problems can be overcome. Economic and social cures should be promised and delivered as carefully as medical cures. Full participation by the leadership of the hospital field can be vital to this end.

It is an endeavor worthy of the devotion of the talents and energies of the management of our nation's hospitals. Commitment of this capability with vision, imagination, drive, and resourcefulness will provide the managerial leadership demanded and needed by our times.

Institution and Area-Wide Planning

This section presents the subject of planning. Planning has been called one of the most important of the managerial functions. Planning is not only pervasive, but is also a prerequisite to the implementation of all other managerial functions. Because of the increasing demand on the health care system, the systematic and rational determination of future courses of action is mandatory within and among health care institutions.

In *THE INTRA-INSTITUTIONAL PLANNING PROCESS*, planning is presented as a managerial tool and process for which the administrator is responsible. Planning can be either formal or informal. In addition, there can be reaction planning, responsive planning, which is controlled by events, or action oriented planning which attempts to anticipate events. Various obstacles to good planning are presented along with suggestions and principles to be considered in establishing an effective planning group within the hospital.

In *AREAWIDE PLANNING FOR HEALTH FACILITIES*, the need for cooperation versus self-interest planning of facilities in the community is presented. Only through cooperation among institutions can comprehensive care and the systematic distribution of facilities be provided at the least cost. The point is made that the future role of area-wide planning must be positive and not be perceived as a threat to individual institutions.

The Intra-Institutional Planning Process

PHILLIP H. GOODWIN AND JAMES D. HARVEY

Phillip H. Goodwin is Assistant Administrator and James D. Harvey is Administrator of Hillcrest Medical Center in Tulsa, Oklahoma.

Planning's importance in the health field is underscored at every level of management whether one refers to governmental or private activities, or national or local activities. Such emphasis on planning is occasioned by rapid changes taking place in natural and behavioral sciences, economics, and theology. The more rapidly change occurs, the more thoughtful one must be in preparing for the future.

Planning has always been one of the major functions of management. Yet, descriptions of how a manager should set about to carry out his planning responsibilities have been sparse in, if not absent from, hospital management literature.

In its most simply understood form, planning represents one's anticipations for the future. In administration these anticipations may reflect what a manager intends to do in response to something which he feels will be imposed either on himself or on elements of his job, or it may be something which he intends to create by himself—or a combination of both. The word "planning" as used in the health field at the present time suggests that it should be considered as a process which produces a scheme of activity as opposed to a scheme of arrangement—as a dynamic rather than a static process.[1]

An administrator always plans, but seldom does he do it overtly. Nearly all of his activities represent results of previously formulated courses of action, which is planning. Frequently, however, he plans as a *result* of forces acting upon his sphere of responsibility. To be sure, he plans to get from a current state of affairs to a desired state sometime in the future. But he focuses on his goal rather than on the process through which he goes to get to that goal. The hazards implied in planning this way are that much wasted effort and perhaps incorrect decisions may result from having paid too little attention to the planning process itself.

[1] Robert M. Sigmond, "The Role of the Medical Staff in a Hospital's Long Range Planning Process" (Long Range Planning Seminar, The Hospital Medical Staff Conference, Estes Park, Colorado, October 1, 1968).

By describing those properties of the intra-institutional planning process which make it difficult for the administrator to plan properly, it should then be possible to develop a planning program for the institution which avoids potential pitfalls.

PROBLEMS IN INSTITUTIONAL PLANNING

Of all his functions, the manager's planning function is least delegable in that, as the top management person in his organization, the destiny of his institution depends in large part upon his own vision and performance. It depends upon his ability to anticipate the requirements of the future and to mold his organization to meet those requirements. Unless the chief executive gives this aspect of his job his concentrated attention, an integrated plan will not result. He is the chief architect for building the bridge between his institution today and the future. He simply cannot delegate the hard work required of the visionary who broadly directs the affairs of an institution so that all its elements are integrated into a mutually reinforcing network of meaningful activities.

One can contrast the function of planning with other management functions such as organizing, controlling, implementing, and evaluating, in that each element of the latter functions can be delegated much more readily and require generally less personal involvement from the chief executive except for the initial and basic considerations to be given to each.

Many of the mechanical aspects of planning can be delegated, but the channeling of all planning forces toward a well-defined objective is basically a one-man job—and it belongs to the top executive because he is the one person in the organization who perceives an occurrence in his institution in its relationship to everything else that is happening. He relates activities in one area to those in another, whereas other management personnel in the organization, although having responsible positions, still operate on a base of particular interests, the sum of which does not add up to the total activities of the institution. These subordinates' perceptions of planning, no matter how objective they try to be, often lack objectivity. This is not to say that these persons wouldn't support the administrator in planning, because they surely must apply the same functions of management to their own positions as the administrator does. The difference is that the application of the planning process to their own realms must be more narrow in order for them to be successful in carrying out their assigned responsibilities.

The question of why planning is not carried out on a more formal basis by chief executives of health facilities is not answered by the fact that it is the least delegable function. The reason it is not generally carried out within a highly structured framework is that there are so many considerations to be given to the subject.

When one attempts to plan for a complex health institution, the factors which bear upon such planning are not easily reduced to formulae. There are hundreds of variables in every institution, and the task of reconciling them so that one may reach a series of alternative conclusions and decisions regarding the future is a most difficult one.

For example, an administrator must possess unusual sensitivity to outside pressures which are constantly brought to bear upon his institution. This one fact probably applies to him a hundredfold more than it would to any other individual in his organization. The effect of external pressures on the administrator's planning activities is very important and does not require eleboration.

PLANNING BY DEFAULT

Paradoxically, considering the difficulties one faces in developing and implementing an orderly planning process, planning goes on in spite of one's intentions. Administrators do indeed plan, but, as previously mentioned, a good deal of it occurs in reaction to things which are happening (or which one thinks will be happening). Too infrequently does the administrator exercise his prerogative to be the prime architect of the destiny of his institution or to help improve, on his own volition, the future health of his community.

Overt, action-oriented planning, in contrast to reaction planning, is a lot more difficult to accomplish. It must be undertaken along formal lines lest it become mired in the institution's rhythm of activity. The administrator must maintain this concept at the surface of his consciousness, reminding himself continually of the process of planning. He should also keep it highly visible before the key persons in his organization, as well as the community. No essential participant should be allowed to forget that planning is continuous and necessary and that it requires wholehearted participation.

Another element which makes planning difficult for the administrator relates to the nature of hospitals and not to the nature of planning; that is, to the necessity for physicians to be involved in the process. Medical staff involvement in planning from institution to institution is neither orderly nor is it broad-based. Planning actions as far as the medical staff is concerned are usually part of the "squeaking wheel" syndrome. Too often the medical staff as a whole does not participate in a broadly-based planning program with the administration—or with themselves, for that matter.

Another property of hospitals which makes planning a difficult undertaking is the existence of a nonproprietary governing board. This body's involvement is necessary but, in far too many instances, sadly deficient. A prime question posed by most top health facility executives is, "How does one enfold trustees into this process in light of their busy schedules and many other interests?" The administrator who can spark response among persons in this category has achieved one of the major characteristics of a successful administration.

Another obstacle to good hospital planning relates to accelerated progress—changes which are being wrought daily in our institutions. This is a direct result of the tremendous quantity of health-related research which is being carried out. There is much concern about the growing gap between the products of research and their subsequent clinical applications. Of particular note is the development of regional planning programs whose avowed purposes are to bring the fruits of medical research into all communities within reach of everyone. These and other similar programs create a fluid state, daily causing shifts in plans in order to make many changes, almost to the point where it makes one wonder whether formal planning is worthwhile.

Pressures to make a change frequently emanate from special interest groups within the medical staff. The reaction time of hospitals to such pressures is usually short, and the response is usually to "give them what they want." Such pressures are almost always disruptive. Certainly it could discourage the person engaged in planning.

Effective organizational planning has gone on for a long time. The armed forces perhaps were the very first to employ it on a grand scale. Planning was and is a necessity because the need for a complex organization such as the Army to remain fluid and act effectively is essential. The space industries also have proved the worthiness of extremely sophisticated planning programs. PERT and critical path programing are two specific examples. Although money has not been a problem in these industries and related government agencies, their astounding successes have been a result primarily of planning, not funding. So should it be for hospitals.

Superimposed upon this confused planning environment in health instututions is the potential impact of such documents as the Report of the Secretary's Committee on Hospital Effectiveness (Barr Report) and Public Laws 89-239 and 89-749, each of which underscores the need for sound programing in each institution. Area and state planning agencies also encourage hospitals to plan, as do numerous third-party prepayment organizations. Much of such encouragement has taken the form of discussion, but not action.

Institutional planning, nevertheless, should come about because the chief executive recognizes that good planning is necessary to make himself more effective, and not because it is required by third-party agencies or is being promoted as something desirable by blue-ribbon committees. Planning should be considered by the administrator as a process which he exploits in order to fulfill his responsibilities effectively.

ORGANIZING FOR PLANNING

Persons in private and governmental sectors alike look to health administrators for more answers than perhaps they are able to give. However, if administrators properly use planning as a management tool they will formulate more solutions and will be able to give answers to those questions being asked by all elements of our society.

This sounds simple, but there are so many roadblocks to good planning in hospital situations that it is no wonder it is so seldom done. It is acknowledged that planning has to be done in conformity with certain external pressures, but it is worth repeating that the administrator, in undertaking planning on a formal basis, should not do so because it's required—but rather that it will be a great help to himself in carrying out his ever-increasing and complex responsibilities.

Planning, therefore, is the vital function of management.

What should be done?

The first thing the administrator should do is to make the planning function a formal part of his job. If he is fortunate enough to be in a position to hire someone to carry out planning tasks, he should make that individual a part of his office. In other words, the planner is in a very close relationship to the administrator. He's part of the box on the organization chart in which the administrator resides. This does not mean that this person is the administrator, but it is a visible sign of the priority which the administrator gives to planning. It also serves as evidence of the hypothesis that it is extremely difficult to delegate the major elements of planning to anybody else. If such a person is available to the administrator he should probably be named Administrative

Assistant and be designated as a part of the administrator's office, rather than placing him alongside such other important positions as the director of personnel or director of data processing. He should be a personal assistant. This will be an important first step.

The second requisite is even more important and relates to the fact that the person who fills the planning slot in the organization should possess a health-administrative background, preferably in both education and experience, rather than have a formal planning background. It is more essential to have the former qualifications because of the complexities and difficulties that the health field presents to a planner. Someone who doesn't understand the varied and changing aspects of the health sector of our society would encounter tough obstacles. It would be much easier to train a health professional in the techniques of planning. This is especially true at the institutional level—perhaps less so in area, state, and federal planning bodies.

The third important approach to intra-institutional planning is to develop full or part-time leadership in the medical staff. It is only through this mechanism that the planning process can be satisfactorily infused into the medical staff, and in turn have the medical staff infuse its tremendous resources and talents into the institutional planning process.

One additional question inevitably arises, "What about the small institution whose budget can't afford additional planning personnel and full-time or part-time doctors to fill medical staff leadership roles?" This is a tough problem and one for which it is difficult to offer specific suggestions. For one thing, the relationships of smaller institutions with larger ones will become much more formal in the future. This act in itself will tend to bring the smaller institution within the framework of a formal planning program. The principles of planning are valid no matter where one may be located within the health field today. The overt, formal approach to planning in a smaller institution is no less necessary than it is in a larger one. The various degrees of involvement described are no less important. It may be that formal planning would be easier to implement within a smaller institution because it is less complex and therefore less time consuming—but it isn't easy no matter how big or small is the enterprise in question.

PLANNING PRINCIPLES AND PROCESS

Keeping in mind the fundamental concepts of intra-institutional planning as previously discussed, it is now possible to examine the essential parts of an institutional planning program. Basic to establishing an effective institutional planning program is to arrive at an understanding of the necessary steps in the process. Fig. 1 illustrates the important steps in an effective planning process.[2]

There are distinct groupings of people which must be involved throughout this dynamic process. On one hand, there is the governing body (board of trustees), which shoulders the policy-making responsibilities of the organization. On the other hand, there is the planning staff, which contributes to the decision-making process by doing the "leg work." Sitting between is the trustee-level planning committee through which information, material, and decisions flow from both directions and which plays a

[2]This chart has been adapted from an article by Perry L. Norton, "The Planning Process," *Patterns for Action Series,* (New York: Executive Council of the Episcopal Church), p. 5.

major role in communications between the planning staff and the policy-making body of the institution. Medical staff representation is implied as being interwoven throughout this process.

The administrator, by implication, walks the thin lines from one side of the chart to the other, being able and willing to travel in both directions. He must be aware, informed, and involved in all phases of the planning process.

The first step in this process is to define a problem, an issue, or a matter of concern. The problem must be analyzed and diagnosed by the planning staff. Once this has been done, a report goes through the trustee committee to the policy-making body. After this report is digested, a statement of long-range goals embodying the solutions to the problem usually follows.

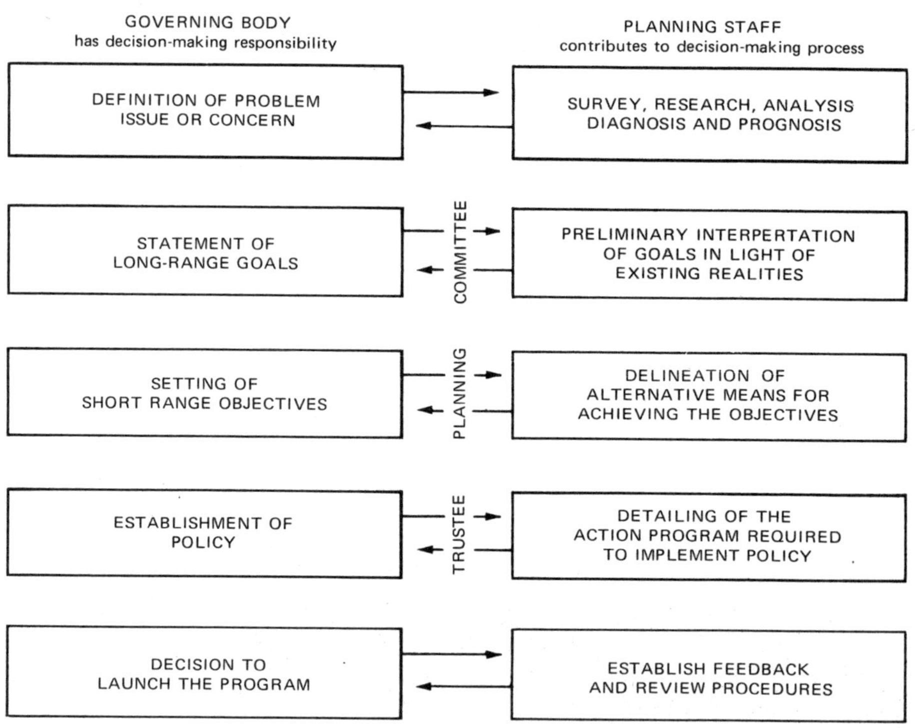

FIGURE 1. A Diagram of the Planning Process

LAYING THE GROUNDWORK

When goals have been established by the governing body, the planning staff then makes a preliminary interpretation of these goals and relates them to facts or existing realities. Once a report has been rendered in this context the board then has the responsibility for setting shortrange objectives to approach the problem. Once these objectives have been set, the planning staff then looks at the desired end result, makes a delineation of alternative means of achieving it, and reports these alternatives back to the governing body. When received, the alternatives are examined and considered by the governing body and a policy is established employing what is considered to be the best alternative. After the policy has been set forth, the planning staff uses it as a guide in developing a detailed action program which would provide for the effective implementation of the policy as established. Once the program has been outlined and returned to the board, it has one final responsibility, which is to act on whether or not the program should be inaugurated. If the decision to institute the program is made, the planning staff has the responsibility for building into the program a mechanism to establish good information feedback and review procedure to insure that, after the program has been put into effect, the people concerned will have at their disposal a method of evaluating the results as well as good visibility of future developments.

The various steps of this process may not always be carried out consciously or in exactly the order listed on the chart. This is reason enough to have a full-time planning program within the institution, because at any given moment the planning staff should be aware of exactly where in the context of this process a particular problem or project lies and whether or not enough preliminary work has been done so that the best method of proceeding is apparent.

A formal planning program can be ineffective if the management framework within which it exists is ill-defined. For this reason, every institution should establish a philosophy and motivational objectives. This is a difficult task, for it requires top-level soul-searching, honest self-criticism, and an accurate appraisal of the institution's place in the community. Once clear-cut statements of philosophy and objectives are established and *distributed* to those who should read them, a set of planning principles supporting the basic philosophy of the organization should be developed. This will be the skeleton upon which a planning program can be built.

BASIC PLANNING PRINCIPLES

There are probably many principles which could be adopted. The uniqueness of each health care institution will dictate what planning principles should be developed. Following are examples of a set of planning principles, most of which will likely be applicable in whole or in part to a typical health care facility.[3]

> **PRINCIPLE No. 1:** *Regional planning is the areawide institutional management.*

This principle supports the concept of areawide comprehensive health planning, but at the same time positively implies that areawide planning can only be effective as long as the basic planning unit is the individual institution within that area.

> **PRINCIPLE No. 2:** *Each health facility should be established, modernized, or expanded only in relation to proven community need for service, education, and/or research, and not based on the history and aspirations of the institution.*

[3]These principles have been adapted in part from principles of planning established and adopted by the Hospital Planning Association of Allegheny County, Pittsburgh, Penn., and the Hospital Review and Planning Council of Southern New York, New York, New York.

This principle calls for awareness of the needs of the community which the individual institution serves and an awareness of its responsibility to the community for expenditure of health care dollars for capital expansion.

> **PRINCIPLE No. 3**: *Each health facility should plan in terms of a specific community or geographical service area which it intends to serve and which may include and/or be shared with other institutions.*

This principle supports the concept of primary and secondary service areas for each institution and calls for each institution to be aware of which areas should be considered primary (the area from which people come directly into the institution for initial services) and which areas are secondary (referral areas) and make itself aware of the distinguishing characteristics of each of these areas.

> **PRINCIPLE No. 4**: *Each general hospital should serve as a center for comprehensive health services through a combination of direct provision of services and coordination with other agencies and institutions.*

This simply states that each hospital should be prepared to see that its patients have comprehensive health care services available. It is impossible for any one institution to provide all the health care services needed by a specific community. It is, however, possible for an institution to be aware of where these various services are available and plan its program so that its patients may have access to whatever services may be needed either by direct provision by the institution or referral to the proper agency.

> **PRINCIPLE No. 5**: *Each health facility should plan for the provision of services sufficient in volume and scope to assure the achievement of high professional standards, reasonable cost, and effective management. The adequacy of the volume and scope must be determined in relation to the location of the institution and its geographic service area.*

This principle means that no health facility should plan to provide services for which it has insufficient demand and which cannot be provided in terms of high professional standards, reasonable cost, and with effective management. If an institution has a demand for such a service but the volume of the demand is inadequate to reach the requirements stated in this principle, then arrangements should be made with some other facility in the community to see that the institution's patients will have these services available.

> **PRINCIPLE No. 6**: *Facility design and administrative policy should consider needs of individual patients and patient groups. For general hospitals this would include provision, supervision, or arrangement for services in rehabilitation, mental health, institutional care of chronically ill, home care, emergency, and ambulatory care for all economic groups and social service.*

This principle states the belief that the services mentioned are basic to general hospital operation and that the hospital should arrange to see that its patients have each of these services available as needed. Again, this may be through direct provision or through cooperative arrangements with other facilities.

> **PRINCIPLE No. 7**: *Health facilities planning for space and personnel must take into consideration the functional program*

of the entire institution when planning for each individual activity.

The best way to restate this principle is to simply say, "Keep everybody informed." Individual departments within the hospital cannot operate as islands unto themselves. Each area must be aware of the programs of every other area and what relationships are needed among them for any given program. Programs within each area of the hospital must be developed in coordination with the total plan of the institution.

PRINCIPLE No. 8: *Each health facility should assume responsibility for public awareness and understanding of its programs of patient care, education, and research.*

This is an area too often neglected. Each health facility has a responsibility to inform the public it serves about what services and programs are available within that institution. Often an institution will establish a program and wonder why the community doesn't respond when, in fact, proper communications were not established between that institution and the community for which the program was established in the first place. The community should be informed not only on programs of direct patient care, but also those programs of education and research in which it (the public) has a stake.

PLANNING PROGRAM DIRECTION

After principles have been adopted, the next logical question is: "In what direction should the planning program proceed?" An institutional planning program should be involved in three basic areas:

a) The Long-Range Plan
b) Internal Program Development
c) External Relationships

THE LONG-RANGE PLAN

Many hospitals today have developed some plan which projects the physical growth of the institution for varying numbers of years into the future. Many of these have engaged the services of consultants and architects in order to develop such a plan, in the hope that, after proper study and preparation, the document will serve as a guide for the physical growth of the institution. The chief executive and his planning assistant must be deeply and continually involved in the formulation of the long-range plan.

One of the primary concerns of the hospital planning department is to evaluate continually the long-range plan to make sure that the projects and programs of today are consistent with the proposed plan, and that the long-range plan does not lose its timeliness as it grows older. These plans should be designed with such flexibility that they will remain contemporary on a year-to-year basis. Many hospitals are currently involved in construction projects relating to long-range plans and anticipate that these will be immediately followed by other projects which have been outlined in their plans. It is important during this period of time to coordinate both the development and delivery of hospital services with the implementation of the physical long-range plan.

Construction of any type is a disruptive process, but the growth and improvement of services rendered by an institution cannot be halted while construction is underway. For this reason it is important that there be coordination so that existing services and physical developments are compatible. This is one area in which the planning department can provide valuable support.

Another area consistent with the concept of long-range planning lies in the development of new services for an institution. Any health service facility which is the least bit progressive will add new services from time to time. These should be planned in detail, keeping the long-range plan in mind, just as the planning for expansion of existing services must have the same relevance to the long-range plan. The function of a planning department in this context is obvious. In all situations concerned with long-range planning for physical and service development, it is very important that the flow of information be timely, adequate, and consistent. A planning information center, preferably located in the planning department, can play a vital role in keeping all concerned informed on the status of various projects.

INTERNAL PROGRAM DEVELOPMENT

Each institution becomes involved in certain programs which are designed to enhance the effectiveness of the organization. The planning department should be involved in developing such programs because, once again, the institution's goals should show the direction such programs take. They should be geared to complement and/or contribute to the development of the total realm of services which that institution's leadership has articulated in a service plan.

An example of how this might work is the popular management process called "goal setting" or "management by objectives." A desirable approach would provide that the institution sets goals periodically which are published and made available to all key individuals within that institution. Each department in turn establishes departmental goals consistent with institutional goals for the period of time under consideration. Department heads would be encouraged to push this process "down" into the organization by involving section heads and supervisors and even the "average" employee. This is no simple task and is not done easily or without a good deal of trial and error. However, once an institution has become experienced in this process, it becomes a very valuable management tool and has the potential to be a highly motivating force for both the institution as a whole and the individuals performing at each level within the organization. One of the biggest problems involved in the goal-setting program, however, is the matter of interdepartmental communications and identifying and examining overlaps and gaps among various departmental goals.

One of the activities of the planning department could be to provide an information clearing house whereby all department heads and members of administration will be constantly aware of not only the total goal program of the institution but how, for instance, one department's goals may affect another department's goals or require the participation of another department or individual. Once such an informational process is implemented, the total goal-setting program will be greatly strengthened and the opportunities for timely accomplishment of individual and departmental goals will be increased. The value of having the planning department in the middle of this process is that a harmonious blend of the institution's short and long range planning will be achieved.

Another internal program where a planning department can offer assistance is in budgeting. Some hospitals go through a very sophisticated process of detailed budgeting by department and service area each year. Other hospitals have done little to date in the way of formal budgeting. Many are just beginning to institute such a program. In any event, a planning department, because of its storehouse of information regarding future programs and the direction taken by the institution—and also because it will be continually accumulating a data base of facts which it will need for long periods of time—can provide an invaluable service to both the budget committee and the individual department head in preparing budgets. Budgeting, no matter how sophisticated, is at best an educated guess. The planning department should be able to offer information and assistance heretofore not available to department heads.

An institutional "services plan" is another program a planning department can handle. A services plan is a comprehensive report on the total services of the institution with an analysis of each individual area within the hospital showing past history, present status, and future projections for each area. This would include such things as budget, number of personnel, type of service rendered, future outlook for services in this department, innovations pertaining to this department and so on. This document should be written and updated annually and when completed should present a comprehensive picture of the total operation of the organization.

Probably the most fertile field for internal planning and program development is the medical staff. This is a subject often talked about—but seldom acted upon. Hospitals and other health care facilities must draw key members of the medical staff into the main stream of institutional operation and planning on a continuing basis. Using this concept, a real and not "in name only" planning committee should be developed which will ultimately represent the focus of all planning efforts carried out within the medical staff. For too long, many hospital governing boards and administrators have regarded the medical staff as "the other side" instead of "the other hand." This has been the situation from the point of view of many physicians as well.

There is every indication today that medical staff members are sincerely interested in the institution within which he practices. There is no denying the importance of physicians' judgments to a health facility's planning efforts for services and programs. Previous reference to the Barr Committee mentioned that group's insistence upon the involvement of doctors in the ongoing operation of the hospital—proof that high-level encouragement is being given to this aspect of hospital and health institutional management.

THE FLOW OF INFORMATION

Another important entity which must be incorporated into the hospital's planning program is the patient and/or consumer (potential patient). Though not representing a formally organized group, the patient should be given the opportunity of expressing views and ideas regarding the programs and service of the institution. There are numerous ways to achieve patient involvement in the institution's planning program, ranging from informal questionnaires to formal committee representation. The methodology of patient involvement is not as important as the fact that some effective means is established which will provide a platform from which the patient may contribute to the institution's planning program.

A hospital chief executive should be ever mindful of the fact that, after all is said and done, the application of his institution's programs and resources are to individual patients and groups of patients (see Principle No. 6). It is only reasonable to assume that the thoughts, ideas, and reactions of the consumer groups should influence the hospital's planning program.

A final example of an area in which a planning department should be active is, in a sense, the sum of the first five areas, and concerns the flow of information within the institution. By keeping itself informed and aware of what is going on in each area of the hospital in terms of services, goals, budgeting, physicians' opinions, etc., the planning department is in an excellent position to be a communications center. This being the case, a hospital administrator should take advantage of the planning department's position to establish a mechanism by which all key individuals and groups are kept advised of developments within each important area of activity.

EXTERNAL RELATIONSHIPS

Today's hospital administrator finds external pressures growing in importance for his institution. This emphasizes the need to work with, become informed about, and achieve representation on state and local area health and planning organizations. Participation in professional groups is also important in coping with external influences. With the relationships between and among various planning, operating, and professional bodies becoming more and more intense and important, and in order to keep abreast of developments in today's rapidly changing health world, at least one individual in each institution should make it his job to be informed on such external activities. It is inconceivable that any institution can develop its plans and undertake to outline its future course without being aware of the influences of these outside forces which now play such a key role in establishing the direction in which the health care field is moving.

The idea of planning is no longer conceptual. It is real. It is imperative that each institution not only be aware of what is happening in planning but be involved in the developments as they occur.

The planning department should be the institution's major link with these outside influences.

Formal planning at the institutional level is not easy to establish nor carry out on a continuing basis. Planning is not something with which one can expect to create sweeping changes. It has been observed that one of the biggest problems within an institution which is attempting to develop a formal planning process is to arrive at a point where the concept of planning is an accepted topic of conversation within the institution.[4] Although this is true, it is hoped that the necessity for formal planning within an institution has herein been established.

Planning, in any form, is not foolproof. A sound planning process properly implemented within an institution will not eliminate the unexpected. It will not avoid the development of pressure points which demand action and which may not have been included in "the plan." However, if a program of formal planning does exist, the institution will find itself in a better position to adapt readily to finding a suitable

[4]Robert M. Sigmond, "Who is the Planner?" (Presentation to the Hospital Planning and Development Course, Columbia University-Center for Hospital Continuing Education, New York, New York, November 27, 1967).

solution to the unexpected when it does happen because the problem will exist within an established planning context which will, at least, have boundaries within which the problem-solving can take place.

Planning must be a creative rather than a reacting process. To be most effective, planning must be voluntary. The control or incentive aspects of comprehensive health planning should come through the involvement and acceptance of planning principles by the various third-party interests. As these third parties recognize, accept, and adopt the processes and principles of voluntary planning, they will establish relationships between planning and methods of reimbursement. As these relationships develop, no effective health care institution should be unable to plan effectively and meet the requirements established by third parties at the same time. As this happens and institutions plan cooperatively, the position of all community elements concerned will be greatly strengthened, and community and regional health care systems will become realities. For this reason, the concept of comprehensive health planning, both on an areawide and institutional basis, is not a concept to be feared but rather a concept to be welcomed.

If there is still doubt on the part of the small health facility administrator about the applicability of the principles and processes outlined herein, let it be stated again that the points presented are valid no matter where one sits in the health field today. The overt, formal approach to planning in a smaller institution is no less necessary than it is in a larger one. The chief executive carries the major burden of responsibility for planning in his institution, whatever size it may be. Although the administrator of a smaller hospital can expect his planning to be integrated into a process from a larger system of institutional planning, he will find that he will more profitably serve his institution and community by delegating more day-to-day activities and concerning himself more with the future as far as his institution is concerned.

It has been implied herein that the planning for health care in our nation starts at the point of its delivery. At every other point in health care planning—be it community, area, state, regional, or national—no actual care is purveyed. Only general planning takes place at these levels. Planning should start where the action is. Instead of the national health planning process converging from the top down, like a funnel, upon the individual institution, the process actually takes on the form of a pyramid where the base of service (the individual institution) is the broad aspect of the planning process and the single focal point at the top represents the nation, with various layers of planning activity located between the base and the top. The planning thrust must be upward in the health care system if it is to reach its ultimate achievable effectiveness. The test of how successful this concept is to be rests on the shoulders of the health care professional who today occupies the chief executive's chair in our health care institutions.

BIBLIOGRAPHY

"Guide and Suggested Procedures," *For Use by a Hospital Long-Range Planning and Development Committee,* New York: Hospital Review and Planning Council of Southern New York, Inc., 1964.

"Hospital Service Areas in Allegheny County," *A Guide to the Analysis of Geographic Areas Served by Short-Term Voluntary Hospitals,* Pittsburgh, Pennsylvania: Hospital Planning Association of Allegheny County, July, 1963.

Hughes, Charles L., *Goal Setting: Key to Individual and Organizational Effectiveness,* New York: American Management Association, 1965.

Norton, Perry L., "The Planning Process," *Patterns for Action,* New York: Executive Council of the Episcopal Church.

"Secretary's Advisory Committee on Hospital Effectiveness Report," Washington, D.C.: U.S. Department of Health, Education and Welfare, 1968.

Sigmond, Robert M., "The Role of the Medical Staff in a Hospital's Long Range Planning," *Long Range Planning Seminar,* Estes Park, Colorado: The Hospital Medical Staff Conference, October 1, 1968.

Sigmond, Robert M., "Who Is the Planner," Paper presented at the Hospital Planning and Development Course, New York: Columbia University-Center for Hospital Continuing Education, November 27, 1967.

Areawide Planning for Health Facilities

CHARLES I. STONE

Charles I. Stone is an attorney and partner in the firm of Perkins, Coie, Stone, Olsen and Williams in Seattle, Washington.

The American hospital system is undergoing some of the most profound changes it has experienced in its entire history.[1] The nation's population is expanding at a rapid rate, hospital employees are demanding professional and economic recognition, and there is an accelerated expansion of medical science and technology. Because of these and other pressures, the provision of organized health services to the community is becoming more complicated. An additional complicating factor is the public's growing concern about both the cost and the quality of hospital care.

VIEWING COMMUNITY NEEDS

Areawide planning can serve to assist the administrator of the individual hospital in resolving some of his communitywide problems. At the same time it can provide information and perspective that will increase the capability of the individual hospital to meet its daily responsibilities. Traditionally, each individual hospital has viewed the community from its own pinnacle, estimated the community's needs, and then proceeded to attempt to meet these needs on an individual basis without consultation or coordination with other community health facilities.

Inherent in areawide planning is the fundamental advantage that viewing the community as a whole results in the consideration of each individual hospital's role in perspective. It is thus possible to develop an overall program designed to bring hospital care to the community on an organized coordinated basis. The situation is one where in the past, competition has been the byword. The future bespeaks a more integrated system for the provision of health facilities care, with cooperation and coordination the guiding principles.

[1] Pattulo, A. Hospitals and the community in transition. *Hosp. Progr.* 47:59 June 1966.

Areawide planning implies a rational system and distribution of facilities.[2] This system must take into consideration all aspects of the provision of health care, including not only acute and long-term patient care facilities, but also the necessary educational systems for medical and paramedical staff. Empirical observation of the relationship between the provision of patient care on an organized basis and the growing shortage of personnel with which to operate the related health care facilities makes it clear that areawide planning must, necessarily, include attention to educational programs.

Today's environment not only is one in which there is growing concern on the part of the community as to quality of care as well as the cost of health care facilities, it is also an environment in which there is an increasing scope of knowledge that can be implemented into a planned and coordinated system of health care for the community.[3] At the same time, we have an accelerating shortage of personnel, most of whom are demanding increased professional and economic recognition.

Areawide planning agencies within the United States are concerned with these problems to the same extent as is the individual hospital administrator. It is apparent that there is need for solutions to these problems, and that the development of new problem-solving and planning techniques will increase the need for, and prove the quality of, areawide planning.[4]

FUNCTIONS OF PLANNING AGENCIES

Areawide planning is still in its formative years, and as such, most of the planning agencies continue to be substantially concerned with justifying their existence rather than with developing a body of knowledge relating to techniques and methods of conducting the planning effort. These agencies are nevertheless emerging into a period during which technical, economic, and social issues are being identified.[5] Implicit in this is the expectation that in the future, organized planning for community health care will fill a more dominant role in the community exercise of self-determination.

There is a growing awareness throughout the United States that the concept of regional organization of hospital services has merits that in the past have been ignored.[6] [7] The impact of the major forces within the community that are working on the hospital environment, such as population increases and medical advances, are altering inescapably the environment within which the provision of hospital care traditionally has been conducted. Hospital administrators are beginning to think in terms of cooperative computer service, centralized laundries, and centralized sterile

---

[2] Lossing, E. H. Areawide planning. *Can. Hosp.* 43:50 Jan. 1966.

[3] Paley, M. A. Areawide planning: tool for orderly development. *Hospitals, J.A.H.A.* 40:79 June 1, 1966.

[4] Hospital planning today. *Hospitals, J.A.H.A.* 40:39 May 1, 1966.

[5] Rosenfeld, E. D. Regional organization of hospital services. *Hospitals, J.A.H.A.* 40:40 May 1, 1966.

[6] Maynard, J. K. Regionalization at work. *Can. Hosp.* 43:51 April 1966.

[7] Haire, E. B. Fitting the individual hospital into the regional plan. *Hospitals. J.A.H.A.* 40:47 May 1, 1966.

supplies.[8-10] As examples of corrdination, these ventures into cooperative activity can expect to have the blessing and encouragement of the areawide planning agency.

Beyond this, the planning group can serve as a catalyst in the development of improved techniques for providing the industrial components of hospital operation, so that such nonpatient-directed functions can be provided to the community at lower cost and in higher quality. The industrialization of the hospital environment daily is becoming more apparent. At the same time, although hospitals must assume many of the attitudes and techniques of industry in the provision of ancillary services, they must not lose sight of patient care—the function that is their paramount responsibility.

PLANNING FOR HOSPITALS

Formerly, planning for hospitals has been confined to the functional organization of the hospital itself. It has been accomplished by hospital architects, hospital consultants, administrators, and boards of trustees. Although the communitywide aspects of such planning were not completely ignored, they received considerably less consideration than the planning for the individual facility. With the advent of areawide planning, it has become apparent that the focus of attention has moved from the individual hospital's needs to the needs of the community as a whole.

COORDINATION

The need for increased emphasis on coordination of planning on an areawide basis has been effectively summarized by E. D. Rosenfeld, M.D., a New York hospital consultant. Dr. Rosenfeld stated: "The absence of sound regional planning and lack of local standards relating to quantity and comprehensiveness of service are too often responsible for the placement, relocation, or retention of hospitals without consideration of (1) population trends and geographic concentrations, (2) developing and projected transportation and excess.patterns, (3) availability of staff and capital funds, (4) controlled land use projects and adequacy of site for future growth and present needs, and (5) adequate operating income potentials and indigent medical care programs."[11]

Dr. Rosenfeld also stated that in our large metropolitan areas, hospital experience has indicated a declining occupancy rate in obstetric and pediatric units and in some instances an increasing need for short-term adult beds. He also indicated that a major stimulus to the development of areawide planning for hospital facilities is the effect this planning will have on costs and quality of service. Again, there was reference by this author to the improved service and lowering of cost that could be achieved through centralization of laundries, personnel departments, purchasing departments, pharmacies, blood banks, ambulance services, nursing school, x-ray therapy departments, and resident, intern and paramedical programs.

[8] Bowden, J. Eight hospitals join in co-op computer venture. *Hosp. Top.* 44:46 March 1966.

[9] Weymes, C. Regional central sterile supply serves a group of hospitals. *Hosp. Top.* 44:139 Feb. 1966.

[10] Rikli, A. E. *et al.* Study suggest value of shared computers. *Mod. Hosp.* 106:100 May 1966.

[11] Rosenfeld, E. D. *op. cit.*

Most of the material published during the past year is devoted to various aspects of the philosophy of planning. Very little of it is involved with the techniques of planning.[12] There is indication of an increasing awareness by government that areawide planning, if properly directed, will play an increasingly important role in the future.[13]

At the same time, the federal government is becoming more involved in the organization and operation of the community hospitals. This involvement has not yet assumed any particular pattern, and only time will tell its extent and direction. If any pattern is beginning to emerge, it would appear to be a growing recognition on the part of the federal government that the delivery and organization of health services to a community should be based upon community concepts and not political divisions.

OPPOSITION TO PLANNING

A review of the published writings of individuals interested in areawide planning suggests that planners are more preoccupied with selling the philosophy of planning than with developing a body of knowledge involving the techniques and tools of planning. Perhaps this is as it should be, because planning is a relatively new concept, and there are areas of opposition to planning as a community tool for improving hospital services to the community. Opposition to planning, however seems to be on the wane, and most boards of trustees and hospital administrators seem to have accepted the rationalization that planning need not materially affect their autonomy. One author stated that planning is a tool for orderly development. The issue, of course, is whether this will be a sharp or a dull tool.

FUTURE OF PLANNING

The future of planning rests to a great extent not so much on the ability and energy of those involved in planning, but rather on the environment in which planning takes place. All too frequently planning has established itself as a body of expertise that exists for the purpose of establishing a framework in which the community health facilities are required to function. In the past this was a comfortable position for planning to take because of its relative immaturity and its relative lack of experience and demonstrated success.

Hopefully, the future will see a change in the orientation of planning, and those involved in planning will grow to recognize that they must establish a working partnership with the individuals who are experts in the field of health care administrations and the furnishing of health care to the community. Once this recognition is achieved, planning will function in an environment wherein the guidelines established by planners for maximum or minimum development will, in fact, be used as guidelines for the future development of the community hospital system-guidelines that will be considered as assistance rather than threat, and that will be accepted voluntarily by the individual health facility.

[12]Drosness, D. L. and Lubin, J. W. Planning can be based on patient travel. *Mod. Hosp.* 106:92 April 1966.

[13]Graning, H. M. Hill-Burton at 20. *Hospitals, J.A.H.A.* 40:43 March 1, 1966.

It is foreseeable that areawide planning agencies will serve in a growing capacity to encourage the development of centralization of certain industrial components of hospital activity as well as the development of a coordinated system for the provision of patient care.[14] Canadians as well as Americans are awakening to the need for reevaluation of methods for providing for the distribution of health services to the community.[15-17] The Canadians appear to be primarily interested in developing a system of regionalization of hospital services, whereas the Americans appear to be primarily concerned with meeting the problems of maldistribution of services, obsolesence, and the low occupancy of certain hospital service departments such as obstetrics and pediatrics.

The 1966 literature relating to areawide planning has shown a growing concern over the need for regionalization of hospital services. It has shown an increasing awareness of the role areawide planning will play in working with hospitals and developing guidelines for their future service requirements. The literature also indicates a maturing attitude toward the planners' own role as a mechanism whereby the community hospitals and related health care facilities can more efficiently and economically meet their future responsibilities.

[14]Cooper, M. S. Hospital PKU screening laboratory serves 65 hospitals *Hospitals, J.A.H.A.* 40:69 Jan. 16, 1966.

[15]Ferguson, R. B. Areawide planning. *Can. Hosp.* 43:50 Jan. 1966.

[16]Neilson, J. B. Areawide planning. *Can. Hosp.* 43:50 Jan. 1966.

[17]Hastings, J. E. F. Current issues in health services. *Can. Hosp.* 43:44 Aug. 1966.

Health Care Policy Issues

This section examines the areas of health care delivery and financing systems. The present environment within which the hospital administrator must operate is characteristic of emerging governmental intervention and changing social values with respect to health care expectations. Presently, the whole health care industry is at a crossroad. Its future direction should be critically evaluated today. The following readings present some of the important policy issues pertaining to the health care delivery and financing systems which will eventually have to be resolved.

In *HEALTH CARE SERVICES AT THE CROSSROADS: ISSUES OF PUBLIC POLICY,* it is indicated that the current patterns of organization and the financing of health care services are in a state of controversy. In addition, the accelerating cost of health care is viewed as a symptom of structural maladjustments in the financing and delivery systems. Various emerging trends are presented. First, the fragmentation of facility relationships has fostered area-wide planning and control. Second, the institutionalization of health care has promoted the hospital facility as the hub for community health services. Third, a managerial revolution is emerging in the operation of facilities. Finally, the trend toward national health insurance is growing along with all of its related issues.

In *POLICY ISSUES IN FINANCING MEDICAL CARE,* the point is made that the methods available for the future financing of personal health care are no longer simple. The passage of the Medicare and Medicaid acts marked the beginning of government involvement in the financing of health care. A number of philosophical questions are also raised as to whether the future medical care financing mechanism should be the welfare approach, social insurance approach, private insurance approach or some combination of any or all three. A treatment of the structural differences between the (1) private versus social and (2) welfare versus social approaches is presented. Issues of importance are coverage, financing, premium and benefit relationships, and eligibility. The conclusion derived is that there is no simple solution. Perhaps, more importantly, resolution of the financing mechanism will require that social value judgments be made.

Health Services at the Crossroads: Issues of Public Policy

HERMAN M. SOMERS, PH.D.

Herman M. Somers, Ph.D., is Professor of Politics and Public Affairs at Princeton University in Princeton, N.J.

Patterns of organization and financing of health services are in a state of turbulence and controversy, as even the casual viewer of the mass media must now be aware. It is still more a tumult of rhetoric than of action. But the signs are ample that the verbal pyrotechnics are a prelude to significant change.

Such movement is reasonably predictable: 1. Because social developments normally follow such a sequence; 2. because the essential discontents which underlie the welter of noise are mainly valid; 3. because there is now virtual universal acceptance that important change is unavoidable. There remains, however, great uncertainty and disagreement on the best methods to correct conspicuous ills and the most appropriate alterations. Needless to say, there are formidable institutional barriers to overcome.

PRICES AND COSTS

At the source of the loud complaints besetting the entire field is the staggering inflation of prices and costs, an inflation unmatched in intensity and duration. When properly analyzed, prices serve as indicators of conditions in the entire system. They may signal imbalance, maladjustments, or structural inadequacies.

It was cost experience, and its accompanying resentments, that focused a bright spotlight on the health care industry. Once the glare began to penetrate the crevices of this complex field it appeared to reveal an array of serious difficulties, such as care arrangements fraught with inefficiency, obsolete organization, social inequities, and waste. All have been increasingly criticized by health professionals as well as laymen, but apparently are intractable to quick or obvious reform.

Indicative of the heights of public concern which the issue has reached, on July 10, 1969 President Nixon forecast a "massive crisis" in health care within the next two or three years unless prompt action was taken. At the same time the secretary of the Department of Health, Education, and Welfare and the assistant secretary for health and scientific affairs jointly stated: "This nation is faced with a breakdown in the delivery of health care unless concerted action is taken by government and the private sector."

The two phenomena—high costs and a disjointed or inadequate delivery system—nurture one another. It has become clear to most critics of high cost that the problem will not be met successfully by dependence on arbitrary price fixing or price ceilings or any instruments directed exclusively at dollar controls, although such devices are not to be disregarded.

The primary emphasis of reform has shifted from direct attack on prices and costs through financial controls to alterations in the health services delivery system—its productivity, its adequacy, its effectiveness. This has enlarged quality consciousness, sensitivity to the wide variations in value of particular services—a problem gradually being shorn of the protective veil of professional mystique. In short, we are now examining the larger question: What are we getting for our money?

PRICES VS PRODUCTIVITY

It may be useful to remind ourselves very briefly of what in fact has been happening to prices and costs. Health care expenditures in the United States during the fiscal year ending June 30, 1969, continued their long and rapid increase and exceeded $60 billion. The growth in one year was $6.4 billion, or 12 per cent, as it was also the year before. *Per capita* expenditures were four times as large as in fiscal year 1950, averaging an increase of 7.2 per cent each year.

Health expenditures for a long time have been rising faster than the nation's total output of goods and services. In fiscal 1950, health outlays were 4.6 per cent of the gross national product; by fiscal 1969, they were 6.7 per cent. In less than two decades health care enlarged its share of GNP by 46 per cent. The rate at which health outlays have been outpacing GNP has been accelerating. By the end of this decade about 10 cents out of every dollar we produce may go for health care.

The elements of rising costs are generally divided into three broad categories: 1. Increases in population; 2. increased utilization of services (which includes increases in the level, or quality, of care); 3. increased prices per unit of service.

All three have been moving up steadily, but at quite different rates. The enormous increase of expenditures between 1950 and 1969, from $26 billion to $60 billion, can be accounted for as follows: Population increases explains 18 per cent of it. Increased services per capita (both quality and quantity) explains another 35 per cent. While *per capita* expenditures increased more than two and one-half times during that 19-year period, less than one half of that increase bought additional real services; the remainder was washed away by higher prices.

Between 1946 and 1969 medical care prices advanced 155 per cent while the index of all prices advanced 88 per cent, an average annual increase of 4.7 versus 2.8 per cent. By far the major influence was hospital daily service charges which increased 592 per cent, almost seven times as fast as all prices, and five times as fast as all services in the Consumer Price Index.

Price and cost imbalances over so protracted a period are, among other evidences, symptoms of structural maladjustments in the financing and delivery system. The most striking consequence (as well as cause) of the maladjustments is failure in productivity. As nearly as can be determined, the productivity rate appears at best to have remained about constant and possibly even decreased, in sharp contrast to the rest of the economy.

The productivity problem in health care is extremely difficult to cope with. Aside from the extraordinary problems of measurement, this is a service industry characterized by monopolistic conditions not disciplined by a competitive market place or regulated by public authority, an industry in which there even appears to be significant built-in disincentives to increased productivity. It is an unique industry for which conventional remedies do not seem appropriate.

There are obviously, however, a wide variety of powerful interests with very heavy stakes in the health care economy and whose welfare is conspicuously threatened by continuation of the present price behavior. These include government, employers, labor, the health insurance industry, the health professions, and others. They have become alarmed and in various ways they are now taking aim at the maladjustments they discern. Encouraging movement is beginning to be visible—some of it is due to social motivation, some to enlightened self-interest, and some to simple fear of what might otherwise befall them. In any case, the unprecedented agitation is having results and change is beginning to emerge.

SYSTEMS AND SERVICE

Among the emerging trends in delivery and financing worthy of attention a few seem particularly significant. Admittedly, for the most part, they represent new probings, experiments, and tendencies, and the evidence regarding their probable outcomes is still fragmentary. Yet patterns may be discerned, and these will be reviewed briefly.

First, is the recognition of the need and the search for systemization, an attempt to arrange the segments of health care resources of communities into coherent relationships to increase effectiveness, maximize productivity of personnel and institutions, and to make possible delivery of comprehensive health services.

Two years ago the eminent Barr Committee (the Secretary's Advisory Committee on Hospital Effectiveness) reported to the secretary of HEW that "The key fact about the health service as it exists today is this disorganization. . . . Lack of planning and control in the health services has resulted in fragmentation and disjunction that promote extravagance and permit tragedy."

In the typical American community the various health resources have little operational relationship to one another. Individual hospitals are autonomous in structure and decision-making. Services and equipment may be duplicated unnecessarily; other needed services may be available in none. Other health institutions in the community—clinics and skilled nursing homes—may or may not have organizational relationship with a hospital or with one another. Physicians may have an affiliation with one or several hospitals (in some cases, none) and for some parts of their practices it may prove to be the wrong hospital. Referral procedures are haphazard and arbitrary. Organization has simply not been adapted to mesh the efforts of increased specializations.

For the patient such fragmentation often means confusion, uncertainty, and incomplete care. Access to an appropriate site and level of care is limited by the dispersion of specialized professional personnel and facilities. Quality is restricted by gaps in available services, lack of a point of responsibility for the patient as a whole, and discontinuity of care. Productivity is curtailed by the inherent waste of such dispersion and lack of integration, and cost is increased.

The objective is to bring together the bits and pieces into a system which relates them to one another operationally, illuminating the gaps as well as the surpluses. At whatever point a patient enters the system through the physician's office, the outpatient department, or a clinic—the organized system should have responsibility for assuring access to the spectrum of services. Preventive, diagnostic, therapeutic, and rehabilitative services should be coordinated to maintain a primary doctor-patient relationship, avoid unnecessary duplication of tests and other services, assure that the appropriate level of institutional care is assigned, and provide centralized complete medical records for each patient.

To achieve this goal, a community must define the different functions of different institutions, from primary care to the specialized sophisticated procedures of a medical center. Such definition in itself is likely to identify shortages or imbalances in existing facilities, for example, inadequate primary care centers and ambulatory services. It could indicate for smaller communities what kind of relationships they must develop with nearby community facilities to supplement their own. It requires that every physician have a professional relationship with a hospital and that the various hospitals and other institutions have a functional relationship with one another.

Such arrangements enable more efficient use of manpower by wider use of paraprofessional personnel. A coordinated system could adopt performance standards for many levels of personnel, instead of sole dependence upon diplomas, and thus effectuate both vertical and horizontal mobility of personnel where none now exists. More effective employment of existing personnel might demonstrate that the magnitude of the current manpower shortage is in large part created by structural frictions.

This kind of rational systemization is in large measure what the proponents of the Regional Medical Program (P.L. 89-239) had in mind. The concept of regionalization primarily connotes systemization plus planning. Most of the regional medical programs established under the legislation initially resisted acceptance of such a goal and for the most part little progress has been made toward it. But they have now moved to wider recognition of its necessity through force of circumstance.

PLANNING AND CONTROLS

Second, we are witnessing a lively groping toward meaningful health care planning. This is still only vaguely defined but is aimed toward effective community control over construction, allocation of equipment and manpower, and balanced distribution and utilization of resources. System demands planning, and planning to be effective requires controls.

Recently, the concept of planning has broadened to encompass the goal of rationality in relationships among the autonomous entities in health care, to move toward a coordinated system of facilities and personnel, to assure the availability of comprehensive services. Instead of just saying "no" to unnecessary facilities, the planning mission is now viewed more as an affirmative sponsoring of the development of an effective mix of services within a broadly organized framework. It should provide a mechanism for allocation of area resources to maximize output and accessibility. As one writer put it, it would create a technostructure for what is now essentially a cottage industry.

Presumably the Partnership for Health legislation enacted by Congress in 1965 (P.L.89-749) was intended to establish machinery in each state for such goals. Health planning councils have been established all over the nation, but generally have been ineffectual. Their functions have not been clearly defined. The councils lack an adequate administrative framework and they lack enforcement powers.

It is now generally agreed that in the absence of a market regulator and discipline, a source of external regulation or control must be substituted. Several states have, in varying degrees, established modest regulatory mechanisms, including New York, California, and Rhode Island.

The American Hospital Association has officially accepted the principle of mandatory planning (although conditioned upon a *quid pro quo* of third-party payers accepting responsibility for capital financing in their reimbursement formulae). Blue Cross plans have said they "will not pay full reimbursement or continue our contract" with hospitals that do not comply with health planning agencies.

MORATORIUM ON NEW BEDS

Commercial insurance carriers have also assumed a sympathetic stance. A recent report of the Committee on Medical Economics, Health Insurance Association of America, says, "While there is not agreement on the 'proper' number of general hospital beds per thousand population, there is agreement that, whatever the number, both hospital administrators and physicians will see that the beds are kept filled. This suggests that a moratorium should be declared on building new hospital beds until the need for more beds, or such an expensive type can be fully justified."

It appears that the parties at interest are ready for effective action, but machinery is sadly lacking. It also seems clear that if the machinery is to be effective, the agencies will have to be given enforcement powers.

Their range of functions will also require changes in existing restrictive legislation in the states. For example, licensing laws and regulations which promote the present rigid guild system applicable to nurse's aides, nurses, and other paramedical personnel, and virtually prohibit occupational mobility, must be changed. Obviously hospital licensing must be made compatible with the standards of the authorized planning agency; franchising may well have to be substituted for traditional licensing. Similarly, the laws in many states which effectively prohibit the development of prepaid group practice plans must be repealed.

An effective planning instrumentality also offers an excellent opportunity for constructively meeting the growing demand for consumer participation in decision-making and consumer education in health care issues. It can also serve as a vehicle for organizational changes to lower the barriers to adequate health services for the poor.

HOSPITAL, THE HUB

Third, we are experiencing increased, and probably inescapable, institutionalization of health care—a continuing expansion of clinics, community health centers, hospital-based medical practice, and similar developments. The first two trends, systemization and planning, as well as the imperatives of new technology, will gradually associate such institutions into an organized network of facilities for a community or region with formal or informal affiliations or agreements. The central coordinating force, the organizational hub, of this network of health services will be the hospital.

This does not imply any diminution in the role of the family doctor. On the contrary, as an integral element within the coordinated network, directly augmented by the facilities, equipment, and organization of an institutional setting, the capacities and importance of the family doctor will be substantially enhanced. True, solo practice will continue to decline as it has for many years, but that is quite a different matter.

Nor does it mean that present hospital authorities will assume a dominating role in community health services, or that more health services will be rendered within the confines of the hospital. The emerging hospital, as the hub of community health services, will be the site where all professional and community needs and values meet and can be reconciled. It will encompass not only the trustees (whose representational character will be significantly altered), the administration, and the medical staff (with which all practitioners will have an affiliation), but also the nursing services, and the satellite institutions (clinics, skilled nursing homes, and community health centers). Established at the core of the planning process it will also reflect the voice of the consumer.

The community health system will probably require fewer hospital beds *per capita* than at present because it will be more practical to emphasize ambulatory care and decentralization, permitting care in lesser facilities for all but those who require the most sophisticated technological equipment and highly specialized personnel. There will be relative expansion of primary health centers, group practice clinics, qualified long-term care facilities, home health services, and first-aid stations in isolated areas.

The trends suggest the most rapid relative growth of neighborhood health centers in urban areas paralleled by small limited service hospitals in rural areas. Neighborhood health centers often are thought of as instruments for serving the poor, and they are admirably suited to meet that difficult problem. But their effectiveness will cause them to spread as resources for primary care in affluent areas as well, although they may be called by different names. In the future all of them will have a working relationship with a hospital.

The economies of prepayment group practice plans have already caused government to encourage their expansion and we may expect to see more aggressive stimulation of such arrangements in the near future through financial incentives and other devices. But experience indicates that such institutions also are most effective when tied in with a hospital facility.

MANAGEMENT AND PROFESSIONALISM

Accompanying the foregoing developments is a fourth movement, a general managerial revolution in the operation of health institutions, a new recognition of the crucial role of efficient management.

Historically, "charity hospitals" have been characterized by their relatively small size, anomalous organizational structures, and other unique features. The result has been neglect of efficient management as an essential feature of American hospitals until recently, with the emergence of a new corps of trained professional administrators. Even these skilled administrators, however, face formidable obstacles in traditions, built-in diffusion, and ambiguity of authority.

Difficulties are both external and internal. The most obvious external factor is the separateness of each institution. About half of all short-term general hospitals are too small (under 100 beds) to warrant or afford adequate managerial talent, for example, skilled personnel managers. This may account, in part, for the notoriously poor relations between hospitals and labor. Incentives for merger are lacking in the not-for-profit sector, but more common among proprietary institutions.

There is little reason, except in tradition and vested interest, that a group of hospitals should not be under a single management, resulting in considerable efficiencies and economies of scale. In some areas arrangements have been made for joint purchasing, joint laundry operations, and the like, which have proved beneficial. But this is not a substitute for unified management. Joint management of institutions would minimize present planning difficulties.

Internally, there have been great improvements, but the authority of the administrator is severely limited and often ambiguous. The physicians, typically not employed by the hospital, are privileged to use its facilities for their patients, and generally determine or dominate important hospital policies. Yet the doctors are in an essentially irresponsible position in relation to the efficiency and financing of the hospital. The administrator does not have adequate authority to cope with the prestige and autonomy of physicians—whose convenience or empire-building proclivities may not be consistent with the welfare of the hospital as a whole—who have no personal financial stake in the results. Excessive equipment and costly low occupancy rates (over 20 per cent of the average hospital beds are normally empty) are frequently the consequence. Administrators are often appalled by a system which uses expensive beds too freely and unnecessarily.

The crucial role of managerial effectiveness is now generally recognized and a source of increased concern and action. A minimum standard of managerial adequacy has been proposed for inclusion among the conditions of participation in Medicare. Others have recommended that management competence be a condition of licensure. A variety of proposals have been made for assimilating the medical staff into an integrated management. The most noteworthy of these was the recommendation of the Barr Committee that the medical staff be directly involved with administration in developing the budget and operating plan and in achieving financial and service objectives as budgeted; and that, once the budget and operating plan are accepted by the board of trustees, the administrator shall have the authority required to enable him to manage the operations of the institution in accordance with the approved budget and plan.

FINANCING AND GOVERNMENT

The spreading alarm regarding the inadequacy of present arrangements for financing health care is generating a fifth development. There is a growing awareness that serious illness can wreck families financially and the need exists to assure universal access to care without means tests. The arrival of Medicare and Medicaid has substantially alleviated the problem but they have also called sharper, more impatient attention to all the remaining shortcomings of financing and access. The experience of Medicaid has brought on general disenchantment with "welfare medicine" and with means tests as a condition for health service.

Private health insurance made spectacular progress during the past two decades and vastly improved access to medical care, especially for employed workers and their families, since the large majority of protection is bought through employe-benefit group insurance plans. Over 80 per cent of the population has some form of health insurance, but some 36 million persons are wholly unprotected, a disproportionate number of them among the poor and among children. The degree of protection provided for most people is regarded as far too meager by current standards.

Many leaders of the industry are acutely sensitive to the problem and are pressing hard to expand the scope of protection. Some further progress can be expected, but insurance is also a victim of medical price inflation. If carriers are to broaden protection, they must raise premiums. But when inflation causes a large increase each year in the cost of the existing package of benefits, it obviously becomes more difficult to tack on still higher premiums for enlarged benefits.

The feeling is spreading that, given the hard economic facts, it will not be possible for private health insurance alone to meet the problem adequately. Consequently, there has been a marked revival of interest in "national health insurance," evidenced by a proliferation of well publicized proposals, increasingly in the form of legislative bills. The dramatic rise in costs has been a major stimulus.

The term "national health insurance" is being used to label a wide variety of quite different programs whose only common factor is their apparent intent that health insurance be made effectively available to the entire population. Beyond this, plans differ in virtually all essentials.

The scope of support for one or another of the array of proposals suggests that the nation is moving toward a consensus that some form of universal insurance is necessary. It is reliably expected that this will be one of the major issues of Congressional debate within the next few years and that some new federal financing scheme will emerge before the close of the decade.

The problem of timing has been disturbing and dividing even those otherwise in agreement on objectives. One group fears, on the basis of recent experience, that unless great corrections are first made in the supply, the vast infusion of demand generated by universal coverage could cause a breakdown of the entire system. They express apprehension that a massive pumping of new money into the system would tend to underpin present arrangements and halt the trend of change described earlier. By removing the current pressures, they feel, we may be removing the best leverage we have for necessary change.

The other side does not deny the dangers of the stringency of supply, but argues that the threat of system breakdown is already here and that only with the authority and incentives of a national program will it be possible to tackle the supply problem meaningfully and adequately.

All this suggests that extreme caution must be exercised in the development of a national health insurance program. We are beyond the simplistic belief of the late forties that more money alone can assure universal access to comprehensive health services. We now know that money alone will not correct the maladjustments and imbalances in the delivery system. Any new program which merely provides government subsidies for present arrangements such as the income tax credit proposals (often referred to as Medicredit) is likely to do more damage then good.

REGULATION AND EXPERIMENTATION

The sixth, and final, trend on the horizon is a corollary of the other five. Any system that guarantees full financing, whether by government or by private instrumentalities or a combination of both, and is uncontrolled by the competitive market place, will inevitably require some form of cost regulation. Such regulation usually demands accompanying standard setting for quality, since price and the nature of the product are not logically separable.

We have already seen that Medicare and Medicaid, which started out with a simple intent to pay the "market price" for physicians' services, were soon obliged to set some limits to payable fees. Private insurers are moving in the same direction. The Medicare and Medicaid formulae for reimbursing hospitals for their "reasonable costs," whatever those costs might turn out to be, are under severe criticism for allegedly aggravating cost inflation. So are the Blue Cross reimbursement formulae.

In its 1967 amendments to the Social Security Act, the Congress authorized the Social Security Administration to experiment with alternative methods of reimbursement. The Department of Health, Education, and Welfare is asking Congress for authority to tie reimbursement to some criteria for reasonable cost control and to limit its payments accordingly. Planning and systemization, if they are to be effective means of producing greater efficiency, will require regulatory authority. It takes only a few non-cooperators to break down a system.

Because the best means of cost regulation have not been determined, we will soon be seeing varied experiments with such devices as incentive payments to hospitals and other institutions, negotiated rates, prior budget approvals, fee schedules, capitation payments, and others. But the best and surest means of containing costs and maintaining high quality will lie in effective rationalization of the delivery system to increase productivity. A disjointed and uncoordinated health care system is inherently inefficient and will continue to generate high costs, whatever regulations may be written, and ultimately the costs must be paid.

CONCLUSION

I have attempted to call attention to what I regard as encouraging movements toward reform. But these, in the main, still represent early probings. Thus far most of them are characterized by lively discussion, earnest hopes, and drawing board plans, more than by solid accomplishment. The crucial question remains, therefore, whether we can and will act rapidly enough.

The public reaction to high costs, difficult accessibility, and uncertain quality has been growing louder and harsher. Unless there is more visible movement toward effective reform, impatience and discouragement may generate inexorable demands for quick dramatic action that may force ill-considered, precipitous responses which could prove damaging to both consumers and providers. It is a not unfamiliar historic pattern: When reform is too long delayed or comes too haltingly, rebellious—often destructive—reaction may set in. The signs of such possibility are not lacking now. Time has become a critical factor in the future of health services—and it is not on our side.

Policy Issues in Financing Medical Care: a Continuing Debate

ROBERT J. BLENDON, SC.D.

Robert J. Blendon, Sc.D., is Associate Dean for Health Care Programs at Johns Hopkins University in Baltimore, Maryland.

Within our present political framework, philosophical terms are changing or losing meanings. Established political party attitudes are being fused or are becoming less relevant [8]. Rapid social and economic change is forcing fundamental rethinking of policies, opinions, and faiths. One issue emerging from the upheaval is a renewed debate on the future financing of personal health services in the post-Vietnam era. The size of our population, the number and heterogeneity of our health-care institutions, the extent of our social problems, and the development of new science and technology have tended to make the issue more complex. Increasingly, it is becoming difficult to debate issues of public policy in terms of clear-cut alternatives because the actual choices are no longer simple, and the present alternatives lack the moral clarity that once existed in earlier battles for social reform [12, 28].

The enactment of the Social Security Amendments of 1965 supposedly climaxed a decade-long national debate over governmentally financed health services for the aged. However, the legislation did not resolve the major philosophical issues in the field of financing personal health services. Rather, it represented a compromise between the major interest groups [35]. Through this legislation, the United States embraced simultaneously *two* philosophically distinct methods of financing health services [7]:

1) Title 18 of the act conferred certain health care benefits on the over-65 population by application of the social insurance principle.

2) Title 19 of the act made health services available to portions of the indigent population on an income-determinant basis, by application of the welfare principle.

The enactment of the Social Security Amendments of 1965 probably marks the beginning, rather than the end, of large-scale governmental involvement in the financing of personal health services. It seems inevitable that there will be a growing future demand for the extension of benefits to groups outside of the aged or indigent categories.

PRESSURES TOWARD GOVERNMENT PARTICIPATION

The trend toward more governmental participation in the financing of health services is motivated by the same forces which brought into being the voluntary health insurance movement during the 1930's. Once again, the precipitating force is that of growing financial pressures on the employed, lower and lower-middle income groups [23]. Year after year, it becomes more expensive to provide health services. Consequently, a larger percentage of personal income is required in the form of insurance premiums. Thus, a greater proportion of the population will encounter substantial difficulty in providing themselves with *adequate* health insurance coverage. They, in turn, will most likely seek some form of financial assistance from the government in order to obtain adequate health services [33]. Likewise, as health care costs continue to rise, the burden imposed upon state and local welfare programs will be enlarged. Therefore, it can be anticipated that considerable pressure will be exerted by these governments to have the national government, with its broader tax resources, absorb an increasingly larger proportion of the administrative and financial load [13, 15]. This problem in the future will become especially critical in the large cities where the tax base continues to decline and the demand for public services continues to expand [13, 16].

With the continuing demand for extension of health service benefits, the hitherto unresolved philosophical question will have to be faced: Should the future expansion of the public sector in the field of financing health services be through an amplified welfare program (Title 19) or should it be through the use of the social insurance mechanism (Title 18)?

The above mentioned controversy is commonly referred to in the literature on social policy as the welfare approach to medical care versus the social insurance approach [4]. In actuality, this tends to be an over-simplification of the issue. With the exception of a few die-hard individualists, very few advocates of the welfare approach to financing health services have been enamoured of the concept of welfare itself, particularly as it has existed in our society. Rather, they have been strongly attracted to the private (voluntary) insurance mechanism with its associated diversity of sources and dispersed economic power. They contend that private insurance can adequately cover the needs of the majority of the under-65 population and will have fewer deleterious effects on the organization of health services than any other method of payment [14, 22]. Only that portion of the general population which is unable to afford the costs of subscribing to private health insurance should receive governmental assistance (welfare). On the other hand, social insurance by its inherent nature must be nearly universal in its range of coverage. The real choice confronting us in this issue, then, is not welfare versus social insurance, both of which are under governmental auspices, but rather private insurance (except for the very low-income groups who will be taken care of by the government) versus social (government) insurance.

RIGHT TO HEALTH CARE?

Another point which requires clarification in the context of the present controversy is the meaning of the nearly universally accepted phrase "the right to health care." Conservatives and liberals alike utilize the phrase, but its meaning is equivocal. The ambiguity stems from the existence of two relevant definitions for the word "right." A "right can be a just claim, whether legal, prescriptive, or moral." It also can be "that which is due to anyone merely by claim." The former is the definition accepted by those with more conservative leanings while the latter appeals to those who tend to be more liberal in medical care matters. The first fits in conveniently with a welfare approach in which the individual and his family are expected to provide for their own health care requirements under normal circumstances, but the community accepts the *moral* responsibility to meet those needs which lie beyond the limited capabilities of the individual and his family [9, 38]. The second definition corresponds easily with the doctrine of social insurance in which illness is considered to be one of a small group of major hazards in the modern industrial society with which the individual and his family cannot adequately cope. Therefore, the collective action of the whole society is required and the provision for universal eligibility for health services becomes the *legal* obligation of the community [4].

Undoubtedly, the financing of the large and apparently increasing *outlays* for health services will become one of the major fiscal problems of contemporary social policy in the United States. In attempting to make the unavoidable decisions on public policy required in a modern democratic society, individuals are commonly confronted by the complexity of the issues for which they frequently have no systematic method of evaluation. The purpose of this paper, then, will be to explain briefly some of the structural differences which exist between the two alternative methods of financing health services. Since the "private insurance—welfare approach" actually includes more than one method of financing, the paper will be divided into two sections: private insurance versus social insurance, and welfare versus social insurance.

PRIVATE INSURANCE VERSUS SOCIAL INSURANCE

To begin with, social and private health insurance resemble each other in at least three major respects:

1) Both private and social insurance are based essentially upon the polling of definable risks over a large statistical population. [11].

2) Both social and private insurance require payment of premiums or contributions although the nature of the relationships between premiums and benefits usually differs between the two types of insurance [11].

3) For persons with insured status, the payment of predetermined benefits under either system does not depend upon the demonstration of individual financial need Instead, it depends upon the occurrence of a specified contingency, namely illness [11].

The differences between the two insurance principles, however, far outnumber their similarities:

1) Private health insurance is customarily voluntary; social insurance is usually compulsory. Under social insurance, individuals have little or no choice as to membership, scope of benefits, or contributions to be paid by or for them [2, 19].

2) Under social insurance, the employed population can be universally enrolled. Private insurance always suffers from an "enrollment gap." By utilizing

the social security system, all employed individuals can be enrolled by legislative fiat [1]. Private health insurance continuously struggles with the problem of enrolling the ill, the partially employed, and the self-employed. However, our present social insurance system excludes from possible coverage those who are not employed: the unemployed and partially employed worker, the retired, and the children of unemployed parents [7, 33]. For these groups to be included, the social insurance system would have to be substantially modified, since these groups do not contribute financially to the program. The precedent for such a policy change was firmly established by the Title XVIII provisions of the Social Security Amendments of 1965. Under this title, all individuals age 65 and over were automatically included even if they had not previously contributed to the social security system [35].

3) The two insurance principles differ in the relationship between premiums and benefits.

Private insurance tends to adjust premiums to the expected risk for various groups of insured persons (experience rating). Within any group, a given premium will buy the same amount of protection [24]. However, one variation in the private insurance principle, such as is found in some Blue Cross plans, is the community rating concept. The community rating plans attempt to charge the same premium for the same benefits to all individuals or groups regardless of their age and sex composition and their past health services usage experience [1]. But, even among the few remaining community rated plans contributions are not assessed on a flat rate but in relation to the subscriber's number of dependents [10].

Under social insurance, the objective of securing adequacy of benefits takes precedence over the concept that each individual should receive benefits in direct proportion to his contributions. Consequently, there exists a potentiality for large subsidies in this system. Such subsidies could come either from outside the system, or from within it, or both [11].

Although private insurance has had relative success in providing some form of health insurance for most of the under-65 population, its success in terms of the extent of protection provided has been less impressive [34]. The proportion of medical expenses paid by private insurance for such increasingly important items—as-out-of-hospital drugs, physicians' home and office visits, out-patient services, nursing home care, and psychiatric and home nursing care has advanced slowly, and probably cannot be increased significantly. In 1966 private health insurance paid 32 per cent of all consumer health care expenditures. In the last eleven years the increase in the medical care expenditures covered by private insurance has averaged approximately one percentage point a year [30, 31]. At this rate, almost 20 years would be required for private insurance to cover 50 per cent of these expenditures.

4) Although it is not an inherent feature, social insurance, in the American tradition, has required the employer to contribute as much as his employees. Under private insurance the contribution varies considerably [10, 25].

5) Private insurance is based on a legally binding contract between an insurance company and the purchaser of the policy. Social insurance is based upon statutory legislation which promises certain benefits to the insured. These

benefits are not the subject of contractual guarantees but are open to legislative modification [11].

6) The insuree under social insurance is better protected from financial losses due to adverse economic conditions or poor management than he is under private insurance. If revenues of the social insurance system become inadequate to cover desired benefits, the government can meet the difference by a direct contribution from general tax funds [11].

7) Social insurance does not require a trust fund of considerable magnitude, and therefore, operates on a nearly "pay as you go" basis. Private insurance requires the maintenance of large reserves sufficient to produce revenues that in conjunction with premiums will fully privide for discharging liabilities to policyholders [20].

8) Many costs that are incurred in the administration of private insurance programs, such as sales and acquisition expenses and surplus to investors, are not found in social insurance [19].

9) Benefits cannot be cancelled with social insurance except by government fiat [10]. This, however, has rarely if ever occurred in any society [32]. Under private insurance the policy can be terminated by the insurance carrier, the employer, or the inability of the insured to pay the premiums [10].

10) With the notable exception of the non-profit voluntary plan, such as Blue Cross, most private insurance companies attempt to limit their benefits in terms of fixed dollar amounts (indemnity benefits) [23], but social insurance is likely to provide benefits in terms of services rather than dollars. This differs significantly from the traditional forms of social insurance (old age and survivors' insurance, workmen's compensation, unemployment insurance) which provide benefits in terms of fixed dollar amounts rather than services [6].

11) Since social insurance provides benefits in terms of services rather than fixed dollar amounts, and since social insurance provides for a near governmental monopoly, the administrators of the program tend to develop considerable leverage and control over the providers of health services throughout the country [37].

Inevitable, the amount of control exerted by the federal government in the field of health services will be proportionate to the magnitude of the federal expenditures for personal health services. Thus, the more substantial the expenditure the more likely the federal government is to exert its power and authority.

Whenever the Congress considers a service so essential to the national well-being that it is willing to distribute it according to the criterion of need rather than on a basis of a willingness and ability to pay then, inevitably, the legislative and executive branches of government become subject to public pressure. This pressure is for the government to assume responsibility for inquiring into the need, for determining whether or not, and to what degree the service actually satisfied the need, and for questioning whether or not the service was rendered as economically as possible [5, 18].

On the other hand, under private insurance, with its many sources of payment, economic power is dispersed and, therefore, considerable freedom of action is enjoyed by the providers of health services in determining quality, quantity, range of services offered, manpower requirements, and distribution of facilities [25].

Likewise, any political opposition to increases in health expenditures is diluted. As long as personal health services remain primarily in the private sector, very few questions are raised directly [1].

WELFARE VERSUS SOCIAL INSURANCE

If the United States should contemplate the future enactment of any new legislation providing for public financing of personal health services, it will have to come to grips with three basic questions: (1) Who should bear the cost of the new program? (2) Who should be eligible to receive benefits? (3) How should the costs of the new program be distributed among the various levels of government [21]?

The two alternative methods of government financing present the following contrasts:

1) Under a welfare program the recipients of the benefits are not expected to pay the costs of their own security. All public assistance programs are of a non-contributory nature. At every level of government, the program is financed from taxes that do not fall solely, if at all, on the beneficiaries. In contrast, social insurance systems require that all, or a substantial part, of the cost of the health insurance program be provided by those who are to be insured. Payment of the costs of social insurance by these beneficiaries is the inevitable consequence of those systems which pay benefits on the basis of past contributions [37].

Under a social insurance system, at least in the United States, the tax on wages and self-employment is of a regressive nature. There are no exemptions granted by reference to any minimum income or to size of family. Also, the tax rate is uniform, whatever the level of earnings, up to the taxable maximum [20].

Under this method of financing, the beneficiaries, as a class, are required to pay for their own security. Thereby, the lower economic groups must pay a higher proportion of their total income for security than for those with larger incomes. The strict application of this program would greatly limit the scope of the benefits that could be financed for those persons whose current incomes are high enough to permit them to pay the necessary taxes and yet retain an acceptable standard of living [6].

2) Social insurance attempts to cover all the employed population, and often many others, within its program. Under this system, the payment of predetermined health care benefits is not dependent upon the demonstration of individual financial need, but rather, rests solely upon the occurrence of a specified contingency-illness [37].

On the other hand, welfare attempts only support to those unable to provide for health care with their own resources. This, then implies the policy of investigating the financial status of the individual requiring care in order to determine whether his income is below the established level for eligibility for the program. The income evaluation (a means test) generally involves detailed reporting of all income and other resources, verification of all statements by house visits, and confirmation of reports from relatives, employers, landlords, and neighbors. After the investigation the agency may use considerable discretion in withholding benefits [7].

In contrast, the legal specificity of social insurance makes recipients less subject to the discretion of administrators than are those who obtain their health care benefits in the form of public assistance. Since the eligibility conditions are set out in considerable detail in the law and are related to objectively ascertainable facts, namely illness, the individual is familiar with his benefit rights under law, and the realm of official discretion is considerably reduced [2].

3) Social insurance is funded entirely through the federal government Welfare programs are funded with a combination of federal and state monies. The more the costs of health service programs are shared with the states, the greater the disparity in the provision for the "medically indigent [7]." The less wealthy state is doubly disadvantaged, because not only is its economic and therefore, its fiscal resources limited, but also, the poorer state will have greater numbers of people with incomes below what is accepted as a general standard of minimum adequacy for medical care. Thus the problem of financing public assistance health services is intensified by the fact that there tends to be an inverse relationship between the needs of the states and their financial capabilities [4]. Therefore, even with federal matching grants favoring the low income states, we continue to find wide differences in income eligibility requirements between the states for welfare medical care programs. Thus, a situation is created in which there is a substantial incentive for indigent individuals to migrate from the low income rural states to the high income urban states, seeking their generally better welfare programs [3]. Often this makes the already difficult social problems of our urban areas more complex.

4) Since social insurance is administered entirely by the federal government, an individual can relocate anywhere within the United States without losing or altering his benefit privileges.

Under public assistance (welfare), where administrative responsibility is carried primarily by the various state governments, an individual's eligibility changes every time he moves from one state jurisdiction to another [6].

5) Recently, there has been a growing public concern about the unresponsiveness and inflexibility of many of our highly centralized social institutions. Without considering in any detail the advantages and disadvantages of centralization as contrasted with localism in the administration of health services, it is appropriate to point out that since social insurance is financed and administered by a single federal agency, the administration of the program tends to be highly centralized [26].

Public assistance (welfare) on the other hand, is administered primarily by the 50 state governments and, as a result, the program administration is considerably more decentralized [37]. Thus, political and economic power is dispersed and much freedom of action is enjoyed by the various local providers of health services.

6) Social insurance with its mandatory employee-employer contributory fund tends to be the best method for insulating any program against the future uncertainties brought about by a change in the political climate [17, 29]. Any governmental program which encompasses beneficiaries

from all economic strata will be better protected from political change than any program consisting primarily of the "poor" and the indigent. Once the middle class is included, the program's political vulnerability declines sharply. One only has to compare the relative political and economic stability of the medicare program (Title 18) with severe financial and political setbacks experienced by the medicaid program (Title 19) to see the validity of this corollary.

7) In all advanced countries teses are relatively high and not easily increased. Although the limits of total governmental expenditures are elastic, it is nevertheless true that at any given time, large incremental expenditures in one area tend to restrict what can be spent in other areas [36]. Therefore, since a social insurance program is likely to be more enduring and less subject to change as a consequence of variation in the political climate than is a public assistance (welfare) program [17, 29], the net effect will be to decrease the potential tax resources available in the future for other social ends. Furthermore, the prospect of increased federal expenditures of any kind have to be considered in the light of (1) persent and future commitments to national security; (2) the likelihood of a growing public pressure for a post-Vietnam tax cut [27]. If present national policies continue, and once again immediate as well as long range priorities are given to expenditures for national defense, the funds necessary to implement an enlarged social insurance program would most likely have to come from the same pool of tax resources potentially available to other equally worthy social programs such as education, welfare, work training, and scientific research [3, 20].

The search for equity in financing social services is one of the most perplexing issues facing our society today [13, 36]. Problems involved in financing health services in particular, pose complex economic, political, and philosophical questions. These questions must be answered if financing methods are to be designed which will bring about a proper, and equitable distribution of costs among groups of people and between various levels of government.

The two alternative methods of financing health services (private insurance—welfare or social insurance) are not necessarily mutually exclusive, but in the future, society will have to decide between the two. It will be difficult to make this choice on purely rational grounds without taking into account the human values to which our society adheres. On the basis of these values, our society must decide:

1) What priority should be given to health services expenditures in relationship to other potentially worthy social programs, and

2) Whether it prefers that the control and management of the health services industry remain primarily within the private sector or whether present needs require that it be moved to the public sector.

REFERENCES

[1] Anderson, Odin W. "Private and Public Action in Meeting Health Needs." *Ann. Amer. Acad. Polit. Soc. Sci.* 337:66, September 1967.

[2] Ball, Robert M. "The American Social Security Program," *Medical Care, Social and Organizational Aspects,* ed. DeGroost. Springfield, Illinois: Charles C. Thomas Publisher, 1966.

[3]Buchanan, J. M. *The Public Finances.* Homewood, Illinois: Richard D. Irwin, 1965.

[4]Burns, Eveline M. *The American Social Security System.* Boston: Houghton Mifflin Company, 1951.

[5]Burns, E. M. *Social Policy and the Health Services: The Choices Ahead.* New York: Columbia University Press, 1967.

[6]Burns, E. M. *Social Security and Public Policy.* New York: McGraw-Hill, 1956.

[7]Burns, Eveline M. "Some Major Policy Decisions Facing the United States in the Financing and Organization of Health Care." *Bull. N.Y. Acad. Med.* 42:1073, December, 1966.

[8]Campbell, Angus et al. *The American Voter, an Abridgment.* New York: John Wiley and Sons, 1964.

[9]Carlson, Valdemar. *Economic Security in the United States.* New York: McGraw-Hill, 1962.

[10]Cohen, Wilbur J. *Health Insurance under Social Security. A. J. Nurs.* 60:505, April, 1960.

[11]Clark, R. M. *Economic Security for the Aged in the United States and Canada: A Report Prepared for the Government of Canada, Vol. 1.* Ottawa: The Queens Printer, 1959.

[12]Dahl, Robert A., and Lindbloom, Charles E. *Politics, Economics, and Welfare.* New York: Harper and Brothers, 1953.

[13]Eckstein, Otto. *Public Finance.* Englewood Cliffs, New Jersey: Prentice Hall, 1967.

[14]Feingold, Eugene. *Medicare: Policy and Politics.* San Francisco: Chandler Publishing, 1966.

[15]*Intergovernmental Problems in Medicaid.* Advisory Commission on Intergovernmental Relations. Washington, D.C., 1968.

[16]"Fiscal Balance in the American Federal System," Vol. 2, *Metropolitan Fiscal Disparities.* Advisory Commission on Intergovernmental Relations. Washington, D.C., 1967.

[17]Folsom, Marion B. "Current Issues in Financing Income Security." *National Policy for Education, Health and Social Services,* ed. James Russell. Garden City, New York: Doubleday, 1955.

[18]Fuchs, V. R. "The Contribution of Health Services to the American Economy." *Milbank Memorial Fund Quarterly* 44:69, 1966.

[19]Gagliardo, D. *American Social Insurance.* New York: Harper and Brothers, 1955.

[20]Gordon, M. S. *The Economics of Welfare Policies.* New York: Columbia University Press, 1963.

[21]Haber, William. "The Problem of Financing Social Services." *National Policies for Education, Health and Social Services,* ed. James Russell. Garden City, New York: Doubleday, 1955.

[22]*Hearings on Health Services for the Aged under the Social Security Insurance System.* U.S. Congress, House Committee on Ways and Means, 87th Cong., August 2, 1961, 1369-1377, 1382-1388. Testimony of the American Medical Association.

[23]Hedinger, Fredric R. *The Social Role of Blue Cross as a Device for Financing the Costs of Hospital Care: An Evaluation.* Iowa City: University of Iowa Press, 1966.

[24]Hohaus, Richard A. "Equity, Adequacy, and Related Factors." *Social Security: Programs, Problems and Policies,* ed. W. Haber and W. Cohen. Homewood, Illinois: Richard D. Irwin, 1960.

[25]Klarman, H. E. *The Economics of Health.* New York: Columbia University Press, 1965.

[26]Laroque, Pierre. "Major Issues Raised by Contemporary Trends in Income Security Policies," *National Policies for Education, Health, and Social Services,* ed. James E. Russell, Garden City, New York: Doubleday, 1955.

[27]McCracken, P. W. "After Vietnam What Next for the Economy?" *Challenge: The Magazine of Economic Affairs:* 33, July-August 1967.

[28]Myrdal, Gunnar. *Beyond the Welfare State.* New Haven: Yale University Press, 1960.

[29]Peterson, O. L. "Financing A Medical Care Program Through Social Security." *New Eng. J. Med.* 265-527, September 1961.

[30] Reed, L. S. "Private Health Insurance: Coverage and Financial Experience, 1940-1966." *Soc. Sec. Bull.* 30:22, November 1967.

[31] Rice, D. P., and Cooper, B. S. "National Health Expenditures, 1950-66." *Soc. Sec. Bull.* 31:19, April 1968.

[32] Richardson, J. H. *Economic and Financial Aspects of Social Security, and International Study.* London: George Allen and Unwin Ltd., 1960.

[33] Rohrlick, George F. "Implications of New Social Insurance Mechanisms for Other Population Groups." *Bull. N.Y. Acad. Med.,* 42:1117, December, 1966.

[34] Somers, A. R. "Some Basic Determinants of Medical Care and Health Policy." *Milbank Memorial Fund Quarterly* 46:25, January 1968.

[35] Somers, Herman M., and Somers, Anne R. *Medicare and the Hospitals Issues and Prospects.* Washington: The Brookings Institute, 1967.

[36] Strayer, P. J. *Fiscal Policy and Politics.* New York: Harper Brothers, 1958.

[37] Turbull, J. G., Williams, C. A., and Cheit, E. F. *Economics and Social Security.* New York: Ronald Press, 1967.

[38] Youngdahl, Benjamin E. "Social Services: Need and Scope," National *Policies for Education,* ed. James E. Russell. Garden City, New York: Doubleday, 1955.

INDEX OF TOPICS